Blessed Motherhood, Bitter Fruit

Blessed Motherhood, Bitter Fruit

Nelly Roussel and the Politics of Female Pain in Third Republic France

ELINOR ACCAMPO

The Johns Hopkins University Press
Baltimore

© 2006 The Johns Hopkins University Press
All rights reserved. Published 2006
Printed in the United States of America on acid-free paper
2 4 6 8 9 7 5 3 1

The Johns Hopkins University Press
2715 North Charles Street
Baltimore, Maryland 21218-4363
www.press.jhu.edu

Library of Congress Cataloging-in-Publication Data

Accampo, Elinor Ann.
Blessed motherhood, bitter fruit / Nelly Roussel and the politics of female pain in
Third Republic France / Elinor Accampo.
    p.   cm.
Includes bibliographical references and index.
ISBN 0-8018-8404-7 (hardcover : alk. paper)
1. Roussel, Nelly, 1878–1922. 2. Birth Control—France—Biography. 3. Feminists—France—
Biography. 4. Women social reformers—France—Biography. I. Title.
HQ764.R68A33 2006
363.9'6092—dc22
2005033501

A catalog record for this book is available from the British Library.

In memory of my mother,
Alice Accampo (1910–1998)

In memory of my sister,
Jane Callaghy (1946–2001)

For my daughter,
Erin Accampo Hern

CONTENTS

Illustrations follow page 107

The research for this book began with a different project in mind. After having studied French fertility decline in the nineteenth century among the working classes, I wanted to find out more about what the French were thinking when they had small families. I began researching the neo-Malthusian (French birth control) movement in the hope of learning what male, and especially female, proponents of birth control were saying about reproduction and gender issues, but I soon discovered that few women numbered among their ranks. One of them, Nelly Roussel, had, however, left an enormous archive.

I am an accidental biographer. As a social historian, it would never have occurred to me to write a biography had not the sources Roussel left behind been so rich. For the first few years of looking at her archive, I tried to avoid "wasting time" reading materials that were not relevant to my project as I had defined it, but I finally gave in to this treasure of personal papers when several friends and colleagues prodded me to write a biography. Many years later, I feel gratified that doing so allowed me to address the questions that had inspired my original project. I have many people to thank for making the final result possible.

First, I owe thanks to the institutional support I received. For my original conception of this project I thank the National Endowment for the Humanities for a Travel-to-Collections Grant and the American Council of Learned Societies for a summer grant. Otherwise, all the support for this project came from the University of Southern California: research grants from Institute for the Study of Women and Men in Society, the Zumberge Faculty Research and Innovation Award, the USC College Award for Research Excellence, and the USC College Faculty Development Award. This funding made travel to France and to conferences possible.

I thank the staffs at the Archives nationales de France, Bibliothèque nationale de France, the Bibliothèque historique de la Ville de Paris, Archives de la Préfecture de la Police de Paris, Laure de Margerie at the documentation department of the Musée d'Orsay, and the staff of International Institute of Social History in Amsterdam. I owe my deepest thanks to Annie Metz, *directrice* of the Bibliothèque Marguerite Durand, and to her staff. She welcomed me, encouraged me, gave me complete access to Roussel's papers, and helped me in ways that can only be described as exceptional. She and her staff sustained me with inspiration, patience, sympathy, and friendship as we negotiated our way through Roussel's less-than-organized collection on each of my annual two-week visits. To say that I could not have written this book without their immense generosity is an understatement.

I received invaluable feedback during various stages of this book at annual meetings of the Society for French Historical Studies, the Western Society for French History, and the Social Science History Association, from audiences at the University of Michigan–Flint, Michigan State University, Western Michigan University, the European History Colloquium at the University of California–Los Angeles, Oregon State University, the Center for Feminist Research at the University of Southern California, and the California Group of French Historians. For feedback, friendship, and support, I thank Susan Ashley, Susanna Barrows, Marjorie Becker, Lenard Berlanstein, Lisa Bitel, Linda Clark, Tom Callaghy, Helen Chenu, Nancy Fitch, Nina Gelbart, Sharif Gemi (one of those who persuaded me to do a biography), Steven Hause, Lynn Hunt, Peg Jacobs, Cheryl Koos, Paul Lerner, Yves Lequin, Andrea Mansker, Ted Margadant, Theresa McBride, Anne Meyering, John Merriman, Leslie Moch, Kristen Neuschel, Karen Offen, Roderick Phillips, Michelle Perrot, Barbara Pope, Lou Roberts, Florence Rochefort, Nick Salvatore, Hilary Schor, Debora Silverman, Bonnie Smith, Richard Sonn, Judy Stone, Ann Sullivan, Mary Lynn Stewart, Patricia Tilburg, David Troyansky, Frans van Poppel, Whitney Walton, and Alan Williams. Although she has not read any part of this book, I am indebted to Joan Scott because her work on gender—as is true of Karen Offen's—has provided a major source of inspiration, as well as signposts for my thinking about it.

Among those who persuaded me to write a biography was my colleague and friend Mauricio Mazón. He read all my early efforts to grapple with this project and spent much time talking to me about it. I am bereft that he passed away before he could see the final product and before I could thank him adequately. When putting together her edited volume *The New Biography: Performing Femininity in Nineteenth-Century France* (2000), Joby Margadant gave me invaluable insight with her feedback on my contribution and inspired new ways of understanding Roussel. Similarly, Vanessa Schwartz's reading of the first half of the book opened perspectives I otherwise would not have had; her friendship has sustained my spirit and determination in the last stages of this book. Jean Elisabeth Pedersen generously shared her own work on Roussel and pointed me to a police file of which I had been unaware. Christiane Demeulenaere-Douyère shared her work on Paul Robin, gave me a photograph of one of Henri Godet's sculptures, and put me in touch with Michel Robin. Michel Robin, in turn, has been generous in the information offered through his memory of the family history; he and his wife, Martine Robin, have been gracious hosts in Paris. I thank Jean-Philippe Schnell, a descendant of Roussel's family. In addition to sharing his side of the family history, he introduced me to Henri Godet's archives in the documentation of the Musée d'Orsay. I also thank graduate assistants Laura Kalba and Megan Kendrick for their expert help, and I thank the staff of the USC History Department, Lori Rogers, Brenda Johnson, and La Verne Hughes for their abiding support and endless patience.

Very special gratitude must go to those who have read the entire manuscript or more than one version of it in various stages of preparation. I thank Henry Tom and the anonymous reader at the Johns Hopkins University Press for astute criticism and affirmation, and Claire McCabe for production assistance, Martha Sewall for assistance with illustrations, and Peter Dreyer for his extraordinarily skillful copyediting. Steve Ross, Lois Banner, and Lynn Dumenil each read the whole manuscript in its final stages and provided invaluable advice, particularly in cutting excess verbiage and antiquarian detail. Rachel Fuchs first drew my attention to Roussel's archive—and encouraged me to do a biography. She has been a mentor, collaborator, colleague, and comrade. Her friendship, intellectual inspiration, and memories of times spent in Paris have sustained me in this project.

Bob Nye has also played a large role in my intellectual growth. His own scholarship has had a major influence on the way I think about things. From my first biographical paper on Nelly Roussel nearly ten years ago, he has read and commented on everything I have since written—not just the entire manuscript, but more than one version of many chapters. His encouragement, enthusiasm, friendship, and belief in this project kept me going on many occasions. He is one of the most intellectually generous academics I have ever known.

I dedicate this book to the memory of my mother. As a social worker, she influenced my becoming a social historian. As an English teacher, she imparted to me a love of literature, the importance of good writing, and what it takes to write well. Even though putting that knowledge into practice continues to be a struggle, her inspiration lives on. I dedicate this book as well to the memory of my sister Jane Callaghy, whose sudden, tragic, and untimely death gave me occasion to reflect more acutely on the impact she has had on my life, my scholarly ambitions, and my professional trajectory. It was she who first inspired my love of all things French—language and food especially. It was because of her that I became a French historian.

I also dedicate this book to my daughter, Erin Accampo Hern, who has made motherhood a joyful experience for me. I thank her for having to endure my absences, mental and physical, in the process of researching and writing this book. She has had to live with it her entire life. I thank her for making me drop everything to go get ice cream, because being with her in those moments—and all moments—reminds me of my true priorities. I hope that we shall have many more such moments as she now launches herself into adulthood.

Finally, my husband Bob Hern knows more than anyone what it has taken to complete this book. He has been there for me every step of the way. I thank him for his support throughout—he has been father and mother in my absences and husband and "wife" to me, often taking on well over half the household chores, especially in the final stages of the writing. I thank him for his enduring patience, understanding, appreciation, and encouragement in what often seemed to both of us a project whose end point continually receded.

Blessed Motherhood, Bitter Fruit

Introduction

Nelly Roussel, "Contemporary of the Future"

In every society, there appear above-average individuals, precursors troubling the general somnolence and pushing the world ahead, often to their own detriment; for it is a dangerous trade, that of the innovator, above all, of the moral reformer, confronting secular prejudices and egotistical interests head-on, rising up against injustice, even when it only affects others. Blessed are these troublemakers, these contemporaries of the future.

Charles Letourneau, L'Évolution de la morale (1887)

As a feminist, advocate of birth control, journalist, and public speaker, Nelly Roussel (1878–1922) would have fitted the "second-wave" feminism of the 1970s better than she did her own time. Roussel argued that women have the right to pursue self-fulfillment—happiness as individuals—regardless of their social, marital, or maternal status, and that they also have the right to avoid pain. These ideas may not seem radical in the context of twenty-first-century Western culture, but they were deeply disturbing to hers. What made Roussel so advanced for her time was her conviction that the means to female emancipation lay in birth control. Her life's mission was to liberate women from unwanted pregnancies, as well as from other forms of pain she perceived as particular to women. She believed that science could alleviate the pain of childbirth, and that social reform could cushion the burdens of motherhood. Roussel's chosen mission was no simple call for civil and political equality with men; she advocated a radical transformation of both private and public life by explicitly associating a woman's autonomy and capacity for full political citizenship with her control over her own body. In connecting reproductive rights to citizenship itself, she departed from the mainstream feminism of her day. This book argues that her message threatened the very foundation of the political culture and bourgeois belief systems that dominated the Third Republic.

No full-scale biography has been written of Nelly Roussel. She has consistently garnered a few scattered paragraphs in histories of French feminism, but she has never held a central place in them, because the majority of feminists in her generation, publicly if not privately, eschewed what she advocated.[1] Yet in her own time she was famous for her charismatic speaking, feminine beauty, warmth, and devotion to her family and her friends. She was widely publicized, deeply loved, often despised, and almost always respected, even by her enemies. Her words and her career provoked extensive debate. In both word and deed, Roussel made private issues public by addressing the taboo topics of female sexuality and maternal pain. Extraordinary in her subversiveness, she also tapped into the ordinary, common sentiments of her audiences and gave impulse to expressions that otherwise would have remained unspoken.

The major purpose of this study is to analyze reactions to Roussel and to her doctrine as a means of elucidating the gender system in France and its relationship to political culture. I have sought to combine the methods of traditional biography with those of the "new biography" in seeking to understand the contradictory forces in French society that inspired Roussel to formulate her uniquely modern version of feminism. I also analyze the conflicts Roussel provoked as she forged and performed her public self, and what those conflicts tell us about French national identity during the fin de siècle, the Great War, and the aftermath of that war.[2] Roussel's most immediate goal was to provoke controversy, which she did to a considerable degree. Examining that controversy allows us to understand better the stake French society had in the prevailing concept of the "eternal feminine." It also reveals the weight of history on French gender relations.

The message Roussel sought to spread, her public career, and the conduct of her private life were partly her own invention and partly a product of the French past. They simultaneously reflected the enduring force of Catholicism and the persistent revolutionary tradition that opposed it. Her life clarifies how the French experienced the transition to modernity, specifically with regard to changing meanings of womanhood. In "troubling the general somnolence," Roussel uncovered the contradictions inherent in a society that sought to protect individual freedoms as a matter of principle but withheld them from a category of people whose exercise of those same freedoms would undermine the social order. Feminism has always exposed such contradictions, and continues to be troubling for the same reason. Even more fundamental than the overall project of demanding equal civil and political rights, however, was Roussel's insistence on the right to control over one's body in an era when the very meaning of reproduction was changing radically—more rapidly, in fact, than in the whole of human history.[3] It is in the context of the relatively sudden emergence of modern birth control movements both in Europe and in the United States and the politicization of demography in Third Republic France that Roussel's disruptive message and unusual life resonate.

Birth Control and Its History

The means to limit human fertility have always existed, especially in the forms of abortion, infanticide, late marriage, prolonged sexual abstinence, extended nursing, and withdrawal. To one degree or another, people have always controlled family size. Moreover, from ancient times to the early modern era, women used contraceptive and abortifacient pharmaceuticals—herbs—that modern science has deemed effective. But in the seventeenth and eighteenth centuries, the conjuncture of economic, demographic, scientific, and political change forged a culture that shrouded these methods in a veil of secrecy, and they became less widely known and used. The natural sciences produced new biological theories that reinforced definitions of male and female as opposite. As opposites of men, and with the knowledge that female orgasm was not necessary for conception, women were not supposed to enjoy sexual intercourse and were expected to be sexually passive.[4] The emergence of industrial capitalism and the removal of work from the home reinforced notions of gender difference, because they required more strictly defined roles for men and women. Men followed work into the public sphere, while women, at least among the middle classes, became domestically and maternally oriented.

Enlightenment thinking about women provided further logical foundation for conceptualizing men and women as opposites. As men used reason to conquer nature for the advancement of civilization, women came to be identified with nature, especially in the unchanging cycles of menstruation and reproduction.[5] Enlightenment thinking thus emphasized women's "natural" role as a vessel of motherhood and morality; any diversion from that role as an unmarried, infertile, or overtly sexual woman was seen not only as unnatural but as socially subversive. Although women did have their "own Enlightenment," in the sense that more of them became published authors, and reading and writing made them more modern, because they began to develop a sense of "self," such women remained in the minority; the prescriptions for "proper" womanhood, moreover, carried legal, cultural, and scientific weight. These assumptions about female nature took on added importance in the era of emerging democracy, in which women were supposed to assume the role of "republican mothers." As such, they were to create virtuous citizens, a belief that in turn imbued motherhood with a social and public importance.[6]

Enlightenment thinking, however, also raised concerns about the laws of population growth. Political economists began to publish treatises about the relationship between the size of a nation's population and its political and economic power. Thomas Malthus's *Essay on the Principle of Population* (1798) argued that unlimited procreation, driven by the sex instinct, would result in a geometrical increase in the population, and that this rate of growth would far outpace the arithmetical increase in food production. Overpopulation would inevitably lead to misery, vice, and war. The only solution Malthus advocated was delay in marriage or permanent celibacy among those who could not afford children. This hugely influential tract had the unintended consequence of inspiring some social reformers to advocate contraception instead of abstinence, because they believed the sexual instinct too strong to curtail. Thus Jeremy Bentham advocated the use of a sponge; the radical dissenter Richard Carlile went a step further by describing its use, as well as that of a male "glove," in the first book published on birth control with the enticingly modern title *Every Woman's book: or What is Love?* (1826). These and other Chartist and Owenite reformers advocated contraception to the working class as a way out of the misery caused by early industrialization. Such propaganda spread from Britain to the Netherlands, France, and Spain in the last third of the nineteenth century.[7]

Advocates of contraception came to be known as "neo-Malthusians" because they departed from Thomas Malthus's reliance on celibacy as the only moral solution to overpopulation. Their pamphlets provided education about female means of contraception such as sponges and, later, pessaries, as well as condoms. Though the birth control movement assumed a somewhat different form in each country, it is important to keep in mind that everywhere its goal was the improved welfare of families or, more specifically, the social advancement and empowerment of the poor, rather than the sexual emancipation of women (the title of Carlile's book notwithstanding). Nonetheless, all the varieties of birth control advocacy caused substantial controversy in the nineteenth century. This was in part because of middle-class sexual prudery, but also because of the perception that avoiding pregnancy, especially with mechanical means, was unnatural. Though it is ironic that these movements emerged at a time of unprecedented sexual repression, especially for women, it is understandable, because the drop in infant mortality created a greater need to limit births. In addition, the role of children changed in the industrial era as they gradually lost their capacity to contribute to the family economy and, at least among the middle classes, became objects of emotional and financial investment.

The French neo-Malthusian movement differed from its counterparts in Britain and the United States, because its founder, Paul Robin, and his disciple Nelly Roussel put women and women's control over their own bodies at the center of birth control doctrine. An irascible and ill man, Robin was eventually marginalized from the movement. But Roussel persisted in pairing feminism with neo-Malthusianism, and this combination proved particularly contrary to prevailing definitions of womanhood at the turn of the twentieth century. Roussel used the familiar argument that fewer births would make for better mothers and healthier children, but women's liberation from motherhood itself, and their right to develop a fully human self, independent of maternal identity, constituted an unmistakable subtext of her campaign. Unlike most of her feminist contemporaries, she believed that sexual pleasure—which she (and others) euphemistically termed "love"—was an important component of a woman's full development as a human being, and therefore her inalienable right. Roussel's neo-Malthusian doctrine thus differed markedly from that of most of her French compatriots, as well as from those in other countries. France's revolutionary past and fin de siècle demography, moreover, intensified the resonance and the contradictions of her message among the French.

The Legacy of Recurrent Revolution

Roussel's doctrines and the public reaction to them played out in a political culture heavily influenced by France's revolutionary past. The perpetual political upheavals beginning with the Revolution of 1789 created a more profound ideological need for incontrovertible "truths" about distinctions between the sexes than in other modernizing Western societies. Women's participation in political demonstrations and acts of violence, their demands for rights (including that to bear arms), and the practice of donning male clothing caused great discomfort among men as war and domestic strife escalated. Their actions gave rise to mythologies about female affinity for violence and "furies of the guillotine" who took pleasure in watching the bloody heads drop from the blade of justice. From the perspective of the new political elite, the Revolution defeminized women and released monstrous qualities from within them.[8] The new social order required republican male virtue, which depended upon women's absence from public life and their nurturing presence in the home. Only an unchanging female sex in her appropriate role would temper and balance men's radical individualism in a republican society and a free market economy. More than any other modern country, the French embraced the concept of *l'éternel féminin* (the eternal feminine, or eternal womanhood) as expressed in the final line of Goethe's *Faust:* "Das Ewig-Weibliche / Zieht uns hinan" ("Eternal Womanhood / Leads us above"). Women, as long as they remained true to their permanent nature, would redeem men from "all things corruptible."[9]

The revolutions of 1830, 1848, and 1871 each produced female participants. They again brought to the surface issues of appropriate gender identity and again produced outbursts against women whose actions seemed unnatural to those seeking to reestablish order.[10] Unlike the political evolution that occurred in the United States, Britain, and Germany, the recurrent revolutions in France forged a republican ideology that held a unique place for women. The most important example of this ideological direction can be found in the writings of Jules Michelet, the famous nineteenth-century historian of the French Revolution. French republicanism was anticlerical and anti-Catholic from its inception, and its ideologues believed that they needed to wean women away from the influence of priests and create a new place for them in a republican cosmology. Michelet became instrumental in this process after the Revolution of 1848, and he exerted a permanent influence on conceptions about gender during the Third Republic (1871–1940). He developed his views most systematically in *La Femme* (1859) and *L'Amour* (1858), both of which had wide readership and several editions. In these works, he developed in detail the familiar theme of woman's unchanging place in nature—indeed, because of her menstrual cycles linked to the stars, sea, and moon, woman *embodied* nature and belonged to a circular time, while man was a historical actor in linear time.[11]

This concept of womanhood not only pervaded the literary imagination but had practical consequences as well. It formed the thinking of leading social reformers such as Jules Simon, Fréderic Le Play, and Émile Cheysson.[12] Revolutionary upheaval similarly infused the imaginations of devoted Catholics for whom, as Richard D. E. Burton has noted, "the spiritual function of woman [was] to weep, bleed, and starve for the salvation of others, to offer herself up as a holocaust to appease a revengeful male deity."[13] This culture of suffering initially held a minor place in Catholic devotional practice, but its influence spread with Antoine Blanc de Saint-Bonnet's widely read *De la douleur* (1849). The doctrine, Burton argues, became more prominent after 1870, when the Catholic hierarchy and writers of the Catholic literary renaissance highlighted the Christlike sufferings of women. The French Catholic and republican cultures thus shared a concept of womanhood as unchanging and self-sacrificing.

The Unique Demographic Profile of the French

If recurrent revolution in France created a need to define woman as rooted in nature, the nation's unusually low birthrate made it a practical imperative. France was unique in its precipitous fertility decline. Dating from the mid eighteenth century, the French transition to a low birthrate preceded fertility decline in other modernizing nations by a century. The national comparisons are striking: from 1760 to 1764, Frenchwomen had an average of 5.2 children, while Englishwomen had 4.9. But by the following decade, the French rate had dropped below that of the English. In the years from 1790 to 1855, it fell to 3.5 children per woman, while the English rate remained at 5 and even climbed to 5.2 by 1870.[14] During the decade of the 1870s, the French produced an average of only 25.4 children annually per 1,000 inhabitants, compared to England and Wales's 35.4, Germany's 39.1, and Italy's 36.9. The Germans and English did not even begin to approach the low birthrate of the French until after World War I, and by World War II, France still had the lowest rate.[15]

The comparison of national growth rates further highlights the unique pattern among the French. In 1789, France had the largest European population, standing at 27.5 million inhabitants. But by 1914, it had only grown by 45 percent (to 40 million), while Italy had grown by 225 percent (to 36 million), England by 450 percent (to 45 million), and Germany by 340 percent (to 68 million). Although territorial loss resulting from the Franco-Prussian war of 1870 contributed to the statistical result, the defeat likewise bolstered the image of France as an anemic, dying nation that could not even defend its own boundaries. Vital statistics darkened the picture further: deaths exceeded births in seven of the years between 1890 and 1914. Even the modest increase of the French population did not come from reproduction (the rate of which produced a loss of five million), but from an increase in longevity and from the immigration of five million foreigners. By 1933, even Italy surpassed France in population.[16]

Yet demographic statistics provide few clues to explain why French fertility declined so early and, in stark contrast to England and other countries, prior to rather than after its economic modernization. Wide regional variation further complicates any demographic explanation for the decline. The most common reason offered for low France's low birthrate—one to which contemporaries pointed—is that partible inheritance legislated during the Revolution of 1789 encouraged the French to reduce family size to avoid breaking up their property among numerous heirs. However, for present purposes, the cause of the decline is less important than its effect on the French mentality. Demographic statistics led politicians, government officials, doctors, social hygienists, and moral reformers to conclude that the numerical deterioration ensued from moral decay and a sense of selfish individualism in the French population, particularly on the part of women.[17] Foreigners as well as French nationals viewed the population as "decadent" and "degenerate." This perception created an even more urgent need to define women as mothers who would regenerate the French "race."

Indeed, that France should have a birth control movement at all appears ironic, in view of the fact that the French were already achieving smaller families without new contraceptive technologies. Why preach to the converted, and why should such preaching be so controversial? The obvious answer to the latter part of this question is that contraceptives would lower the birthrate even further and, according to the pronatalists, weaken France, especially with regard to its military potential. But the more complex answer, as my study of Nelly Roussel's career will show, is that this preaching to the converted was less about family limitation than it was about female sexuality.

From Eternal Woman to Eternally Sacrificed Woman

The weight of France's past and its demographic present were hardly monolithic in their influence during Roussel's lifetime. Her generation experienced unusually rapid social and economic change with the second industrial revolution, educational reform, and massive transformation in modes of communication and transportation. In 1900, Charles Péguy concluded that "Europe had changed more in the previous thirty years than it had since Jesus Christ."[18] Among these changes was the new science of sexology. Although even in the nineteenth century, sex manuals written by doctors acknowledged women's right to sexual pleasure within marriage, and some were explicit about how to achieve it, most marital advice manuals through World War I presumed that "normal" women had a weak sexual instinct.[19] The new theories about sexuality, however, began the process of acknowledging and normalizing female sexual desire by linking it to women's development as individuals. They laid the groundwork for redefining sexuality as a form of pleasure central to human identity, rather than an exclusively reproductive function. A greater acceptance of female sexuality was apparent in forms of popular entertainment such as burlesque and other eroticized stage performances. In the words of Stéphane Michaud, "the end of the century was aquiver with the discovery of sexual energy."[20]

Other cultural changes—the rise of mass consumerism and new forms of entertainment—drew women further into public life and defied any notion that their nature was "eternal." Women also entered higher education, became professionals, engaged in body-strengthening gymnastics, rode bicycles, and wore bloomers. Instead of embracing qualities associated with motherhood, especially self-sacrifice, the New Woman sought self-fulfillment. In doing so, she demonstrated that sexual difference, rather than being fixed, was "contingent and precarious."[21] Precisely because they sought fulfillment independent of marriage and motherhood, the image of these New Women—which was far more pervasive than they themselves were in reality—inspired more fear and concern than did mainstream feminists, who glorified motherhood to advance their cause.

Nelly Roussel's career path exemplifies the possibilities of the New Woman countercurrent even in a culture whose prevailing morality attempted to retain traditional ideals of womanhood. Creating a public space for herself was more like carving through limestone than cracking the granite monolith of a public that disdained "public" women. But such carving nonetheless required exquisitely honed tools. Roussel might have made it on her own had she never married, though it is improbable. She owed her success largely to the meticulous counsel of her husband, the sculptor Henri Godet, who provided indispensable infrastructural and emotional support for her speaking tours. Moreover, through his own art, he helped create a maternal image of her that facilitated her ultimately antimaternal message. Her life was filled with other ironies arising from the times in which she lived: in particular, she deployed traditional feminine tactics to promote her radical stance. While spending extensive time away from her own children, she deliberately utilized her status as wife and mother to portray herself as uniquely qualified to pronounce on all issues of motherhood and to legitimize her advocacy of women's personal, political, and sexual autonomy. In her multiple images (mother, public speaker, journalist, tragedian), Roussel may not have resolved what feminists in our own generation have defined as the "liberal paradox" of equality versus difference, but she transcended it in her unselfconscious evocation of equality *and* difference, and in the way she manipulated and embodied shifting definitions of masculinity and femininity current during the Belle Époque.

The New Woman became a phenomenon in every modernizing country, but in France she drew special scrutiny because bourgeois republicans—including many women—had a stake in the traditional femininity of *l'éternel féminin*—

whose core was self-sacrifice rather than self-fulfillment.[22] Roussel converted *l'éternel féminin* into an embodied *l'éternelle sacrifiée,* or "eternally sacrificed" woman, the title of her most famous lecture. Woman was eternally sacrificed, not by God or by nature, but by republican society itself. Pain, in fact, was the overarching theme in Roussel's private life and in her work. Her discourse focused on three sources of pain: maternity, disease, and war. Her own maternal pain was the most important experience that transformed her consciousness: in addition to fearing that motherhood would cause her to lose her sense of self as an individual, the physical ordeal of childbirth traumatized her. She protested the silence that tacitly sanctioned pain in the labor of birth, and she proclaimed that child rearing ravaged women's bodies and minds, because the Church, the government, and the economy did not afford women the means to have dignity or selfhood as mothers.

Disease also preoccupied Roussel. As with the majority of her contemporaries, she was often ill. In her case, ill health culminated in tuberculosis. Most intriguing about this personal struggle, unlike her others, is the silence that surrounded it. Like maternal pain, open discussion of tuberculosis was largely taboo; moreover, female suffering from this disease took on the added meaning of self-sacrifice and redemption.[23] But she and others also misunderstood the nature of her illness. She suffered for twelve years with symptoms not related in their appearance to pulmonary tuberculosis, and no one, including her doctors, understood what ailed her. They concluded that her work made her ill. But in keeping with her own battle against the notion of "woman always being sacrificed" by something unnecessary, she pursued every scientific and "alternative" cure she could.

War, the third source of human pain that concerned Roussel, caused particular agony for women as "creators of life." Her hatred of any pain she deemed unnecessary made her a pacifist early on. Unlike most pacifists, even on the Left and even among feminists, she did not join the "Sacred Union" that so compelled the vast majority of French people across the political, social, and cultural spectra in the patriotic fervor of 1914. Her beliefs and commitments during the war remained consistent with those prior to its outbreak, a stance that subjected her to censorship and persecution.

Roussel once made fanciful reference to the "intimate correspondence of Nelly Roussel published after my death," suggesting that she deliberately saved her papers for posterity. She preserved a wide variety of materials, an act that in itself constitutes a form of autobiography and reflects the very modern process by which she constructed herself as an individual and as a feminist—a self that she apparently hoped others would see. Hundreds of letters she exchanged with her husband Henri Godet, family, friends, and colleagues offer a view of her interior life and subjective self. In addition, from the beginning of her career in 1904 through 1922 (with two years missing), she kept agendas in which she listed her daily activities. Though referred to here as "diaries," these agendas are similar to the account books from which modern diaries originated—at day's end, Roussel recorded how she had spent her time (rather than money), using only single words or brief phrases. They contain no self-reflection or emotion. Roussel also preserved materials that provide a view of her exterior, public self. The mass press, as with the Dreyfus Affair, made her into a "phenomenon." She clipped every newspaper and journal article written either by or about her—which numbered in the hundreds—and pasted them in notebooks. These have proved an invaluable source, especially because they criticize, ridicule, and shame her, as well as honor, praise, and glorify her.[24]

Some modern readers will be unfamiliar with Roussel's neoromantic, Victorian style of speaking and writing, which went out of fashion in the 1920s. But this style and her message were compelling to audiences of her era, and her message continues to resonate in our own. In quoting her words, I have retained her dramatic emphases and indicate the rare occasions where I have added my own. Roussel traveled alone throughout France and parts of Europe (map 1), taking her doctrine to huge audiences of men and women of all social classes and backgrounds. Slight in stature (about 5 feet, 3 inches, and 110 pounds), she was arresting in the beauty of her dark hair, pale skin, and piercing eyes, and when she mounted the podium, restless audiences fell silent as they became swept up in her charisma. "Today, motherhood is only a source of misery, impotence, and humiliation," she would say. "In marriage the mother is annihilated, her sacred rights unrecognized; outside marriage, the mother, abandoned, succumbs to public contempt. It is in the name of her maternal function that laws and morals subjugate Woman. And what makes the mother bee a queen renders the human mother a slave. Has M. Édouard Drumont ever asked if it is not a bit for these reasons that conscientious women refuse to have children?"[25]

Drumont, an infamous nationalist author of anti-Semitic publications, was one of her detractors. With such rhetorical tactics, Roussel gave her own interpretation of the "depopulation crisis" and justified women's apparent lack of desire to bear children. Her logic and imaginative metaphors flustered her detractors. In the end, however, they had the law on their side; in one lawsuit in which Roussel was involved, the court ruled—proving her point—that if they engaged in sexual activity, women did not have the right "not to suffer."

The purpose of this book is to understand Roussel's experience as a New Woman in a culture that was undergoing tremendous change, as well as to analyze the reactions to her and to her doctrine. As one newspaper put it: "Applauded by some, attacked by others, she pursues her mission, obtaining the most desirable of successes: that which consists in being controversial. Silence, in effect, is the most dreadful enemy for anyone who writes or speaks and wants to have an impact on the public."[26] Roussel was persecuted, but never by silence. Audience reactions reveal the force that stereotypes about womanhood continued to exercise on the French political imagination. And while her broader impact in fighting this stereotype cannot be measured precisely, examples of it abound. The lives she changed or indirectly influenced ranged from those of humble working-class origins, such as Charlotte Davy, to bourgeois intellectuals such as Simone de Beauvoir. The former became a feminist, socialist, and collaborator of Roussel's; the latter, too young to know her personally, felt her influence. De Beauvoir's *Le Deuxième Sexe* (1949) helped inspire second-wave feminism and challenged the trope of *l'éternel feminin* very much the way Roussel had.[27]

Those of us who came of age in the 1960s, let alone those who have followed, have perhaps failed to appreciate the very different sensibilities of the past. The opposition to Nelly Roussel cannot simply be interpreted as a function of the masculine will to preserve patriarchal power, for even dedicated feminists opposed her. Her life recorded a remarkable historical moment in which female sexuality began to be separated from reproduction, when sexuality began to become a legitimate part of a woman's identity. This historical moment is but a blip in human history, and its implications not only remain controversial but continue to become more complex with the ongoing revolution in reproductive and nonreproductive technologies. My hope in writing this book is, not only to do justice to a life worthy of attention, but to provide some historical perspective to changing definitions of womanhood and cultural perceptions of motherhood, sexuality, and pain. My hope as well is to offer a deeper understanding of the relationship these definitions and cultural perceptions had—and have—with national politics. These issues remain relevant. The birth control pill and the sexual revolution that ensued solved some problems but created a host of others that need no enumeration here. Even with reproductive choices, including the choice not to have children at all, reproduction itself continues to define women and to limit their rights in many of the same ways Roussel protested.

CHAPTER ONE

Conversion Experiences

General Rule

Everywhere and always, a young girl must seek to attain this purpose: to conserve and safeguard her modesty, her sincerity, and her
innocence. Thus, in whatever circumstances you find yourselves,
Mademoiselles,

> N'écoutez pas, ne dites rien,
>
> Baissez les yeux, vous serez bien
>
> [Do not listen, do not say anything,
>
> Lower your eyes, and you will be fine]
>
> —*Nelly Roussel, grade-school notebook, c. 1890*

Nelly Roussel was born on January 5, 1878, into a France that was sharply
polarized between the heirs of the Revolution of 1789 and those of the counter-
revolution. On one side stood republicans who welcomed the new possibilities
offered by science and modernization, embraced egalitarianism in civic life, in
principle, if not in the practice, and viewed the Catholic Church as their enemy.
On the other stood moral conservatives who embraced traditional hierarchies,
ardently supported the Church in public as well as private life, and opposed secular republicanism. Bourgeois families on both sides of the great political divide
felt insecure about their tumultuous world, one that, particularly from a Catholic
viewpoint, was fraught with danger for young girls. The admonitions that Roussel meticulously penned on the inside cover of her grade-school notebook, capture what so many adults felt on behalf of girls.[1]

Roussel was born into a proper bourgeois family that was, for the most part,
on the right-wing side of the great divide in French political culture. Although
she was raised as a devout Catholic, she nonetheless became one of the most
radical feminists France had ever known. Why and how did this occur? Part of
the answer lies in her innate attraction to theater and performance, and even her

religious devotion itself. The answer also lies in the political culture within which she came of age in the 1880s and 1890s: the legacy of the Paris Commune and the tumultuous events of the Dreyfus Affair.

The Paris Commune in 1871 had permanently deepened political fissures and increased moral fears in France. In this brief but bloody civil war, left-wing, antireligious, and predominately working-class Parisians patriotically resisted the French government's surrender to the Prussians and attempted to establish an independent municipality with far-reaching goals of radical social reform. Their resistance to the national government (temporarily located in Versailles) from March 18 to May 28 culminated in a siege of Paris by the latter. An estimated 20,000–25,000 people died in the fighting, and much of Paris burned, including some of its most venerated and symbolic buildings, such as the Tuileries, Hôtel de Ville, Palais Royal, and many others. The Communards' violent acts included taking hostage and executing the archbishop of Paris. In revenge, the government troops brutally tortured and killed many of their prisoners when they finally took control of Paris after a week of bloodshed.

Despite its brevity, the Commune bequeathed to France and Europe a legacy of deep bitterness and fear of class warfare. It also left an enduring image of the horrors that could result from women's participation in public life. Communard women not only demanded rights for themselves but participated in violence against government troops. The revolutionary Louise Michel and her associates wore men's clothing, formed battalions, and built barricades. But the most enduring image—one that made its way into Third Republic textbooks—was that of the purported female incendiary, the *pétroleuse,* who was everything a woman ought not to be: she represented liberated women who would "forget their femininity, devour their (male) children, and destroy civilization."[2] The *pétroleuse* was the product of magnified and distorted memory of women's actual activity. In the popular imagination, female arsonists of the Commune had demonically crept around Paris setting fires with petroleum-filled bottles, targeting in particular the basement windows of bourgeois homes. Contemporaries imagined that by engaging in violence—which women had indeed done, but not "insanely"—they unleashed their worst female instincts and threatened civilization itself. On both sides of the political spectrum, women's participation in the Commune left an enduring mythology, which, like the mythologies of previous revolutions, reinforced perceptions of the need to restrict women to their proper roles.[3]

The memory of military defeat, violent civil war, and mythical tales of the horrific *pétroleuses* of 1870–71 contributed to a widespread bourgeois belief that France was suffering from national decadence and degeneration.[4] A number of other developments—universal manhood suffrage, legalization of trade unions, intensified working-class unrest, and the emergence of mass culture and consumerism—reinforced this notion. Department stores, the "spectacular" attractions of Haussmann's wide boulevards, the growth in the number of theaters and *cafés-concerts*, and public spectacles such as world exhibitions that attracted millions of visitors brought men and women of all social classes into new public spaces. Economic and gender boundaries that had previously separated these public spaces melted away. New enticements—"dream worlds" and "dreadful delights"—gave bourgeois parents and teachers of young girls all the more reason to advise them to lower their eyes when in public.[5]

Adolescent girls and young unmarried women of the bourgeoisie lived under the constant scrutiny of their parents. The French bourgeoisie of the nineteenth century particularly feared women's innate sexuality and its potential for disrupting society. The "rules" appearing in Roussel's notebook illustrate a typical example of the moral education imposed on female students. Dangers lurked in every corner: the "principal subjects of perversion reside[d]" in the public spaces where young people exited from school, work or amusements. But they were also present in private spaces, "in bedrooms, receptions, conversations, reading and visits." Explicit instructions were given on how to appear in public: what to wear, how to be escorted, how to walk ("walk with a calm and light step, gloved hands joined, eyes lowered, the face imprinted with an expression of modesty and innocence . . . and veiled, with no holes for the eyes").[6]

Despite her apparent effort to commit these instructions to heart, at some point during her youth, Roussel raised her eyes. What she observed ultimately caused her to cross the battle lines from the Right to the Left; she became a freethinker, a Freemason, and a feminist. Her heroes came from the Communards and members of the First Communist International. Indeed, by her early adulthood, thanks to her marriage, she found herself surrounded by people who had participated in the Commune. Louise Michel, the ultimate "virago" of this event, became her most venerated heroine. The divisions and contradictions in French political culture and in the French gender system played themselves out in Roussel's life, helped shape her personal identity, and made her career.

Youthful Dramas

Nelly Roussel (figs. 1 and 2) was the first of two girls born to Louise Nel Roussel and Léon Roussel, who were, respectively, twenty and twenty-four years old at the time of her birth. Both parents were of bourgeois background: Louise was the daughter of a railroad engineer and the granddaughter of a physician. Léon Roussel, a building contractor, was the son of a wholesale dealer in colonial produce. Léon died at age forty, in 1894, when Nelly was sixteen. Although one friend referred to Roussel's "cult" of his memory, her father remains curiously absent from her personal papers and from the memory of his grandchild. On the other hand, Nelly was close to her mother, Louise Nel, "a sensible and timorous woman" (fig. 3). Andrée was born two years after Nelly, in 1880. Although the sisters were close friends most of their lives, they were extremely different from one another. Nelly became a serious intellectual with a passion for social causes. Andrée was self-absorbed, frivolous, and immature throughout her adulthood.[7]

Although Roussel received a traditional religious education for girls and embraced religion with passion, she also developed a love for the theater and for acting. Like the competing left- and right-wing forces in French culture at the time, her two passions were at once interrelated and at odds with one another. Her religious devotion should have produced a "modest, sincere, and innocent" young woman, as stated in the "General Rule." But the "melodramatic brilliance of [the Church's] rites" instead fed her passion for drama.[8] Her maternal grandfather, Thomas Nel, in whose "villa" the family lived at 73 avenue de Saint Mandé, in the twelfth arrondissement, further cultivated her love for the theater, as well as for reading, playwriting, and acting. Nel, a well-off railroad engineer at the Gare de l'Est and member of the Engineering Academy, was forty-five when Nelly was born. They developed an extremely close relationship, particularly around their mutual taste for literature. Nel introduced his granddaughter to the theater. He had the greatest admiration for the famed actress Rachel (pseudonym of Elisa Félix, 1820–1858), who revived Corneille and Racine, seventeenth-century playwrights who became Roussel's own favorites.[9] In addition to introducing Roussel to literature, Thomas Nel wrote plays, which the entire family acted. Nelly took up this hobby and wrote her first play at age six. Her transition from acting as child's play to serious commitment as an adolescent caused the first misunderstanding with her parents.

Most of the fiction Roussel wrote during her childhood and adolescence is uninteresting from a literary viewpoint, for it lacks originality and imagination. But her stories and plays do reveal an intellectual precociousness. They also contain recurrent themes that preoccupied her throughout her life.[10] In only one of the twenty-some manuscripts preserved in her personal papers does an adult male figure appear; he is a greedy landlord who suffers because he does not take the advice of his wife. Almost all the narratives assume the form of a fable. They feature a young girl or a young woman, usually of Roussel's own age at the time of writing, in a position of moral righteousness. The various heroines rescue boys or young men from moral or physical peril. Occasionally, a mother is present, and she too is rescued by the young heroine in some manner. But the children and young adults in these stories are more often orphaned. Some of the narratives suggest an acute social conscience in their graphic descriptions of poverty. All of them are set in a religiously inspired, morally unambiguous world. They often end with adages such as "avoid pride and seek simplicity," and "a good deed is never lost." They emphasize female modesty, hard work, studiousness, Christian piety, patriotism, and always the importance of honor.

These recurrent themes come to full fruition in the plays of Roussel's late teens, such as "La Soeur de Comte Jean ("Count John's Sister"), which she composed in December 1896, just before her nineteenth birthday.[11] The setting is Paris during the Middle Ages, in the reign of Charles V. Blanche d'Estrées, nineteen years old, lives with her brother John, who is twenty-two. Orphaned, Blanche has become the mother figure in John's life. Blanche is dying of an unnamed disease (probably tuberculosis) that involves slow degeneration—she is expected to live another one to three years. Concern and love for her brother give Blanche the will to stay alive.

John and Blanche live in mutual adoration, but there is one problem around which the plot develops: John leads a life of debauchery, despite Blanche's efforts to set him straight. He attends intemperate "orgies," from which he returns "with a fevered head, haggard eyes, troubled spirit," a state "not worthy of a gentleman." Blanche succeeds in persuading her brother to give up his "mad passion for pleasure," but he breaks his promise to her and attends one more banquet, which proves fateful: he argues drunkenly with another young man and ends up thrusting his sword into his opponent's chest, unintentionally killing him.

John returns home shamefacedly, feeling that he has lost his honor. He is no longer worthy of the name d'Estrées. When informed that the king may pardon him, John reacts indifferently, convinced that he has "lost his manhood," and that nothing can restore his honor. Upon hearing the news about her brother, Blanche's illness becomes critical. John believes that she is dying because of the dishonor he has brought to her and to the family name. On her deathbed, Blanche's Christian love prevails. She tells John that he must suffer for both atonement and reparation. He must renounce his licentious life and perfidious friends and engage in prayer and charity. But his life also has a more heroic purpose: the king and the *patrie* need him to bear arms. He must sacrifice himself for the health and glory of the country. In pressing these duties upon him, she evokes the memory of the Crusades. As Blanche dies, her last wish is that John, through valor and devotion, "earn for himself the right to raise his head again."

Similar themes emerge in "La Passion du jeu" ("The Passion for Gambling"), also written in 1896, which is set in contemporary Paris.[12] In this play, a sister again serves as the moral guardian of her brother, whose addiction to gambling causes him to lose the family home and his portion of the inheritance. As in the previous play, the brother laments losing his honor; the sister responds with Christian love and forgiveness and offers to preserve the family honor by pay-ing off his gambling debts with her own inheritance. Themes of Christian piety, codes of honor, and feminine modesty and female self-sacrifice dominate these plays. An interesting irony also runs through them. Women, excluded from pub-lic life, do not have the liberty to become debauched or to gamble; rather, they rescue irresponsible brothers who are the bearers of family honor yet bring dis-honor to the family. Roussel's heroines are selfless, and they reflect prescribed roles for women in the 1880s and 1890s—except for the fact that none of them ever marries or expresses any wish to do so. Her themes also imitate those in female-authored domestic novels of the nineteenth century.[13]

These narratives suggest Roussel's girlhood attachment to traditional social and cultural values. She also revealed this traditionalism in her notebooks of *confidences,* or "secrets," kept as part of a popular form of parlor entertainment in which family members and friends recorded their preferences with regard to contemporary cultural tastes. In 1889, at age eleven, she listed "piety" as her favorite virtue. Henri IV and Louis XVI were her favorite "real-life" heroes, and Joan of Arc and Marie Antoinette were her favorite heroines. In a man, she most valued courage, patriotism, and loyalty; in a woman, gentleness, friendliness, and charity. Reading was her favorite activity, and her literary tastes included Racine, the comtesse de Ségur, and Jules Verne. Several of these "favorites" persisted through the next decade, reappearing in a subsequent notebook of "secrets" re-corded in February 1898, just after her twentieth birthday, and just after she met her future husband, Henri Godet.[14]

Roussel's youthful tastes at first sight suggest devout religiosity and veneration of France's monarchical past. But they also reflect countervailing tendencies of a nascent independence. Her plays follow the patterns of her favorite playwright, Racine, who portrayed human nature as self-seeking, impulsive, and weak. She applied these negative qualities, however, only to men. Her stories repeatedly emphasize female strength and wisdom in the face of male weakness—even stupidity—and loss of honor. Women often appropriate the honor abandoned by fathers and brothers. Her favorite authors suggest a further ambivalence: the comtesse de Ségur penned highly popular books for young people—*Les Malheurs de Sophie* is a sample title—which were read by middle- and upper-class girls of Roussel's and later generations, but Jules Verne wrote about an exclusively male universe of travel, escape, adventure, exploration, and a belief in scientific progress and the infinite possibilities of modernity.

Roussel's tastes suggest contradictory influences on her character, at once feminine and masculine, the first encouraging conformity to a conservative feminine ideal, the second, independence of mind and strong will. Her family and her education provided both forces. Her "timorous" mother imposed a strict Catholic education and religious observance on her. In both Catholic and secular schools, textbooks taught that the ideal woman was "gentle, patient, modest, charitable and reserved." She bore hardship with "joyous resignation." One of these hardships—apparent in Roussel's stories—was the loss of one or both parents, something not infrequent even in the late nineteenth century. When such losses occurred, young girls were expected to take on the adult roles of parenting and housekeeping. Underlying the content of Third Republic textbooks was the supposition that "women found self-fulfillment only by serving others." Characters in the textbook stories emphasized sacrifice as the "source of the best joys."[15]

The curriculum also stressed patriotism as a sentiment that girls had to learn so that they could transmit it to their future husbands and sons and encourage them to fight for France and fulfill their duties to the *patrie* by being brave. Textbooks also provided material on Roussel's chosen heroes, celebrating Joan of Arc more than any other Frenchwoman and even providing "flattering vignettes" of Marie Antoinette. Roussel's literary tastes and personal heroes largely reflect these themes. Her passion, spirituality, and, most important, her sense of justice derived from her Catholic education.[16]

Popular culture reinforced the conservative curriculum for Roussel and other Catholic girls. Joan of Arc became a pervasive icon after Prussia defeated France in 1870. Local festivals were held in her honor, and statues of her were erected in towns throughout France. Her image appeared on postcards, souvenirs, almanacs, and in commercial advertising, while hotels and other enterprises took on her name. But this armor-clad, sword-wielding amazon, who defied both Church and patriarchal authority, hardly embodied the image of ideal womanhood that both the Church and the Republic sought to foster. Children, and girls in particular, learned about her through a popular children's book, *Histoire de notre petite soeur Jeanne d'Arc* (The History of Our Little Sister Joan of Arc) by Marie-Edmée

Pau (1874), which recounted Joan's story only up to the time she left home. It portrayed her as obedient and pious, rather than as the unfeminine warrior she became.[17]

The Virgin Mary also enjoyed a surge in popularity after 1870. She too embodied the "good" feminine qualities of "chastity, humility, and maternal forgiveness" that Roussel learned in school, and that she wrote about in her stories and plays. French Catholics used her as a unifying national symbol in an effort to atone for the sins that had caused military defeat and civil war in the Paris Commune. Moreover, the Church used modern means of mass production and the mass press to popularize her image. Their efforts became particularly intense from the 1880s on—Roussel's formative years as a schoolgirl—when the Assumptionists founded the daily newspaper *La Croix* and utilized all possible tactics in their defense of tradition against the evils of the modern world. Emmanuel d'Alzon formed the religious order called the Augustins de l'Assomption in 1850 as a response to France's repeated experience with revolution. The "rights of man" had been won, but he wished to make certain that "the right of God" would not disappear. *La Croix* became a key Assumptionist weapon in this task and enjoyed widespread influence among Catholics. Its circulation grew from 14,000 in 1884 to 168,000 in 1892, and prior to World War I, it reached 180,000.[18]

Although Roussel's writings and tastes reflected the weight of her Catholic education and the cultural icons that reinforced it, they also have a subversive quality. One of the most important teachings in girls' textbooks—and indeed in article 213 of the Civil Code—was the moral, psychological, and legal subservience of women to men. Husbands were supposed to rule over wives, while fathers represented "authority, force, and work."[19] But authoritative, hard-working men have no place in Roussel's fiction. Their absence allowed her to reconcile the blatant contradiction in a society that set women up as repositories of virtue, while placing all authority—especially legal authority and citizenship itself—in the male. In their emphasis on female strength and wisdom in the face of male weakness, Roussel's stories implicitly challenged women's exclusion from citizenship.

Roussel's independence of mind received encouragement from the most important male influence in her life, especially during her teens: her maternal grandfather, Thomas Nel, who encouraged the "male" side of her personality by giving her access to his library and encouraging her playwriting and acting. Like many other bourgeois Frenchmen in the nineteenth century, Nel was not a practicing Catholic, and he provided a crucial counterpoint to Roussel's formal education with the books he made available to her. Moreover, the popular icons that symbolized conservative moral values also represented their opposites. If Joan of Arc and the Virgin Mary—and even Marie Antoinette—presented adolescent girls with powerful patriotic imagery of martyrdom and self-sacrifice, they also contained contradictory symbolism, as well as mixed messages about femininity and motherhood. Joan of Arc heroically defended "truth" with her body like a man, not to mention rejecting marriage and motherhood. While admired as the "most powerful and ideal of mothers," Mary hardly represented the realities of motherhood. Inasmuch as her child, Jesus, was immaculately conceived, she was *both* a virgin *and* a mother, an ideal girls could not possibly fulfill. Moreover, her most common iconographical representation, similar to those of Joan of Arc, had Mary standing over the crushed snake of sin, with arms outstretched, projecting an image of militancy and defiance.[20] Marie Antoinette, although not portrayed in textbooks as such, had been vilified in her lifetime as a sexually licentious "bad mother." Added to these three powerful images in French culture was a fourth, Marianne, the iconic representation of the Republic itself. A complex symbol with multiple meanings, Marianne represented a nurturing "motherland," but she also represented revolution, independence, liberty, and democracy.[21] Young girls and women were thus continually exposed to female representations not only replete with internal contradictions but different from the ideal of womanhood that both the Church and the Third Republic intended to promote. Thus the "conservative" influences in Roussel's life supplied her with weapons for her future militancy: in subsequent years, she would deftly employ the images of the female martyr and the female warrior, both supplied in her youth.

Female education and French popular culture in the 1880s and 1890s could thus influence girls in a variety of ways, either in conformity with or subversive of "ideal" womanhood. In Roussel's case, personal experiences when she came of age finally tore the veil from her eyes. Her religious faith began to weaken in the early 1890s. This disaffection corresponded with events that brought anger and personal tragedy to her life as she completed her formal schooling. Her parents did not permit her to continue her education beyond age fifteen (1893), when "honest girls" terminated their studies. This deprivation, which Roussel's daughter later described as a form of "castration," became her first perception of the "injustice that favored boys." That same year, she lost a good friend to typhoid, and the following year, 1894, her father died. Her mother somewhat scandalously remarried barely a year after Léon Roussel's death. Her new husband was Antonin Montupet (fig. 4), a wealthy shipbuilding engineer and family friend, a grand bourgeois "who made quite a to-do with his automobile, coach, and Sunday walks in the park." Neither Nelly nor Andrée ever warmed to their stepfather, and they frequently expressed contempt for him. After her mother's marriage,

Nelly spent more time in Marseille, where her grandfather Nel had moved, "devouring" his library. Letters she wrote to him from Paris manifest the special connection with him that freed her from the conventions of her own family.[22]

A hunger for the theater dominated Roussel's life. Considered "remarkably gifted for tragedy," she desired more than anything to pursue an acting career. In this era of Sarah Bernhardt's celebrity, actresses became more accepted as public figures. A greater acceptance of women who were "ambitious, achieving, and public" permitted actresses to become rich, famous, and consequential, which, in turn, offered new models of womanhood. But the stage nonetheless eroticized women, and actresses did not make "honorable" wives in conventional marriages; some, in fact, became courtesans.[23] That Nelly's mother and stepfather refused to let her pursue an acting career is therefore hardly surprising. It made sense in their world, for no bourgeoise of proper upbringing would take such a path.[24] Disconsolate at having her ambitions denied, Roussel devoted herself privately to theatrical performance in playwriting, directing, and acting, particularly when she was with her grandfather, friends, and other family members. Letters to her grandfather reveal the degree of their collaboration, the seriousness with which she took her own theatrical projects, her love of costume, and the power she felt in directing plays. In 1896, she described the activities of the little troop of friends she had recruited to perform one of her plays:

> I hope that our new drama is taking shape in your brain; the sight of great quantities of sapphire must be germinating noble and grandiose ideas within you. I recommend giving Charles VI a magnificent role, with fits of madness sometimes furious and terrible, sometimes painful and poignant. Let your genius soar, and glide into brilliant spheres!
>
> As for drama # 1, we rehearsed all day last Thursday; all went very well, Juliette carried off the conception successfully; Renaud was full of fire; Rodolphe was better than usual.[25]

Roussel's dedication to traditions and personages from the Middle Ages and the moral content of the plays she wrote in her late teens indicate that religion continued to inspire her. She considered the Church her "other theater, [her] place for facing obscure forces, but also [a] temple for discourse, [the] place of the spoken word, which fascinated her."[26] But two events in 1898, just after she turned twenty, radically transformed her life. The first was the reopening of the Dreyfus case; the second was her introduction to Henri Godet, a sculptor, freethinker, and Freemason fifteen years her senior. The conjuncture of events occurred just as Roussel was ripe for taking on a new, very different role than that which she could play out within the parameters her family had established for her. Becoming involved with Godet just when the revived Dreyfus Affair shook the foundations of French political and cultural identity gave their relationship more personal and political poignancy.

Marriage: A New Curtain Rises

Henri Godet was barely an inch taller than Roussel, but with his shock of dark hair, beard, and irrepressible wit, he was an imposing presence (fig. 5). He had been born in the Belleville district of Paris in 1863, and by the time he met Roussel, he had for many years been living at 58 rue du Rendez-vous, a mere three hundred meters away from her home. They were introduced in January 1898, at a party given by mutual friends. In a later memoir, Godet wrote that their meeting produced in her "a whole new dawning of ideas, as well as the complete blossoming of her own faculties."[27] The subject of conversation the night they met must surely have been the Dreyfus Affair, for it was an unavoidable topic, whose intensity was peaking that same month. This event left an indelible mark on French history and transformed countless lives, including those of Nelly Roussel and Henri Godet.

Alfred Dreyfus, a Jew from Alsace, was a captain in the French Army assigned to the General Staff. In 1894, a clique of monarchists in the army accused him of having delivered confidential documents to France's most hated enemy, Germany. Though evidence of his guilt was weak, anti-Semitic presumptions about the likely disloyalty of Jews resulted in his being court-martialed in December 1894 and sentenced to imprisonment on Devil's Island, a penal colony in French Guiana. Dreyfus's family organized a protest, initially to little effect. It took three years before the case drew the unsympathetic attention of the French National Assembly, at which point the press stepped in and turned the case into an *affaire*.

Henri Godet numbered among those who sympathized with Dreyfus's plight. Initially labeled "revisionists," those who backed Dreyfus wanted the case retried, because it had been so badly conducted. They believed that because judicial procedure had been compromised, France itself—an exemplar of republicanism—was being compromised and was risking its international reputation. Those who opposed reopening the case—and Nelly Roussel may initially have been among them—believed that the army and its justice were "sacred," and that questioning Dreyfus's conviction would seriously weaken the nation and its defense. For the sake of its security, France and its military had to be above doubt. But many in this camp firmly believed in Dreyfus's guilt because he was Jewish, on the anti-Semitic assumption that Jews were treacherous by nature, and that he was part of a conspiracy. The virulent anti-Semitism that provoked the initial accusation stemmed from a number of complex factors located in social, cultural, and economic changes that were taking place throughout Europe during this period. In France, Édouard Drumont—one of Nelly Roussel's future enemies—fanned the flames of hatred in his five-hundred-page best-seller *La "France juive"* (Jewish France), published in 1886. In 1892, he founded an anti-Semitic newspaper, *La Libre Parole* (Free Speech), whose circulation quickly peaked at 100,000, and did much to inflame anti-Dreyfusard sentiment.[28]

On January 13, 1898, Émile Zola published his article "J'accuse," an exposé of the military court's errors and their cover-up, which galvanized both Right and Left into camps of bitter opposition. These events were unfolding when Nelly Roussel and Henri Godet met that same month. A few weeks later, on February 20, Henri joined a group of elite intellectuals, artists, and members of the liberal professions to form the League of the Rights of Man, whose membership grew to 8,000 by the end of the year.[29] The League's purpose was to discover the truth about the case and to convey it to the reading public; members committed themselves to ensuring that the Declaration of the Rights of Man and Citizen of 1789 and 1793 was put into practice, and they agitated for the separation of church and state. From early 1898 on, the republican, freethinking, intellectual Left was enthusiastically Dreyfusard and actively involved in the Affair. Its polemics rocked France for a year and a half and became a permanent feature of both parliamentary debates and street politics, deepening and consolidating the "war of religion" between Left and Right. Dreyfus was finally retried by a military court in August 1899 and again found guilty. But by this point, France had a new president, Émile Loubet, who pardoned Dreyfus. Though the pardon resolved the immediate crisis, it did not end the Affair—the nation was left embittered, scarred, and further divided than ever. Anti-Semitic sentiment, moreover, had come into its own in the mass press.

Had Nelly Roussel never met Henri Godet, she probably would have supported Dreyfus. Like many French, she might not have paid much attention to the case until the publication of Zola's "J'accuse" in January 1898; but then her inherent logic and intense sense of justice would have politicized her. Godet, as noted above, retrospectively assumed responsibility for Roussel's political conversion in his memory of the night they met. He had, after all, long been political and was attempting to integrate art and politics. Writing in the third person and using Marxist language, Godet described himself at the time of their first encounter as "a sculptor in love with his art, . . . also, which is rare in an artist, a militant of socialism and of freethinking. He suffered from seeing that art was always only employed as an opiate for use by the people to better subject them. He dreamed of a social art, liberating the brains and moralizing the individual, put in the service of the proletariat, which he would improve and make capable of founding the society of tomorrow."[30]

Godet exhibited his sculptures annually at the Salon des Artistes français from 1893 to 1923, and by the time he met Roussel, he had achieved some renown. He received a third-prize medal for a piece entitled *La Fable et la verité* (Fable and Truth) in 1893 (he is standing in front of it in fig. 5). Another sculpture, *Le Lierre* (Ivy) earned him recognition for his technique, unusual for the time, of sculpting from a photo rather than from a live model, which enabled him to represent an unusually difficult pose. But it is difficult to see from most of his pieces how his art was "social." Indeed, despite Godet's avant-garde political stance and his bohemian lifestyle, his sculptures were classical portrayals of the female body and motherhood—in an era of rapid change in the art world. For the most part in his art and in his other cultural tastes, he remained conservative. Long after his death, many of his smaller works in the art nouveau style would command high prices. *La Maternité* (Maternity), which, like many other sculptures he did, glorified motherhood, is perhaps one of his most overtly "moral" works (fig. 6).[31]

Up to the time of their meeting, Godet recounted, Nelly "hardly dreamed of marriage . . . her perspective from the milieu in which she lived made her consider it improbable that she would meet a man capable of understanding her and sharing her ideas," because her ideas were "considered madness." Godet, thirty-five years old at the time, was fifteen years Nelly's senior, and only five years younger than her mother. He had also given up hope of meeting anyone who would suit his "ideal," or of having a family. He had found no one who in any way responded to his own moral aspirations. He would, after all, have to find someone who would consent to a civil marriage, for as a freethinker he was staunchly anticlerical and antireligious, and "it wouldn't occur to him for a single instant" to enter a church.[32] Indeed, civil marriages were among the most important symbolic actions freethinkers could take in order to demonstrate their liberation from any religious imprint.

Upon their meeting, Godet was immediately struck "by the intelligence radiating from [Roussel's] huge brown eyes, and above all by her voice, so pure, at once serious and harmonious." It was probably the political fervor of the Dreyfus Affair that gave her the opportunity to demonstrate her "serious and thoughtful air" that so impressed him. Her black hair, pulled up and back, showed off her beautiful face, and he considered her "an inaccessible beauty."[33] She dazzled him with her "independence of mind" and by how she was making "the most difficult moral evolution" entirely on her own, without any support or assistance. This process required "the hard necessity of ripping from her heart everything [she had] been taught to love, without knowing if all this could be replaced by something else." From that first meeting, Godet imagined Roussel to be "morally repressed." He envisioned himself "tearing her elite intelligence from the clerical influence that surrounds it, which still prevents it from being completely liberated."[34] In fact, her reading tastes (such as Jules Verne) and her acting ambitions suggest that Nelly was more modern and aesthetically progressive than her future husband. He did provide her with the opportunity to realize her own selfhood, but he would soon discover that he played more the role of a servant who released the genie than a Pygmalion who remade the woman.

Godet was hardly the husband Roussel's conventional bourgeois family would have envisioned for her, if, indeed, they could imagine any husband for their unusual daughter. Not only was he an artist, a Freemason, and passionately anticlerical, he was the son of Jules Godet, a Communard and a former member of the First International, who made a living as an engraver of jewelry. Perhaps even more of an impediment for Roussel's family, Godet's mother, Adelaide Gans, was a Jew, making him Jewish and his pairing with Roussel consequently a scandalous event in her social world—especially in the anti-Semitic climate of the Dreyfus Affair. But Henri's friends "forced him to overcome his timidity." Perhaps Roussel's family accepted him because they feared their daughter would never marry, as she herself believed.[35]

The "secrets" (*confidences*) that Godet and Roussel recorded in February 1898, shortly after they met, reveal interesting tastes. Some seem surprisingly conventional, especially for the freethinking Godet. Nelly listed patriotism as her favorite virtue. Her real-life heroes, with the exception of Marie Antoinette, remained the same as at age eleven: Joan of Arc, Henry IV, and Louis XVI. Her response to the two separate questions asking for preferred male and female qualities demonstrated a hint of feminism, for she collapsed her answer for both sexes: enthusiasm, dignity, elevation of ideas. What troubled her most deeply were "narrowness of mind" and prejudice, while theater gave her the greatest pleasure. Perhaps because of the Dreyfus Affair, she listed "honor and fatherland" as her current "state of mind." Henri's conceptions of gender seem to have been more traditional. He listed bravery as his favorite virtue, sincerity as the best male quality, and sweetness (*douceur*) and kindness as the best qualities in a woman. Mothers, as already suggested by his sculpture, were his greatest real-life heroines. He and Roussel shared literary tastes in Victor Hugo and Corneille.[36]

Godet and Roussel became engaged about a month after they met, on February 28, 1898, and they were married the following June 6. Given her independence and his habituation to bachelorhood, it is not surprising that Henri described their period of engagement as one that had "a few quarrels, for each of us wanted to marry a person in perfect conformity of opinion with him- or herself, which seemed to lead us to a rupture. But we slid quickly on the slope of mutual concessions because we loved each other."[37] Indeed, Henri compromised his principles—and not for the last time on her behalf—by having a religious wedding celebrated in the Church of the Immaculate Conception. "Who would not accept it at this moment?" he rationalized. He was "physically and morally in love," with "the clear vision that he [would] never find anywhere a girl responding better to his ideal, a soul completing so well his soul."[38] From that point on, for the next twenty-five years, Godet claimed, their "perfect accord" was never troubled by the least dispute. "Our collaboration was complete in all the domains: Nelly knew how to interest me in the unjust fate done to women by prejudice, religion and laws . . . I showed her the absurdity of all dogmas."[39] Upon marrying, Nelly and Henri moved into an apartment at 179 rue Michel Bizot. It was just around the corner from her family home and from the ground-floor apartment on the rue du Rendez-vous where Godet had been living and where he would continue to have his sculpting workshop. That he employed several workers and paid annual rents of 900 francs and 1,200 francs respectively for his home and workshop suggests that he made a fairly good living as a sculptor.[40]

Roussel retained her maiden name and was only rarely addressed as "Madame Godet." And although she also retained a bourgeois façade in her appearance and longtime social relations, this "marriage of feminism and freethinking," as Godet called it, anchored her in a radical, bohemian milieu of leftist culture and politics. No doubt because of her husband, Nelly joined a mixed Freemason lodge, La Grande Lodge symbolique écossaise, whose members included Louise Michel, Madeleine Pelletier, and Céline Renooz, as well as Henri Godet; it became known for its anarchist, socialist, feminist and neo-Malthusian sympathies. The members of this lodge gave lectures at *universités populaires* (popular universities).[41] There, Roussel quickly discovered the power of her voice and a talent for public speaking when she began doing literary readings and giving lectures.

Like the League of the Rights of Man, popular universities, originating in 1896, rapidly expanded throughout France after 1899 as a result of the Dreyfus Affair. They became a movement whose goal was to unite workers and bourgeois intellectuals for their "mutual education." The audience they targeted consisted of youth in the ages between leaving primary school and entering military service or full-time work. Depending on one's viewpoint, the purpose of these schools was to divert youth in these "dangerous years" from the "traps" of either socialism and revolution or clericalism and nationalism. In principle, they were supposed to offer courses in a large array of subjects, ranging from the hard sciences to the social sciences and aesthetics. But in practice, education took the form of individual lectures, often on practical matters, such as public health, the family, the role of women, alcoholism, and the applications of electricity. They existed in all the arrondissements of Paris, meeting in public spaces provided by the municipalities. Because they brought together two elements excluded from the formation of the Third Republic whose combination was potentially subversive—intellectuals and workers—some public officials viewed popular universities with great suspicion. The right-wing considered them the dangerous work of Freemasons, Jews, and Huguenots.[42]

Both Roussel and Godet actively participated in several of the popular universities, especially in the Masonic "Diderot," located in their own arrondissement, the twelfth. There they held readings, discussions, and literary lectures, many of which were from, or about, Victor Hugo. As an administrator of this particular popular university, Henri allegedly issued free personal invitations whenever an "interesting lecture" was being presented—probably one of his wife's. For this reason, and because the police distrusted these institutions, Roussel and Godet came under police surveillance. Roussel reveled in her experience with these institutions, for it quickly made her realize that public speaking was her true calling, one more "noble and interesting" than the theater, because it was based on conviction and authenticity rather than on the performance of fictional identities. She never, however, abandoned her interest in playwriting and performing, which she eventually integrated into her political mission.[43]

Conception of a Child, Birth of a Mission

Nelly took enormous pleasure in doing readings and discussing excerpts from Victor Hugo at the popular universities, where for the first time she "performed" in front of public audiences. Within the first year of her marriage, however, she became pregnant, which not only interrupted her public activities but transformed her in ways she had not anticipated. In June 1899, approximately three months into her pregnancy, she felt profoundly confused about the new life growing within her. In manuscript ruminations she entitled "Impressions d'un jour de mélancolie" (Impressions of a Melancholy Day), she realized that the prospect of a child threatened her sense of self. Like other memoirs she and

Godet wrote, she composed this one in the third person, as though to step out-side herself to examine her own identity. As the following excerpts show, this un-published memoir offers a candid expression of her feelings about motherhood that subsequently inspired her political evolution. It begins with the description of a young and pretty bride sitting in her room contemplating her fear of child-birth, one that has become "an obsession, a haunting dread, a hardship that un-nerves her, and raises in her . . . a strange impulse to cry. In barely six months, the awaited and dreaded event will have happened. Certainly, she is resigned a little from all sides; readings and conversations have taught her more or less how things happen . . . but what good are words and theories before the troubling anxiety of the unknown?"[44] She goes on to express confidence that all will go well. However, Roussel also knows that in spite of everything, "creation always remains . . . a dreadful thing." She entertains the "secret hope" that what she has heard about childbirth is exaggerated; she finds it impossible that nature would be so unfair and illogical as to make something necessary to the human species "into a torture." She expects to suffer, she tells herself, and suffering does not frighten her, "because she is a woman." Her pride and self-respect will give her courage.

Nelly Roussel was not alone in her dread of childbirth, for it was common among women of her era. Most of them were deprived of knowledge about their own bodies, but they knew about the high rates of maternal mortality. Though she had learned "more or less how things happened" from "readings and conver-sations," such education was unusual in her generation. Even by the end of the nineteenth century, many if not most Frenchwomen remained ignorant about their bodies, sex, and childbirth. Girls and women spoke about them among themselves, but they usually only succeeded in terrifying one another. Mothers avoided discussing childbirth with their daughters because they did not want to frighten them, but ignorance inspired even more fear.[45]

Death in childbirth was common enough that for many women going into la-bor was like "going off to war." In Roussel's day, maternal mortality—defined as the number of deaths during pregnancy, labor, or the lying-in period—fluctuated from .25 percent to 6.6 percent, but sometimes rose as high as 9 percent in ly-ing-in hospitals. Most deaths occurred from puerperal fever, a highly contagious streptococcal infection spread by birth attendants who went from patient to pa-tient. While antisepsis and asepsis reduced the incidence of puerperal fever from the 1880s on, the rate nonetheless remained relatively high, because the strepto-coccus remained unidentified until 1934. Puerperal hemorrhage and hyperten-sive disease in pregnancy were the other leading causes of maternal mortality.[46]

Although childbirth was not the most common cause of death among women—tuberculosis held that place in Roussel's lifetime—its tragedy had symbolic importance because of the "deeply held feeling that mothers should not die in the course of the normal process of reproduction."[47] Roussel recognized this contradiction and went on to suggest in her memoir that the courage to overcome the fear of childbirth was inherent in womanhood—her own apprehension notwithstanding. Fear of pain and death, however, was not all that troubled her, for she continued to explain that she was dominated by "the voiceless and bitter revolt of all her instincts for justice against the destiny of Woman, against all the pains of which her existence is made, and above all against indifference, unpardonable ingratitude of Humanity toward [the mother] who lives and suffers only for it!" Society aggravates nature's burden by "adding humiliation to suffering." It strips the "female Creator" of the respect, admiration, and recognition that she deserves. Roussel then declared that her revolt does not "make her a criminal," because she does not have the "guilty desire to escape from her duties." Yet the moral task of rearing a child also fills her with fear. A "troubling anguish" grips her as she thinks about "the long slavery, the exhaustion, the cares and anxieties of each day." And then "her young face becomes hollow . . . and in her fixed eyes, full of thought, tears well up, burning."

Thinking she had found the courage to endure the pain of childbirth with dignity, Nelly's thoughts uncovered a contradiction within herself: she felt a strong urge to rebel against women's "inevitable destiny," and yet her own sense of honor made her feel that she should not desire any escape from maternal responsibilities. Her words are laden with regret for her inevitable transformation from a "young bride," finally free from familial constraints, to a hollow "slave" emptied of her selfhood. Fear of a metaphorical death in the loss of personal autonomy once a child is born has been common among women.[48] As noted above, in Roussel's day, according to both religious dogma and textbooks attempting to establish gender roles for the Third Republic, women were not supposed to have an autonomous sense of self; they were expected to sacrifice themselves for their families and in the name of civic duty. Moreover, advice manuals available to Roussel's contemporaries emphasized the pregnant woman's moral influence on the fetus and counseled "against sadness or any other bad feelings during a pregnancy" that might harm it.[49]

Nelly's sadness and implacable sense of self thus made her guilty and ashamed. The next passage in her memoir indicates that she tried to lose this selfish side by melting it into something bigger than herself: "Suddenly overcome by remorse, ashamed of her weakness, she pulls herself together, recalling her energy, and forcing herself to look to the future with confidence. . . . no, this is not for herself, for she is but a humble drop in the ocean of Humanity. It is for her entire sex, for the mass of her sisters, the majority of whom are less favored than she, that's why she's so indignant!"

Though denying it, Roussel's desperate tone here does suggest a wish to escape her duties, about which she felt guilty. The woman of Roussel's memoir was a talented tragedienne of superior intelligence, whose pregnancy rendered her ordinary and threatened her with the same fate as most women—including her own mother, who had been the same age as Nelly at the time of her first pregnancy. But in the process of writing this memoir, Nelly took that sense of ordinariness and reinvented herself. Upset that this pregnancy was foiling her life's calling as an actress and public speaker, she converted her anger into "everywoman's" pain and fear. She thereby gave birth to a new "mission" of her own even before giving birth to her child. By giving voice to a "voiceless and bitter revolt" of all women, she could at once vindicate her private feelings and absolve herself of guilt.

In the next passage, she clings to what makes her marriage extraordinary. She is certain that she will receive the "gentlest compensation" for the "inevitable torments of her existence as a woman" in the knowledge that she is deeply loved. Enduring her suffering with courage will perhaps make her husband love her even more. With this realization,

> Her serious face brightens with a smile; and her thoughts, full of emotion, calmed down, turn toward him, who, in her contempt for men, she distinguished as an exceptional being, in order to vow to him a tenderness that will grow ceaselessly, all the more as his superiority over so many others appears more striking. Yes, he will always be for her, whatever happens, the perceptive and devoted friend who supports, encourages, and consoles, because he understood, she has no doubt, all that there is of glory and sacrifice in the sublime Work of the Woman.

Thus Nelly found in her husband a savior from the indignations to which society condemned motherhood. As her devoted friend, Henri not only would understand the "Work of the Woman," but he would encourage her in the other work that she conceived for herself in that very moment.

These ruminations seem a sharp departure from her identification with the young self-sacrificing heroines of her earlier plays. Although she had constructed "maternal" relationships for her fictional characters, these relationships did not derive from biological motherhood. As self-denying maternal-type heroines, moreover, they did not suffer humiliation and disdain. Instead, they were the true possessors of honor. And the men who committed misdeeds suffered punishment. But in the actual world Roussel inhabited, men who mistreated women went unpunished, while innocent women who devoted themselves to motherhood suffered the undeserved retribution of pain and disregard. Ruminations about her own pregnancy thus revealed to Roussel a new source of injustice.

In resisting her female destiny, Roussel also rebelled against notions about motherhood current in Third Republic France. The country's low birthrate turned the attention of physicians, reformers, and demographers to motherhood, but not the sort of attention that glorified it. In its attitudes toward motherhood, nineteenth-century French society "displayed one of its major contradictions: on the one hand, it orchestrated a fervent and lyrical exaltation of motherhood, and on the other, it did not dare to prepare future mothers for their task with any candor. Motherhood was at once idealized and discredited . . . as though the human species wanted to deny its animality" in an age of scientific and technical accomplishments.[50] And, as Roussel already knew, science had done nothing to alleviate the pain of childbirth. Catholic educational and religious precepts held that "pain was considered inevitable and even necessary" and a source of redemption.[51] Pain has always been a feature of childbirth, though its degree and duration have varied historically, culturally, and individually. Nonetheless, the anticipation of agony in childbirth crosses cultures, primitive and modern, and is common enough to have been incorporated into most, if not all, theologies.[52]

The Judeo-Christian tradition has always held that sacrifice is inherent in female nature. It derives from Eve's sin in taking the apple from the serpent and giving it to Adam to eat, tempting him into the Fall. Pain in childbirth is Eve's redemption from the sin of this act. The necessity of female pain and risk in childbirth has long played an important role in French Catholic culture. The renowned churchman Jacques-Bénigne Bossuet (1627–1704) said that "fecundity is the glory of woman . . . it is only at the peril of her life that she is fertile . . . the child cannot be born without putting its mother in danger. Eve is wretched and accursed in all her sex."[53] Both the Bible and Church teachings emphasized the redemptive role of pain in childbirth. The "prayer of the pregnant woman awaiting her confinement" that appeared in seventeenth- and eighteenth-century texts suggests that women were encouraged to accept pain as their only source of redemption. And it must be remembered that death from childbirth remained a statistically significant threat until the twentieth century. That fact made Bossuet's preaching and the "prayer of pregnant women" retain their relevance.[54] Even as France became secularized, it did not lose its Catholic sensibilities, especially among women who remained believers. The assumption that women had to suffer was translated into the notion that they were self-sacrificing "by nature."

Christian theology also developed a more nuanced stance toward martyrdom and suffering. Christ, after all, had performed healing miracles, and the development of medical science provided new possibilities for the alleviation of pain. By the end of the nineteenth century, scientific medicine, the Enlightenment heritage, and modern secular outlooks gave priority to eliminating pain. Drugs such as morphine became available in the early nineteenth century, and efforts to alleviate the pain of childbirth began in the 1840s with the use of chloroform and ether. But the Church resisted eliminating the pain of childbirth and attacked chloroform as "a decoy of Satan, apparently offering itself to bless women," that would instead "harden society and rob God of the deep earnest cries which arise in time of trouble for help."[55]

Queen Victoria gave the use of chloroform high visibility and moral sanction with the births of her seventh and eighth children in the 1850s, however, making it popular in England. A few French physicians adopted it, but its acceptance across the Channel was far slower, in part because of Empress Eugenie, wife of Napoleon III, who, in 1856, suffering a delivery with forceps, refused chloroform, deliberately expressing a "Catholic and Latin morality in which suffering is meritorious and permits the sublimation of the individual."[56]

Indeed, despite the progress of secularization in France, when it came to moral attitudes about the pain of labor, French culture remained traditional, but with a modern republican twist that had roots in France's revolutionary past. Women as well as men during the Third Republic were expected to exhibit civic courage for the *patrie*, in the context not only of the expected future war against Germany, but of the war against depopulation.[57] The best opportunity for them to do so was offered by the "battlefield" of motherhood, where pain assumed a secular meaning. In her study of childbirth in the early twentieth century, Françoise Thebaud points out that the culture remained *doloriste*, embracing the doctrine that pain has utility and moral value. She cites doctors who used the mother's screams during labor to measure its progress. A survey of midwives indicated that within their culture—which at once reflected the medical world and the broader society—pain was considered inevitable, that it was the price one paid for pleasure, and that "woman is a suffering subject." Until the interwar period, French doctors generally did not intervene to reduce pain during labor, because they feared it would do more harm than good by interfering with contractions, resulting in the use of forceps and possible toxicity as a consequence. The only time they resorted to chloroform was when the mother's agitation interfered with the labor itself.[58]

Frenchwomen interviewed about their experiences in the early twentieth century—Roussel's generation—said that "childbirth was lived in the anguish of death, as a violent aggression which caused the loss of all human dignity" and that provoked "inhuman screams" like the "shrieks of injured beasts." Nor did postpartum care bring dignity or relief from pain. Improperly treated perineal tears caused exhaustion and became a deterrent to having more babies.[59] Pain in childbirth was collectively taken for granted, as a plight common among women; even feminists—Madeleine Vernet, Madeleine Pelletier, Henriette Alquier—spoke about the pain of childbirth as "inevitable." It was (and is) also forgotten by many individual women, because in its most extreme form, pain cannot be verbally translated, and the brain thus does not store a precise memory of it.[60] Outside the tiny and specialized milieu of women physicians, no precise demand for prevention of pain in childbirth arose, nor even any coherent public discussion about it. Nelly Roussel would become the one exception in making such a demand and in talking about it publicly.

CHAPTER TWO

Mother and Missionary

The Ideological Foundations of an Unorthodox Feminism

In my confinement, strengthen my heart to endure the pains that come therewith, and let me accept them as the consequence of your judgement upon our sex, for the sin of the first woman. In view of that curse, and of my own offences in marriage, may I suffer the cruelest pangs with joy, and may I join them with the suffering of your Son upon the cross, in the midst of which He engendered me into eternal life. Never can they be as harsh as I deserve, for although holy matrimony has made my conception legitimate, I confess that concupiscence mingled its venom therewith and that it has urged me to commit faults which displease you. If it be your will that I die in my confinement, may I adore it, bless it and submit to it.

A pregnant woman's prayer in Antoine Godeau, *Instructions et prières chrestiennes pour toutes sortes de personnes (1646)*

While Nelly Roussel pondered her unwanted fate as a future mother in June 1899, a large number of Frenchmen—demographers, politicians, government officials, doctors, social hygienists, and moral reformers—were contemplating the future of motherhood itself, albeit in a world of knowledge far removed from that of mothers and mothers-to-be. What concerned these professionals was the inexplicable decline in the French birthrate, especially since 1870. Not only had the rate fallen, but in 1890, 1892, and 1895, deaths had exceeded births—by 18,000 in the 1895 census—indicating that the French population was in a state of absolute decline. Many of them concluded, moreover, that this numerical deterioration ensued from physical and moral degeneration. Their concern was so intense that they produced approximately 250 books on the subject from 1870 to 1914, as well as hundreds of articles in the mainstream press and in feminist and socialist journals, such as *La Revue socialiste, La Fronde, Le Droit des femmes,* and *Le Journal des femmes*.[1] And the same year that Roussel agonized over having her first child, Émile Zola—ever more famous for his role in the Dreyfus Affair—published *Fécondité* (*Fruitfulness*) a widely read novel that contained a scathing social critique of couples, especially Parisians, who decided that their lives would be better with few or no children. Concern about population decline made for some unusual bedfellows.

In their quest to understand the country's languishing birthrate, French demographers refined methods for analyzing fertility in the 1860s and 1870s. J. Matthews Duncan and Louis-Adolphe Bertillon devised "fecundity" rates enabling them to measure, not just the actual birthrate, but the birthrate proportional to the number of married women of childbearing age. In 1877, Bertillon published data revealing that while for every 1,000 married women between the ages of 15 and 50, England produced 248 births, Prussia 275, and Belgium 279, Frenchwomen provided a paltry 173. Such statistics were subsequently deployed to condemn the "selfishness" of married women, rather than to call attention to the economic and cultural reasons for France's low birthrate.[2]

In response to this crisis in the birthrate, Bertillon's son Jacques, also a demographer, formed the Alliance nationale pour l'accroissement de la population française (National Alliance for the Growth of the French Population) on May 29, 1896. Within a year, this group had grown to almost four hundred members, most of whom were businessmen, industrialists, lawyers, doctors, and professionals. They exerted pressure on the French parliament, organized numerous conferences, and made public proclamations about how depopulation resulted from the predominance of individual interests over those of the nation. The Alliance became the most important representative of pronatalist sentiment in France, and the French natalist movement as a whole became the strongest in Europe.[3]

How would the Bertillons and the members of the Alliance nationale have responded to Nelly Roussel's "Impressions d'un jour de mélancolie"? At the time he founded the Alliance nationale, the younger Bertillon blamed men for France's falling birthrate, because he believed, in accordance with the theories of Frédéric Le Play, that men did not want family patrimonies to shrink as they became divided among children. Oddly, he ignored the role of women in reproduction, perhaps because, in keeping with the nineteenth-century bourgeois conception of womanhood, he imagined them as passive, asexual objects of their husbands' desires. In short, he believed husbands controlled whether or not their wives became pregnant.[4] But the contemporary rise of the New Woman and feminist demands for legal reform indicated that many women had interests beyond motherhood, which caused great consternation. Pronatalists also responded to the newly founded birth control movement, whose primary purpose was to distribute reliable female contraceptives.

In 1899, given their approach to the fertility problem, the pronatalists would undoubtedly have found Roussel's musings symptomatic of the individualism and selfishness of French wives. They regarded women only through the lens of biological reproduction, rather than motherhood in all its dimensions. Hence, they lacked understanding of, let alone compassion for, the situation of women. Roussel accordingly made it her mission to enlighten, not just these professionals, but men of all social classes about the practical experiences of mothers.

Motherhood, Feminism, and Pronatalism

Roussel gave birth to her first child, Mireille, on October 5, 1899. She left no documentation of this event and what it meant to her, and it is doubtful whether at this time she thought of her own experience with motherhood in the context of pronatalist politics. She did, however, manifest her complete alienation from the Church and her freedom from her family's conservative morality in not having her daughter baptized. This decision represented a dramatic departure from her state of mind when she had a Catholic wedding. In lieu of the sacrament, two months after Mireille's birth, Nelly and Henri hosted a banquet for their friends. They sent out invitations announcing the "Unveiling of Mireille, living statuette of Henri Godet and Nelly Roussel." Following the model of political and club banquets so crucial to associational life in the nineteenth century, the invitation named an "honorary president"—in this case, Thomas Nel, Nelly's beloved grandfather—and indicated "decent dress obligatory . . . at least until the champagne."[5] But Mireille's actual entry into the world had been far less whimsical than its celebration. Godet would later claim that this painful experience had "accentuated [Nelly's] feminism," and one of her friends later asserted that this birth, which "revealed to [Roussel] all the painful grandeur of the maternal function," was what led her to commit her feminism to the "inalienable rights of mothers."[6] We know, however, from her "Impressions of a Melancholy Day," that she had conceived of this commitment even during her pregnancy.

Yet Roussel's first published thoughts about feminism reflect no obvious concern about motherhood, even though the prevalence of populationist rhetoric had already profoundly influenced the direction of French feminism. Karen Offen has divided early Third Republic feminism into two categories, "relational" and "individualist" (or "integral"). The former orientation, which had its roots in the Saint-Simonianism of the 1830s, had come to dominate most feminisms in France by the turn of the century as a strategic response to the nationalist and populationist political climate. Rhetoric about depopulation had profoundly influenced these feminists; they found that they could attract more support if they stressed women's position as mothers and wives serving national interests, rather than as individuals seeking equal rights. They supported "sexual complementarity," and during this period of intense nationalism, they equated motherhood with patriotism.[7] "The mother makes the race. It is she who gives it vigor, intelligence, and the foundation of instruction; the stronger and more intelligent she is, the more noble her character will be, [and] the more potent the [French] race will be," Dr. Henri Thulié, a Freemason and municipal councilor, wrote in the feminist journal *L'Harmonie sociale* in 1893. Feminists deployed such proclamations about the "primordial" role of women in their demands. Facing fears of "degeneration," they argued that it was the responsibility of mothers to "regenerate the race," not just by bearing children, but by abandoning wet-nursing and bottle-feeding and returning to breast-feeding. Articles by doctors recommending breast-feeding filled feminist journals, but laywomen weighed in as well. The novelist Harlor (Jeanne Perrot, 1871–1970), one of Roussel's future collaborators, wrote an article entitled "Maternité totale" (Total Motherhood), citing the works of Eugène Brieux and Émile Zola to advocate breast-feeding.[8] French feminists thus used motherhood as a basis to lobby for social reform without the benefit of the vote. They took great care when articulating their demands not to seem to threaten women's functions within the family. In short, they used motherhood as a basis for their claims to citizenship. The Feminist Congress of 1900 affirmed that motherhood was women's "primary function" and declared that university education should be open only to an "elite" of exceptionally talented women.[9]

"Integral" or "individualist" feminists viewed women as individuals with rights equal to men's; they did not consider women to have a special nature, with inherent qualities that justified a different public or private status from that of men. They sought equal opportunity and self-determination for women regardless of their functions in the family.[10] Their feminism, however, fell into the liberal "paradox": if women were inherently equal to men, they could not base their claims on their own womanhood.[11]

The categories "relational" and "individualist" help us recognize differences among the various feminisms, but it is important to keep in mind that these are the terms of modern historians, not those of Roussel's era. Her contemporaries often embraced a combination of the two models, and many of the feminist groups had members representing both viewpoints. Moreover, other issue-oriented factors—such as the vote—could override ideological divisions in determining the membership of any particular feminist group. Roussel's rhetoric exemplifies a combination of relational and individualist orientations, although her ultimate agenda and her own behavior placed her squarely in the individualist camp. Her first feminist article, "Sur l'éducation des jeunes filles" (On the Education of Young Girls), appeared in the literary journal *Paris qui passe* just three weeks after Mireille's birth. Ignoring the more conciliatory strategies of mainstream feminism, she used both a violent male language of military metaphor and the language of victimization. "The whole future of feminism" depended on the "revolt against the absurd education of girls," she argued. "It will be necessary to wage a battle against antiquated traditions, secular prejudices, against Routine, the eternal enemy of Progress! No matter! Let us dare to rebel!"[12]

Roussel's battle cry against antiquated traditions, routine, and enemies of progress especially targeted the Church, enemy of the Third Republic. "Secular prejudices" however, referred to the exclusion of women from the Third Republic itself, a republic of men. For Roussel, men on both sides of the French clerical/anticlerical divide constituted the enemy. But in order not to alienate those without whom she could never attain her goals, she suppressed the contempt she had already articulated in her private memoir as she anticipated motherhood. In her closing plea to promote the development of human potential, she expunged the issue of gender. "I have no intention of preaching rebellion, [or] contempt for paternal authority: but I dream that this authority will be more enlightened, less opposed to the free development of the person [male or female]."[13] Nonetheless, this first article demonstrates that Roussel was already willing to take a stand apart from the majority of other feminists by attacking republican men. "Relational" feminists were less inclined to do so.

French feminism(s) spawned more than one hundred organizations during the Third Republic. They defy neat categorization, since their memberships overlapped. Conflicts among them also manifest unstable and ambivalent definitions of womanhood. The contested nature of its meaning became apparent at the International Feminist Congress in April 1896, when Nelly Roussel was eighteen. Though she did not attend, dramatic confrontations occurred that set the stage for her feminist participation. The Congress gave way to conflict between the more radical old guard and new recruits who embraced bourgeois femininity. Old-guard radical feminists believed women would have to renounce the "marks of femininity, of which coquetry is the most demeaning."[14]

The radical faction prevailed, but some of the younger feminists hoped to combine bourgeois femininity with radicalism. The most famous of these was Marguerite Durand, a former actress, known for her beauty and her blond hair, who converted to feminism at this Congress. In December 1897, she started a feminist newspaper, *La Fronde*. According to rumor, Gustave de Rothschild, a prominent Jewish banker, financed it. *La Fronde* covered all of the daily news; staffed entirely by women, it gained immediate attention. Durand recruited "women of letters," some of whom were uninterested in female emancipation. Like other feminist newspapers, it carried articles extolling motherhood and encouraging breast-feeding, and recommended books on child care that contained guides to breast-feeding. But from its inception, *La Fronde* was also militantly pro-Dreyfus, and it earned considerable attention with its daily reporting on Dreyfus's retrial from August to September 1899.[15]

Roussel began publishing in *La Fronde* in 1900, shortly after Mireille's birth. It was her first feminist affiliation, and it brought her into contact with Parisian women whose interests and lifestyles appealed to her, some of whom would become lifelong friends and collaborators. One of them, Marbel (Marguerite Belmont), founded the Union fraternelle des femmes (Fraternal Union of Women, henceforth UFF) on New Year's Eve, 1901, which Roussel joined. The UFF was considered "the daughter" of Marguerite Durand's *La Fronde,* and its purpose was not to compete with other feminist organizations, but instead to create a new platform, like *La Fronde,* exclusively for women. Its group identity formed around shared left-wing politics (pro-Dreyfus, anticlerical) and literary ambitions. Most of its members wrote articles, poems, novels, or plays, which they shared with one another. Hellé (Marguerite Dreyfus, 1870–1966) belonged to this group, as did Parrhisia (Blanche Cremnitz, 1848–1918; her nom de plume means "Free Speech": "parrhisia en grec signifie liberté de parler [*parrhisia* in Greek means freedom of speech]," Victor Hugo wrote in *Notre Dame de Paris*), the novelist Harlor, and Harlor's mother, Amelie Hammer. The UFF's multigenerational character and literary focus made it easier to include family members and friends, but the group also had a radical feminist orientation. It held large monthly meetings, with public lectures and discussions, whose topics ranged widely and included an internationalist bent.

Although fifteen years Nelly's senior, Marbel became one of her most devoted feminist friends. Like many unmarried feminists, she lived with her mother, also a feminist, and earned her living teaching English. Marbel sustained the UFF with considerable support from Nelly, and it lasted through World War I. The UFF was less a political group than a "circle of cultural action, devoted to the propagation of the 'feminist idea.'" It remained small, and it focused on the implications of feminism for relationships in private life. The UFF's orientation provided a sympathetic environment for Roussel to voice her feminist concerns, especially the unorthodox ones that emphasized women's right to self-fulfillment.

Paul Robin: The "New Christ"

Around the same time that Nelly Roussel became involved with *La Fronde*, she also met the man who would have the single most important influence on her feminist thinking, her sense of self, and her career: Paul Robin (1837–1912). Robin had founded the neo-Malthusian (birth control) movement in December 1896, about seven months after Jacques Bertillon founded his association to increase the French population. Nelly came to know Robin because Henri Godet's sister, Juliette, married Robin's son Fritz in 1900. As though in answer to Henri's query about what would replace religion in Nelly's life, Paul Robin became for her, in her own words, a "new Christ, . . . [a] Savior."[16] The analogy was appropriate, for Robin's ideology made her a "missionary" of a new "religion." His neo-Malthusianism lent her feminism a scientific foundation and logic that infused her speeches and writing.

Robin came to neo-Malthusian theory after having studied science and Darwin at the École normale supérieure, and after having become disenchanted with what he termed the "miniscule revolutionary efforts" of socialism.[17] A member of the First International, which was erroneously believed to have been implicated in the Paris Commune, he was exiled to England in 1871. While there, Robin came into conflict with both Bakunin and Marx over doctrinal issues; Marx expelled him from the executive commission of the First International. He then turned to the study of Malthusian economics and came under the influence of the leading British neo-Malthusian pioneer, Charles Drysdale. But prior to spreading this doctrine in France, he founded and directed a progressive coeducational school in the orphanage of Cempuis from 1880 to 1894. There he practiced what he called "integral education," in which he sought to develop the physical, intellectual, artistic, affective, and moral faculties of his students and to harmonize manual pursuits with those of the mind.[18] He also believed that all human bodies—male, female, poor, or rich—could reach perfection. Boys and girls in his school lived together and studied the same curriculum in the same classes. Robin advocated his principles of gender equality at the International

Congress of Primary Education in 1889, arguing that female teachers should receive the same treatment as their male counterparts, and that all teachers should instruct both sexes.[19]

The progressive nature of Robin's school proved too shocking for the members of the conservative press, who fabricated a scandal based on false accusations of sexual misconduct. The press vilified him, indeed demonized him, and continued to do so long after the "affair" of Cempuis.[20] From that point forward, Paul Robin was known as "the man of Cempuis." Every time he made a public appearance, there was a feeding frenzy in the right-wing press, causing most leftists to distance themselves from him. Dismissed from his post in 1894, Robin then turned his full attention to his neo-Malthusian concerns. For Robin in particular, controlling population growth was a matter, not only of food, wages, and prices, but also of the potential for human perfection and freedom. In 1896, he formed the League of Human Regeneration, whose stated purpose was to assure the liberty of parents, but "above all the liberty of the woman." Robin advocated teaching physiology, the social sciences, and the laws of population growth, as well as distributing information about birth control methods and their practical application.[21] Although other aspects of Robin's doctrine touched on eugenicism, individual autonomy was the cornerstone of his thinking, and female sexual emancipation was central to that autonomy. Robin believed that individual liberty could not exist without individual control over reproduction, and that women's bodies were the focal point of that process.

The name of Robin's league, and that of its periodical, *Régénération*, reflected his own concerns about the "degeneration" of the human race through unconscious "breeding"; it also offered a remedy to the fears of degeneration and cultural decadence that preoccupied so many Europeans in the fin de siècle. Based on biological, medical, and psychopathological theories advanced in the 1860s, the concept of degeneration held that the nation and its people were comparable to an organism no longer capable of evolving or of realizing the hereditary struggle for survival. Without permanent regeneration, the species—and in the minds of nationalists, the French nation itself—would become extinct.[22] Robin fervently believed that thoughtful reproduction and contraception would result in human beings of higher quality and enable a permanent "regeneration" of the species.

Since Henri's Godet's father had been a member of the First International and a Communard, the Godet and Robin families may have had ties dating back a generation. Moreover, Henri and Robin had both belonged to groups of socialist artists, and Robin moved in Freemason and freethinking circles, which had defended him during the Cempuis affair. Robin also spoke frequently about the neo-Malthusian cause at the popular universities, where Roussel surely had contact with him.[23] Robin's polemic against the populationist propaganda galvanized Roussel, but it also placed her in a delicate situation, for the majority of feminists opposed birth control. Almost none of the League of Human Regeneration's support came from feminists, and few women adhered to the movement at all. Robin's impassioned and explicit rhetoric clashed head-on with mainstream "relational" feminism.

Outright feminist hostility toward Robin became manifest when he attended the April 1896 meeting of the International Feminist Congress. There, he not only accused the government of making prostitution a state institution by regulating it but argued that marriage itself amounted to prostitution, because it delivered the woman to a tyrant who could impose "rotten social conventions" on her. The remedy for this malady, Robin bluntly argued, was free love and complete liberty in motherhood.[24] The journal *Débat* observed that his interventions at the Congress incurred cries of "down with Robin," and split the attendees into "pure feminists" and "impure Robinistes." "The tumult reached its height," this article recounted, "when M. Jules Bois vigorously attacked Robin's ideas, recalling that he was an apologist for abortion. The ex-director of Cempuis jumped onto the platform and threatened to 'spit in M. Jules Bois's face.'" At this point, one of the delegates demanded that Robin leave, because as a neo-Malthusian, he was not "worthy of talking to mothers." Stamping his feet and unable to make his voice heard above the din, Robin was forced out. As feminists feared, his very presence at their Congress discredited them. *Le Grand Journal* blamed this "man of Cempuis" for "all the scandals that had occurred over several days in this tumultuous assembly." That the "ladies" at this feminist gathering, "who are neither very patient nor very gentle," put up with his presence suggested that the Congress itself could no longer be taken seriously——it was instead a "corner of Paris where one could find cheap amusement, where students met because there were women, not because of serious philosophical problems."[25] Even though feminists publicly shunned Robin, he succeeded with them in the sense that he provoked ongoing discussion about his doctrine in feminist groups such as Solidarité and the UFF.[26]

Robin caused turmoil well beyond feminist circles. From the outset, the League of Human Regeneration aimed to provide access to contraception, and particularly female contraceptives, through the distribution of a translated Dutch brochure titled *Moyens d'éviter les grandes familles* (Means of Avoiding Large Families). Inadvertently helping spread the word, the press described Robin's cause as a "contagious disease" and a "contaminating foreign influence." *Le Temps* referred to it as the "League for Depopulation." *Le Peuple français* called Robin's doctrines "indelicate," especially when he tried to present them to feminists, who could not listen to his blunt speech "without feeling appalled." "These doctrines are going to be carried into every house," the newspaper declared, "in the form of a Dutch brochure entitled *Moyens d'éviter les grandes familles*," and it would especially "demoralize" the agricultural population if it were to "penetrate" the countryside. Distribution of the brochure attracted the attention of the foreign press, which created further consternation about France's international image. The publicity it garnered also increased support for the League. In less than a month after its publication in 1896, Robin received more than 500 letters from all over France requesting copies, and the League received 150 new subscribers.[27]

Moyens d'éviter les grandes familles contained specific instructions for contraception, justifying it as a panacea for most social ills. It argued that economic conditions could never improve if the number of births did not "diminish considerably," and it listed further reasons for having smaller families: numerous pregnancies following closely upon one another harmed the mother's health; infants born into already-large families could not receive adequate care, because of increased expense, sickness, mortality, and demoralization of family life; a lower birthrate would permit workers to demand higher salaries, since there would be fewer of them. The ability to avoid conception would permit young people to marry earlier and consequently diminish the need for prostitutes. Fewer children would further reduce prostitution, because mothers would be able to keep a closer eye on their daughters' behavior, and a higher standard of living would prevent young women from being tempted to sell themselves.

The brochure then enumerated ways to prevent conception, with careful and graphic instructions on how to employ these methods, and with detailed explanations of the advantages and disadvantages of each. Coitus interruptus appeared first, and then the condom, followed by a sponge to be inserted in the vagina, an "irrigator" (douche), and finally, best and most recently invented, the occlusive pessary, a cap fitting over the cervix to prevent the penetration of sperm. In particular, the brochure provided specific instructions on the use of irrigators, sponges, and the more complicated cervical cap, with warnings that the latter two devices had to fit properly and be rigorously cleaned. The last three methods required precise explanation, not only for their use, but of their relationship to the female anatomy. Illustrations at the end of the 16-page brochure provided graphic representation of the three contraceptive devices for women.[28]

With *Moyens d'éviter les grandes familles*, the League of Human Regeneration offered the French public the first technical and explicit manual for female contraception. Because the French birthrate was already so low, the reaction against these methods on the part of pronatalists was predictable. But it was not just pronatalists who reacted negatively: men and women across the political spectrum became intensely uncomfortable with the introduction of female forms of contraception. The most common method of contraception prior to World War I was coitus interruptus. Angus McLaren has argued that although "withdrawal" can be considered a "male form" of birth control, women were actively involved in the process and were often the ones to urge their partners to "be careful." But this method required a specific emotional relationship between partners that certainly eluded even affectionate marriages some of the time, let alone abusive marriages, especially those plagued by frequent drunkenness. In any case, the physical act of control rested with the man, regardless of social class, especially given his greater physical strength, a point neo-Malthusians emphasized.[29] The failure of the method, moreover, is attested to by the frequency of abortion, the only truly effective, albeit illegal, female form of birth control at the time: abortion rates surged at the end of the nineteenth century, reaching from 100,000 to 500,000 as against 900,000 live births per year. Women who wished to prevent births often had no choice other than abortion.[30] Seeking to empower women by giving them control over motherhood and the possibility of greater sexual pleasure, the League and its propaganda provoked great alarm. The police carefully observed the movement to find evidence that it was spreading "pornography," which was the only means they had to initiate prosecution. One undercover agent reported that the graphics Robin used to illustrate contraceptive methods were "daring, although spoken about with a serious air that removes any pornographic character, but that conveys so much more," implying that knowledge of female physiology and contraceptive methods for women was actually more dangerous than pornography.[31]

Robin's Feminist Disciple

Nelly Roussel came to know Paul Robin at a time when she was already a feminist but had not yet converted her feelings about motherhood into a political ideology. His crusade gave her the means—which extant feminisms did not offer—to translate her private anguish into a feminist campaign; but incorporating his doctrine into her own feminism brought her into the treacherous domain of female sexuality and the "nature" of womanhood. A number of his proclamations shaped the direction of her ideology, particularly his argument that female control over reproduction was the "first step, the essential point of female emancipation, and therefore [the emancipation] of the whole race."[32] The notion that women's control over births would offer them material and social independence, raise their dignity, and make them equal to men spoke to her aspirations and sense of self and justified her pursuit of a career. Also influential was the importance and potential of science in the League of Human Regeneration's mission statement, published in the first issue of *Régénération*. According to this statement, the organization planned "to apply the positive knowledge of the physiological and social sciences" in order to prevent "the unwanted fruits of thoughtless passion [that result] from the chance of spontaneous sex. . . . It is up to the men of science, to the positivist philosophers . . . to force humanity to take the first and the most serious step in the path to its emancipation, to make the woman acquire FREEDOM of MOTHERHOOD."[33]

Roussel delivered her first feminist speech in 1901 at the "Diderot" popular university. In her "Talk on Feminism," she for the first time treated the subject of motherhood, and she appealed to the socialist Left by claiming that feminism and socialism were inseparable. Because liberty, justice, and human rights were the foundation and raison d'être of socialism, one could not claim to be socialist if half of humanity were excluded from those rights, especially if one claimed those rights "only for the half of humanity that oppresses the other [half]." Echoing her sister feminists' concerns with the protection of motherhood, she argued that a mother should not be obligated, as men are, to work "in order to earn her bread," forcing her to neglect her children against her will. "Natural law," she said, did not order women to earn wages, but gave them the work of creating life and continuing and "perfecting" the species. But in apparent contradiction to this statement, she also asserted that if a woman were "irresistibly drawn" to professional work, or if "as a result of chance or of *will* [my emphasis], she is not a mother, [then] she is permitted to give a purpose, an orientation to her life. Motherhood must not be, cannot be imposed on her. It must not be an obligation for everyone." Roussel then made a most unconventional claim. One of the "crimes of society," she said, was that the mother was "too often forced to subject herself to the needs of her family."

Roussel then addressed the issue of sexual difference. According to her logic, man and woman are *different* morally and physically; but "different" has never been synonymous with "unequal." They are destined mutually to complete one another, each of the two having, in general, the qualities that the other lacks.[34] She thus readily admitted that nature assigned to men and women different tasks—indeed, different "natures" or states of being—and she insisted that she had no desire to "liken men and women to the point of confounding them," or to "masculinize" women.[35] But she opposed any notion that biology was destiny. If women did become mothers, she wanted the tasks of motherhood to be acknowledged and to be supported socially, economically, and morally; indeed, she wanted them to be glorified. In an egalitarian society, mothers would naturally receive such recognition. If women did not choose motherhood, they should have the freedom to pursue any career they desired. Feminism would allow women to make their own choices according to their temperaments, aptitudes, and tastes. But two obstacles impeded women from fulfilling their greatest potential and achieving equality with men: the law and social prejudices. If the former were changed and the latter destroyed, women would be able "to blossom."

By calling for equality and at the same time recognizing difference between the sexes, Roussel took up an argument dating back to Mary Wollstonecraft and the eighteenth-century origins of modern feminism, which has been a "paradox" ever since.[36] She evaded the feminist paradox by refusing to make biology the foundation of gender difference; difference, rather than being "essential," was highly fluid. In her view, women were fully human, and human nature—as well as its potential—transcended the nature of sexual difference. She understood that if the law excluded women from citizenship on the basis of their "natural" physical differences, it also influenced the way in which nature was perceived and defined. The elimination of prejudice would thus transform the meaning of "natural."[37]

Embracing both equality and difference allowed Roussel to broaden her audience and to permit individuals to hear what they wished. She directed different meanings to different auditors, bridging established discursive fields (motherhood) with new ones (maternal pain and the choice of not being a mother). Women who wanted to avoid motherhood, or at least reduce its burdens, found in her a spokesperson; women who felt their identity authenticated through motherhood received validation, and indeed, vindication. Men could hear that the sexes were complementary and thus feel their own sense of masculinity reassured. Indeed, she gained a number of ardent male supporters, including a senior military officer, Colonel Jean Converset, who would later become a devoted friend. He said that he had been "completely converted" upon hearing her talk on feminism at one of the popular universities in 1900.[38] Though Roussel nuanced her rhetoric, her end goal was subversive and radical, and it would become ever more so, because she refused to abandon her principles as the society around her grew more conservative.

Given her deep ambivalence about her own motherhood and her awareness of women's reproductive plight, it is no surprise that Robin's doctrine spoke to Roussel's innermost being. It provided her with a language, a bold political stance, and a confidence to intellectualize—in a larger framework—feelings that she had previously understood only in personal terms. Although she did enjoy the companionship and confidence of her husband, he did not yet share her views about reproductive rights and felt embarrassed by her public discussion of such issues. Henri told her to leave to Robin and other neo-Malthusians the advocacy and explication of contraceptive devices, as well as most of the discussion about the laws of population growth.[39] At his urging, she agreed to treat the so-called "moral" side of the issue, conceptualizing motherhood in a broad social framework. Ironically, by pursuing that aspect, she developed a message more subversive than simply women's right to contraception; she questioned whether the pain of childbirth and the burdens of motherhood were truly dictated by nature. In short, she questioned the very nature of womanhood as her contemporaries understood it.

Robin's influence is evident in Roussel's article "Feminism et fécondité" (Feminism and Fecundity), written in response to Senator Edmé Piot's pronatalist brochure *La Question de la dépopulation en France*, which attributed primary responsibility for depopulation to wives.[40] Roussel accused Piot of not having done thorough research and of ignoring the interests of those who alone "bear the burdens of reproduction." How could he judge women if he knew nothing of their experience with motherhood? Implicitly referring to her own experience, Roussel posed an obvious but trenchant question: "How can anyone be astonished that the young mother, anemic . . . [and] depressed by a first birth, would be put off at the prospect of another ordeal?" If Piot wanted to encourage motherhood, Roussel reasoned, women should have more physiological education, so that they could face motherhood with greater knowledge and less fatigue and suffering. Finally, on the "moral" issue, she complained to Piot that this "civilized, depopulating country" had only indifference and disdain for "the female producers of children." He should promote the moral and legal reform that would bring dignity to motherhood.[41]

In this article, Roussel took the first step in "de-naturalizing" motherhood and laid out many of the themes that she would repeat throughout her career, particularly with regard to what she perceived as a brutal, humiliating lack of respect for mothers, even among those who called for a higher birthrate. She also argued that one way to dignify motherhood would be to compensate it with a salary. Roussel was not the first and certainly not the last feminist to demand that mothers receive pay. But raising this issue in the context of female control over reproduction suggested that motherhood was productive labor that contributed to civilization, rather than labor derived from the dictates of nature. Economic remuneration for the work of motherhood would place it in the same category as civilized (male) productive labor that conquers, cultivates, and manipulates nature rather than being subject to it.

Bitter Fruit

In addition to literary readings, Roussel delivered six lectures or talks on feminism in Paris in the course of 1901, mostly at popular universities. She became pregnant again in the spring of that year, only about fifteen months after Mireille's birth. We do not know whether she practiced what she preached with regard to contraceptives; given her rhetoric, her dedication to her speaking career, and subsequent events, it is doubtful that she and Henri planned this pregnancy. It did not, in any case, initially interfere with her career. Through the first half of October, Nelly continued her active participation at the League of the Rights of Man and lectured at popular universities. She gave her last lecture when she was quite visibly pregnant at nearly seven months, thus violating the bourgeois convention of concealing a pregnancy and going into seclusion after the fifth month.

Roussel gave birth to a son on December 3, 1901, and named him André, after her sister. This birth nearly killed her, and she remained ill with unspecified symptoms long afterward.[42] Unfortunately for the biographer, Roussel's private papers reveal no direct information about exactly what happened either to her or to her son. We can only imagine that she suffered from one of the three most common causes of maternal mortality: puerperal fever, pregnancy-induced hypertension, or hemorrhage. Whatever the cause, she suffered weakness, depression, and ill health for months afterward. References to pain in her subsequent writings suggest that the birth process itself was traumatic and may have damaged her baby. On April 20, 1902, André died at the age of four and a half months of undisclosed causes in Coubron (Seine-Saint-Denis), about fifteen kilometers from his parents' home. Given Nelly's state of health, the baby had more than likely been put out to a rural wet nurse (a practice that was on the decline at this time), which would have further reduced his chances for survival.[43] André's death compounded and deepened Nelly's suffering.

In the short term, Roussel immediately resumed her activities with the League of the Rights of Man and the popular universities. But she also fell into a state of severe depression and ill health. In July, she left Paris to spend two months with Jeanne Supply, a close friend since childhood, in Revin (Ardennes), near the Belgian border. Henri remained in Paris, and he and Nelly corresponded regularly. Unfortunately, he had not yet formed the habit of saving her letters, and only those that he wrote to her during their separation remain; they nonetheless open a window onto their marriage, as well as onto their broader family relationships and household dynamics. His missives are full of affection, terms of endearment (such as "pauvre petit coca malade"), humor, news from home, and detailed instructions on how to care for her health. They also indicate a strong mutual dependency. Henri worried endlessly about Nelly and felt the strain of their separation. He was deeply saddened by the loss of their son and by Nelly's precarious health and mental fragility.[44]

In his wife's absence, Henri continued to sculpt and tried unsuccessfully to sell his works. He even took them to Reims Cathedral, but the bishop did not think his art appropriate for an ecclesiastical context. Although his sculptures were traditional in form, they had no religious content, and given his atheistic views, his conviction that art should serve social and socialist causes, and his contempt for the Church, his trying to sell them to a cathedral reflects simple desperation.[45] He also carried on his routine social life with friends and maintained close relations with family, upon whom he was utterly dependent for meals and childcare. He spent a large portion of his time with Nelly's grandfather, Thomas Nel, and "les petits"—her younger sister Andrée and Andrée's husband, Paul Nel, the sisters' first cousin. The couple had wed the previous April, and they shared a large apartment with Thomas Nel a few doors down from Nelly and Henri on rue Michel Bizot. To Henri's great irritation, the newlyweds constantly bickered like siblings. They argued about the pros (Paul) and cons (Andrée) of having children, as well as about issues of far less substance. Although fond of them, Henri was disgusted with their childishness, and on one "lugubrious evening," with the customary bickering, he had to bite his tongue when he compared legitimate causes of physical and moral suffering such as his and Nelly's with the way Andrée and Paul created their own pain so needlessly. And yet at the same time, Henri wrote of how he regretted they could not live with "les petits"—presumably, as subsequent letters suggest, because Andrée and Paul could help care for two-year-old Mireille. Mireille, meanwhile, was staying with Nelly's mother and stepfather, but Henri saw her often.[46]

Henri begged Nelly not to tire herself out while she was recuperating and admonished her for planning to deliver a public talk in Revin. But he also advised her on its content, urging caution on "the subject," and expressing his distaste for its potentially offensive, if not scandalous, nature. Robin's reputation as the "man of Cempuis" and the inherently controversial nature of neo-Malthusianism made Henri fear for his wife's reputation. Reflecting his own commitment to freethinking, he urged Nelly to speak to her audiences in Revin about their "intellectual emancipation" (as opposed to sexual emancipation), which they could achieve through organizing lectures and circulating books. He urged her to "make them understand that it is in studying the exact sciences that one best makes war against preachers of inexact dogmas." He also told her to make them understand that they should form syndicates (trade unions) and join freethinking societies. But the best thing, he implored, would be to "do nothing" for the sake of her health. He urged her to take advantage of her stay with their friends so that he could at least have this one consolation for his solitude: "that you will return happier and better armed for the battle of existence," instead of, one might read between the lines, her political battles.[47]

When Nelly informed Henri of the lecture she planned to give, he expressed disappointment, which in turn disappointed her: "And this lecture?" he said, "Isn't there a way of doing something without appearing too shocking to friends?" He advised her to announce that she was simply giving a lecture on Victor Hugo and then intersperse works on feminism or socialism in between readings of Hugo; he added, "you must do this [lecture] while I am there," suggesting that his presence would legitimize her message. He told her he would publicize her talk by sending notices of it—and the fact that he would be there with her—to newspapers, and especially to *La Raison,* which published his literary contributions. Godet did arrive in time for her talk. He complimented her in a loving if patronizing manner, with his own brand of humor: "I am reminded that I am married to a very pretty person who strolls about the banks of the river Meuse, where her speeches, full of juvenile enthusiasms, are very capable of stopping the backward march of this aquatic-metallurgical-mountainous land's celebrated crayfish, and even making them march forward."[48] Henri's moral support for Nelly had no limits, but he also attempted to shape the nature of her message as well as her public image.[49]

Henri's letters reveal another element of household dynamics: the family's utter dependence on domestic servants. He wanted very much to bring Mireille to visit Nelly, but their domestic, Josephine, was about to return to her native countryside for a vacation. Henri could not imagine coming to Revin without her, because someone would have to "amuse" and keep up with Mireille—and to his incredulity, Jeanne did not have a domestic—a further source of anxiety for him, because that meant that Nelly was without one too. In August, the situation with domestics in Paris deteriorated, revealing Roussel and Godet's less-than-generous attitudes toward the underclass of domestics, despite their commitment to egalitarian ideals. Godet came to believe that Josephine was stealing from them and from Andreé as well. He set up an elaborate scheme to "catch the animal in the act," which failed, he thought, because domestics had an "agreement" among themselves and she had been informed. Godet fired Josephine without explanation, telling her to pack her bags. She protested bitterly, claiming to be the victim of injustice.[50]

Firing Josephine, however, made Nelly's return home impossible, especially because within two days of Henri's return to Paris, Jeanne wrote that Nelly had relapsed into ill health and depression, news that deepened his agony and nearly obsessive concern. For his own needs, Henri had to "borrow" his mother-in-law's domestic, and he used one of his employees to run errands; Louise Nel offered to keep Mireille for another two months so that Nelly could remain in the Ardennes to take more time to recover.[51] Leaving Paris for purposes of health cures or for summer vacations away from husbands was common among women of her social class, but in her case, she also needed to escape maternal obligations. Godet apparently saw nothing abnormal in her separation from Mireille; on the contrary, the toddler would interfere with Nelly's cure.

From Martyr to Missionary

Roussel returned to Paris in mid September 1902, having been away from her family for nearly two months. She immediately threw herself into a flurry of activity. Along with Marguerite Durand, she attended meetings of the Diderot lodge, served as a member of the executive commission of the Association of Freethinkers of France, and taught diction as a "professor" at the Conservatory.[52] She participated in literary readings at popular universities and resumed her speaking career with a new fervor. But she now drew even more on her own experience, infusing her speeches not only with the memory of pain and trauma but with drama, for she also returned to acting. At the end of December in Villeneuve–St.-Georges (Val-de-Marne) not far from Paris (for the departments of France, see map 2), she presented an analysis of Jean Racine's *Andromaque*, a tragedy concerning four people locked in relationships of unrequited passion, and then participated in a two-hour performance, playing the role of Hermione before an audience of 300. Roussel, according to the president of the local popular university, who had invited her, "performed without an error, without the smallest of lapses, without the slightest failure of memory; everything, both her gestures and spoken word, were beautiful. I shall not hide from you that I was *de mon 'lingot,'* as one says in the world [of theater], and I was not alone."[53] Though Roussel was able here to taste her old ambition of performing as an actress before a sizeable public audience, her return to acting was also a rehearsal for a new phase in her speaking career, in which she further developed her talent.

While Roussel suffered from poor mental and physical health in 1902, the League of Human Regeneration, which had suffered from financial and leadership problems since its inception, received new direction under Eugène Humbert, a young anarchist worker. Humbert's background was a prototype of the very situation Roussel would come to cite often in her lectures: his mother, Maria Humbert, was a cigar maker from a family of textile artisans who, according to Humbert's biographer, "would have been able to live in honest comfort if they had not had so many children: five boys and five girls," each of whom had to leave home at an early age because of the family's poverty. Maria, typically naïve in her provincialism, met Eugène's father just after arriving in Metz from her natal village. After failing to recognize Eugène when he was born out of wedlock in March 1870, the father went off to "seek glory under other skies" in the Franco-Prussian War, never to return.[54]

Shortly after Eugène's birth, Maria settled in Nancy, where, still unmarried, she had a second child and was once again abandoned by the father. Eugène was placed with an uncle as an apprentice shoemaker, and in that capacity, he became exposed to anarchists and their theories. Self-taught, he became an avid reader and created a working-class newspaper. While in Nancy, he caught the attention of the police as a "dangerous anarchist." His reputation followed him to Paris, where he moved in 1896. There he continued to work as a shoemaker and frequented anarchist milieux. He had known about Paul Robin's educational theories prior to coming to Paris. Although initially not persuaded by neo-Malthusian arguments, Humbert became a convert. Meeting Robin in person was the "capital event in the history of French neo-Malthusianism." Robin hired him in 1902 to oversee the publication of *Régénération*. Humbert became the League of Human Regeneration's first paid employee, and he abandoned all other work. Having appeared only sporadically up to that point, *Regeneration* was published monthly for the next six years. Humbert also organized a team of charismatic speakers who could attract large audiences: the ex-convict Liard-Courtois (a.k.a. Auguste Courtois); Sébastian Faure, battle companion of Louise Michel; and Nelly Roussel. From that point on, Humbert became the real leader of the movement. His background and education, not to mention his winning personality, earned him considerable success in drawing other anarchist supporters to the movement. By 1903, the League's growing team of propagandists fanned out into the provinces, undertaking long speaking tours in the southwest, the north, and in the east.[55]

To Henri's consternation, Roussel began speaking on behalf of Paul Robin's cause to ever-larger audiences and contributing articles to *Régénération*. As one of the few women involved in the neo-Malthusian effort—and the most articulate—she did more than anyone else to infuse women's issues into a movement that considered social reform its primary goal. In January 1903, she published an article entitled "Amour fécond, amour stérile" (Fertile Love, Sterile Love), using language more physically and sexually graphic than in the past (though still tame by modern standards) and echoing the personal pain she had so recently felt. Roussel referred to motherhood as a "mission of sacrifice" and boldly legitimized female sexual desire: "The glory of childbearing goes less to the bruised and aching female creator than to the happy father for whom the entire task has been limited to the collaborative work, a few moments of pleasure. . . . Sterile love is neither guilty nor ugly. Is love ever sterile? Love does not only produce works of the flesh. It produces many other creations." She then attacked the Church for "placing the human being between the suffering of complete chastity and [the suffering of] unlimited fertility."[56]

As a follow-up to Roussel's article, *Régénération* published a "manifesto for women," urging them to understand that one had the right and duty to abstain from pregnancy if one's health or material situation did not warrant bearing a child. "This depends entirely on you, you are mistresses of your destiny . . . you must not be ignorant of the fact . . . that science has emancipated you from the dreadful fatality of being mothers against your will." Two Republican newspapers, *La Patrie* and *Le Rappel*, quoted the article at length and expressed profound discomfort at the notion that women should have such emancipation. *La Patrie* characterized the manifesto as "a veritable challenge to decency and good morals." The article in *Le Rappel* cited Zola's novel *Fécondité* as evidence that artificial means of limiting births were "contrary to the health of the body and the health of the mind" and argued that "voluntary motherhood would be a social scourge—it would not only result in rapid depopulation, but it would arrest the social development of *le peuple* and the progress of civilization itself."[57] Although the League of Human Regeneration did not enjoy a massive following, its activities and its journal, including Roussel's contributions, stirred debate throughout the Paris and national press and drew renewed scrutiny from the police, who also carefully followed League-sponsored lectures. Meanwhile, Godet wrung his hands over the legal status of the newly invigorated League and insisted that Nelly refuse Robin's request that she join its administrative council.[58]

Through 1903, Roussel gave more than twenty lectures, speeches, and talks on feminism, motherhood, and the relationship between feminism and freethinking. She delivered them at the popular universities, at the prestigious Hôtel des Sociétés savantes, at the Masonic lodge of the Grand Orient, at the wedding of a friend, at the municipality of the suburb of St. Mandé, and at public meetings of freethinkers. Many of the titles imply her stance on birth control (such as "Maternity and the Revolt of Mothers").[59] At the behest of the League, Roussel gave a speech in March 1903 on *liberté de maternité* (freedom of motherhood) to an audience of 400 neo-Malthusian supporters at the Salon de l'Harmonie. Assuming the important role of *présidente,* she thanked the organizers for having a woman chair this session, since exclusion from the right to vote also excluded women from the world of politics. She acknowledged that the organizers had placed her in this position because she brought "nothing other than the sincerity and ardor of her convictions"—qualities, she pointed out, not normally credited to the female sex, because it was adorned with the "ornaments" of *"modesty, self-effacement . . . insignificance";* indeed, the very qualities she had learned in school. She then turned to the central subject of this opening speech "On the strike of mothers," a concept coined by Marie Huot the previous decade with the term *grève des ventres* (wombs on strike). Again equating reproduction with productive labor, she said, "The poorly paid worker refuses his work; the 'right to strike' is no longer contested today. . . . Aren't we [mothers] the poorest paid of all workers? And what strike will be more legitimate than ours?" Focusing on the pain and indignities of childbirth, Roussel then addressed herself caustically

To despicable religions that say to us, "You will have children in pain, without respite, without rest, and without glory! Profane love is a stain, and your sufferings as a mother are necessary in order to punish the crime of the [female] lover!" And [to] the ferocious society that says to us, "Do your work, O woman, I need soldiers, I need slaves, I need men to eat!" To our eternal oppressors, to all the prejudices, dogmas and conventions, to all the false morals, to all the doctrines of constraint and servitude, to all those who crush us, who torture us, we shall respond with a war cry! . . . and we shall stand up, indignant, trembling, in the face of all those who dare to speak to us of *work without pay,* and of *duties without rights.*

We are allowed to give our life drop by drop! We are allowed to carry in our aching wombs sons who will later learn to have contempt for us, or daughters destined to the same life of sacrifice and humiliation! . . . . Let us go, all my sisters . . . without hesitating, toward those who today bring us. . . *the doctrine of emancipation of the flesh,* which makes us mistresses of our destinies. It is not only Wisdom, it is *Revolt* that takes us there.[60]

The two undercover police agents, who noted that 150 women were in the audience, hardly knew what to make of Roussel. Their comments reflect their own ideological bias about the role of a woman at such a meeting. One of them asserted that she had simply come there to "prove herself" and wrongly dismissed her lecture as pushing the "minor work" of the elder Robin.[61] Her speaking ability had already won acclaim; a month earlier, after she had lectured in Mantes (Yvelines), a newspaper described her "great oratorical merit." She developed her subject "with soul, with passion . . . she made every heart quiver . . . [and] raised her audience to a burst of applause," after it had already interrupted her several times with applause during her talk.[62]

As Roussel's speaking career accelerated throughout 1903, she once again wrote a play of her own, a short "symbolic scene" (*scène symbolique*), or didactic playlet, which she first performed on April 18, 1903, at the popular university of the ninth and tenth arrondissements. *Par la révolte* offers a particularly rich example of Roussel's use of allegory, both religious and military, as well as the persistent memory of her personal pain. With three actresses personifying respectively the Church, Republican Society, and Revolt, the play opens with "Eve" plaintively seeking someone to free her from her slavery (figs. 7 and 8). She turns to the Church for comfort, but she is told that because she has sinned, she must suffer in silence and humility. She then turns to "Republican Society," which is "born of the blood of heroes." Society responds that the words "liberty, equality, and fraternity" do not apply to her. Woman's duty is to procreate, for Society needs citizens. "Revolt" then appears on the scene, identifying herself as "the sublime daughter of pain." She is proud, draped in scarlet, hair blowing in the wind. "It's not on knees that one marches to justice," she announces. Revolt breathes power into Eve, who then stands up and defies Church and Society, telling them to be silent. Eve admonishes her "sore flanks" to close themselves "until the hour of triumph; the glorious hour when the antiquated fortresses will crumble beneath my exasperated shouts! I shall enter this last conquered place, trembling from heroic battles, in order to make love and beauty germinate there."[63]

Through *Par la révolte,* Roussel channeled her former religious sensibilities into an anticlerical diatribe, deftly turning religious allegory on its head; her "Eve" is victim rather than sinner. She escapes her condition rather than resigning herself to it. "Revolt," the daughter of "sublime" *maternal* pain, in her scarlet robe represents the perpetual bloody mutilation of a woman who is always sacrificed to relentless childbirth, as Roussel herself had been. "Revolt" might also symbolize revolution and the republican icon Marianne. Roussel employed multiple images and discourses, mixing them in unexpected ways in order to forge alternating female identities, while transfixing her audiences and disturbing the assumptions they held. She presented this twenty-minute play frequently over several years, either reading it alone or performing it with friends such as Marguerite Durand, always to enthusiastic response. It was published in the form of a 16-page brochure, with a preface by the famous anarchist Sébastian Faure and a photograph of a bas-relief by Godet of a scene from the play as the frontispiece (fig. 8). *Régénération* announced that the brochure could be purchased from Godet's workshop for 50 centimes.[64]

In August 1903, Roussel again visited her friend Jeanne in Revin. There she continued to prepare talks, while Henri performed secretarial duties for her in Paris and ran numerous errands on her behalf. In his correspondence with Nelly, Henri regularly recounted his conversations with friends and relatives. One of his stories seems exceptional, not only for what it reveals about their social relations, but as an indication of his continued efforts to control the content of her lectures. On the occasion of dining at his sister Juliette Robin's with his eighteen-year-old niece Angèle and their close friends the Wolfs, Henri had the temerity to broach the topic of childbirth and its pain—a taboo subject among the respectable bourgeoisie, especially in mixed company, and hardly appropriate for dinner conversation. Poor Angèle's "eyes grew large and round" as they spoke. Wolf protested that it was their duty not to frighten anyone, especially women. Henri persisted nonetheless with an odd but significant remark: propaganda about childbirth and motherhood, he argued, should be made by men, "just as women can more effectively combat militarism, [because women are] more disinterested in the question, at least in a direct way." He then criticized his brother-in-law Fritz Robin for his ignorance about the dangers of childbirth and for his "unshakeable will to reassure everyone" that it was safe. Henri compared Fritz's attitude to what "the administration of Martinique was doing prior to the eruption of Mount Pelé—as all the administrations today do during times of epidemics . . . [such reassurance] multiplies the disastrous consequences a hundredfold."[65]

Henri's metaphor of natural disaster suggested that Nelly's experience with childbirth would have been different had she known more about physiology. But in recounting the conversation to her, Henri also expressed his own convictions that propaganda about maternal pain—the topic that Nelly was embarking upon in her public talks—was better left to men, in effect, to Paul Robin and his team of speakers in the League for Human Regeneration. Only a day earlier, Henri had received the program for a lecture she was scheduled to give in September at the popular university of Belleville, which listed her title as "Neo-Malthusianism." He complained to her: "you know what I think of the title you have given your lecture . . . I am persuaded that thus presented it can hurt you by making you ridiculous, I hope I am wrong, but it will amuse me not to attend . . . tackling certain subjects in this manner requires the age and authority of the *père* Robin."[66]

Nelly Roussel, "Enfant Terrible"

Neither Henri's cautions nor his romantic attentions tamed Nelly's ambitions to treat sexual subjects in public or led her to refrain from entering into the thick of public controversy. She delivered her talk—listed in her daily agenda as "Lecture on feminism"—on September 17, 1903, at the popular university in the working-class neighborhood of Belleville. But as Henri predicted, the title listed in the program—"Neo-Malthusianism"—produced a scathing reaction in the popular right-wing, anti-Semitic newspaper *La Libre Parole*. A. de Boisandré explicitly addressed "M. Piot, senator and apostle of repopulation" in an article that condemned the curriculum in popular universities, which Boisandré claimed were run by "the Trinity" of Freemasons, Jews, and sectarian Huguenots, who formed a "bloc," and whose purpose was to capture the "malleable brains" of adolescents just leaving school. He claimed that this "bloc" cast a vast net over France, "an immense extinguisher under which the anemic and agonized national spirit is killed." The subject of Roussel's talk, he noted, "needs no discussion in a newspaper such as this." But what "stupefied" him was that a woman would choose such a subject: "If young men are going to hear her that is bad enough; but, what do you think, M. Piot, . . . of the young girls at these strange evening schools, of the perilous coeducation of the two sexes?" Seven other newspapers throughout France published this same article.[67]

Roussel immediately wrote to Boisandré to insist that she had not given a lecture on neo-Malthusianism in Belleville or anywhere else, but added: "I could have done so, and perhaps one day I shall . . . for this question of *thoughtful procreation* is among those that interest me to the highest degree. But I would not give it the title "Malthusianism," a word that I don't really like; I would simply call it: *La Liberté de maternité*." Professing herself astonished at Boisandré's "stupefaction" over a woman's having chosen such subject matter, Roussel proclaimed (contrary to her husband) that she "did not understand very well what the sex of the orator could have to do with the question treated" and that she "had not known that there were any subjects reserved for women or prohibited to them." But if she were to admit for an instant that certain subjects should be reserved for women, nothing would be more relevant to them than "the question of *Maternité libre*." Boisandré published her letter in *La Libre Parole* and then accused her of not addressing the issue at hand. Further exchanges followed, and Boisandré finally concluded that he did not have the "bad taste to disgrace himself" with a discussion of *"maternité libre,"* a matter best left to (the pronatalist) Senator Piot. He feared, however, "that these theories, poorly understood, poorly digested by minds less robust and less balanced than that of Mme. Roussel, would drive us rapidly enough to dangerous and even criminal practices for, in the end, from *maternité libre* to the right to abortion, there is only the distance of a new audacity."[68]

Indeed, though Roussel did not publicly defend abortion, during the same month that the controversy in *La Libre Parole* began, she did publicly link "freedom of motherhood" with infanticide. In late October, she and Henri attended a banquet and ceremony honoring Paul Magnaud, a reformist judge and president of the tribunal in Château-Thierry (Aisne) who believed that society played a role in the crimes that certain individuals committed. Henri had sculpted a bust of the judge (fig. 5, center), paid for by subscriptions, which was unveiled with great fanfare at this event. Nelly and eleven other prominent freethinkers, including the journalist Séverine, gave speeches honoring Magnaud. Before an audience of 800, Roussel called the judge a "feminist" and praised him for having acquitted a *fille-mère*—an unmarried mother—of infanticide, which she called an act of justice rather than one of clemency: "The true murderers of the baby are first the father and second the society. The murderess herself is a victim, and pardoning her only causes more injury—*we* should ask *her* pardon." She also criticized the use of the term *fille-mère*, because of its inherent indignity. This, like her other talks, began in an unassuming, self-effacing tone, and then escalated into a full-scale acrimonious attack on "society" and men. While acknowledging that men could be good to women, she also called them "egotistical and unfaithful seducers."[69]

This celebration received wide and mostly supportive coverage in the press. Two conservative papers, however, criticized Magnaud and the homage to him; they directed their attacks particularly against Roussel, because she had called him a "feminist" and praised his acquittal of the mother who had committed infanticide. They suggested that her logic, if accepted, would lead to mass murder. These attacks also cast her once again as an enemy of Senator Piot's repopulationist campaign. Roussel had become what the neo-Malthusianist Jeanne Humbert later described as the (beloved) enfant terrible among the editorial staff of *La Fronde,* "where she never let any attack go by without reacting, and her ripostes were always scathing, tinged with an irony that filled us with joy."[70] Poor Henri. This sort of publicity hardly brought joy to him, for it was precisely what he feared would tarnish his wife's reputation. Because this publicity also further established Roussel as a direct opponent of Piot, Henri feared that his wife would be ridiculed. Ridicule would not only taint her feminist goals but dishonor him as well.

If Henri Godet was displeased with the publicity his wife's remarks received in the conservative press, he must have been still more so with their characterization in their own left-wing neighborhood daily paper, *L'Avenir du XIIème*, just a week after the Magnaud banquet and in the midst of the Boisandré polemic. A stinging squib titled "Féminisme!" began: "Promenaded by her husband in petticoats [*balladé(e) par son époux en jupon*], the divine Roussel has swept across almost all the floors in the arrondissement. After having appeared at the popular university, where her feminism seemed rather disordered, here she serves in the [Masonic] Lodges and the League of the Rights of Man. There is nothing but her. I am scientific, she says modestly, and my desire is to produce myself everywhere." She "sounds like an overused phonograph [record]," the author exclaimed and added that if she wanted to have all the rights and privileges of men, Roussel should be prepared to defend herself against insults "like a man"—that is, to fight a duel, if it should come to that, since her effeminized husband could not: "la charge la plus commune aux hommes, c'est de se faire bêcher" (the commonest fate of men is to take knocks).[71] Since women did not fight duels, ridicule became the weapon of choice against feminism.

But Roussel forged on with both feminism and neo-Malthusianism. On November 16, 1903, she spoke at and chaired a neo-Malthusian meeting, featuring the well-known, charismatic anarchist Sébastian Faure. The event attracted from 1,200 to 1,500 people. There was standing room only, and the audience overflowed into the corridor. It included "both sexes," a point the police always noted, among whom were "artisans, bourgeois (at least by appearance), employees, functionaries . . . revolutionaries, friends of [neo-Malthusian] propaganda, and adversaries who did not breathe a word."[72] By way of introducing Robin and Faure, Roussel gave her boldest public presentation yet, casting the issue at hand as a "sexual question" whose discussion had been prohibited by a "deplorable residue of Christian atavism." As if sending a message to both Boisandré and her own husband, she insisted in this lecture that "everything *can be* and *must be* said in public." According to the "repopulators" who decried France's low birthrate, women were "not conscious or free beings, but a sort of machine for fabricating 'cannon fodder' . . . or a reproducing animal whose suffering counts for little." Feminism had to proclaim freedom of motherhood in order to release women from sexual slavery. "Emancipation of the flesh" was as important as that of the mind. Roussel also attacked the Church, calling its doctrine cruel and tyrannical. "Motherhood . . . must not be made the unique reason and *excuse* for Love [Sex]," she said. "Love carries within itself its own beauty, and has no need for an excuse"![73] She acknowledged the connection between emotional fulfillment and carnal pleasure, asserting the right of women to experience the latter. This claim distinguished her as a public speaker and as a feminist. Not only did she speak in front of a huge audience—something still uncommon for women in her day—but she spoke about sexual matters while attacking men, whether of the Left or of the Right, freethinker or Catholic. *La Fronde* reported that the audience "listened in reverential and solemn silence . . . [to] the categorical declarations that Mme Nelly Roussel uttered with a clear voice in impeccable language, sure and sober like her movement, as majestically worthy as her bearing."[74]

By the end of 1903, a number of interrelated themes and rhetorical tactics had emerged in Roussel's lectures and writings.[75] Her words challenged the prevailing secular and religious conceptions of women's relationship to nature that formed a basis for their "slavery" and the unspoken assumptions underlying pronatalism. Her most fundamental tactic in her challenge to pronatalists was to emphasize the realities—especially the physical ones—that women experienced as mothers. A second rhetorical tactic addressed those who believed that all aspects of motherhood derived from nature. Taking that notion to its logical extreme, she likened "unconscious," uncontrolled reproduction to the behavior of animals, a comparison she used more in later talks. Roussel's third tactic was to argue that science could alleviate the social and physical ills of motherhood, making the labor process less painful and damaging and dignifying it. She also believed fervently that science should serve to educate women about their bodies and help them prevent unwanted pregnancies, at a time when women still died relatively frequently from childbirth. Not only would such intervention result in better, healthier mothers and children, but it would also improve marriages by freeing women to "love without fear." This last point, of course, was the most unsettling, for not only did the idea of sex without fear of its consequences "denaturalize" motherhood, it also implied that women were sexual, sentient beings. It thus challenged the prevailing conception that proper women had no desire for sexual pleasure. All these themes especially challenged the Church's view of motherhood and womanhood. Thus a fourth tactic Roussel adopted was to manipulate religious myth and metaphor in order to undermine Church doctrine, as she had already begun to do in *Par la révolte*.

Feminism and Free Thought: Confronting Left-Wing Misogyny

Roussel's ideology developed not only within the context of feminism, neo-Malthusianism, and her personal experience with pain, but within the doctrines and network of freethinkers to which Godet introduced her. The winter of 1903–4 was a propitious time for her to escalate her campaign and affiliate with the freethinkers, whose swelling ranks were the political legacy of the Dreyfus case. Societies of freethinkers sprang up throughout France, both in large cities such as Dijon, where membership numbered 200, and in communes of a few hundred people. Victor Charbonnel, the defrocked priest who edited the anti-clerical *La Raison,* to which Godet subscribed, succeeded in November 1902 in federating the societies into the National Association of Freethinkers of France. Its executive commission included all the leading Dreyfusards, and its stated purpose was to protect the "freedom of thought against all religions and all dogmatisms, whatever they might be, and to assure the free search for the truth by methods of reason alone."[76]

The statutes of all the local societies of freethinkers defined their mission as battling "all dogmatisms and all intolerances, with the firm resolution that we shall never give rise to a new dogmatism or a new intolerance."[77] Generally, local statutes recognized the right of women to belong to these societies, stating specifically that "each adult person, without distinction of sex, enjoying civil rights, can be part of the society."[78] In addition to establishing its opposition to Christianity as the "enemy of all life and progress," the National Association of Freethinkers proclaimed itself pacifist, internationalist, and supportive of female emancipation. The Association in turn inspired the formation of the Fedération des jeunesses laïques (Federation of Lay Youth), which met for the first time in Paris in November 1902 and included branches throughout France.[79] The growing movement of freethinkers found further ideological inspiration and organizational structure through the press. In March 1903, a group of young radicals and freethinkers founded a mouthpiece for their politics, *L'Action.* In declaring its main purpose to be anticlerical combat, the new newspaper reflected the tumultuous politics of the Dreyfus era. Soon it established itself as the principle organ for freethinkers. Henri Godet collaborated with the editors and contributed articles from newspaper's inception.

Roussel found in the doctrines of free thought, as well as in the societies of freethinkers, a welcome source of support and a platform from which she could launch her speaking and writing career. Freethinkers' ideas about science, nature, freedom, and anticlericalism fitted her feminist ideology. The anticlerical prime minister Émile Combes, who had come to power in 1902, fostered a political climate in which Roussel could refine a feminist stance that sought to emancipate women from the influence of religion. Moreover, freethinkers should have been naturally open to advocacy of birth control, the most unorthodox element of her feminism, because it directly attacked the moral hegemony of the Church. But to her chagrin, she also discovered contradictions among freethinkers, which led her to confront and expose the fundamentally misogynist attitudes among the men of the Left. Many of them hesitated supporting—and some opposed—full political equality for women, because they presumed that Catholicism had permanently corrupted female loyalty to the Republic. Indeed, women's relationship to the Church served as a primary rationale for denying them the vote throughout the Third Republic, for left-wing legislators feared women would follow the counsel of their priests and vote the Republic out of existence.[80] Finally, Roussel distrusted freethinkers' commitment to women's emancipation, because they had simply replaced God with "nature" as a source of truth. Freethinkers' glorification of nature also reified woman's place within it. Spellbound by the "eternal feminine," most of them believed womanhood could never be free of nature's dictates.[81]

Roussel's immersion in the world of freethinkers led her to develop a critique of left-wing men as acrimonious as her attacks against "repopulators" and clerics. Thus in the lecture she gave in November 1903, she took aim at unnamed "sociologists" on the Left who believed that unlimited fertility would be both possible and desirable once material needs had been met. She called this notion a "monstrous error" on the part of "egotistical men" who thought only of their own material well-being, and she asserted that in a future society, woman "will understand that her body belongs to her, and *that she alone* has the right to make use of it as she wishes." She elaborated on the ways motherhood ravaged women's bodies, weakening them to the point that they could not even make "a gesture of revolt," and she attacked the "new religion of Nature," popular among some freethinkers. "Nature is too often for us not the tender mother about whom poets have sung," she declared, "but a blind and cruel stepmother, against whom we find ourselves obligated to battle." This religion of nature was the "triumph of *Instinct* over *Reason* and *Intelligence!* . . . Civilization is only made by man's conquests of Nature. The role of science in mitigating laws is to reduce errors, to tame and direct unconscious forces . . . and it is Science that distinguishes us from animals and savages. . . . Science . . . is the affirmation of human power; it is the victory of the *Mind* over *Force* and over *Matter,* and of *Will* over *Fate.*"[82]

Roussel had yet further reason to be wary of freethinkers. In the summer of 1903, while she was visiting her friend Juliette in Revin, Henri passed on the news that Marguerite Durand had decided to fold *La Fronde* into *L'Action.* Nelly responded immediately, expressing fear over the loss of feminists' journalistic autonomy. Henri urged her to "salute this new orientation" of *L'Action* by writing a feminist article on religion, but Roussel believed strongly that another feminist newspaper should be established, independent of *L'Action*. Henri thought that it would be a very "impolitic" moment to do so, since another feminist journal would create competition for *L'Action* when its readership had not yet developed.[83] Nelly became all the more determined to establish feminism firmly within free thought.

In December 1903, Roussel gave a major address at the National Congress of Free Thought, which took place at the headquarters of the leading French Masonic obedience, the Grand Orient de France. In her address to the Congress, she reproached men "for conducting themselves as egoists" and for not accepting women as their equals. She said that the freethinking "priest eaters" had attitudes toward women no better than the clerics they attacked, because "the alleged 'irreligious' are still completely impregnated with the old Christian morality" and "fierce 'anticlericals' have . . . in spite of themselves, preserved the most *clerical* of all prejudices, *masculiniste* prejudice." Roussel conceded that the Church had made women subservient. Christian resignation had "put their dignity to sleep." But the fusion of feminism and free thought would make women blossom in their intellectual, political, and physical development. Moreover, freethinkers needed feminists to achieve their ends. Men lacked an "education of the heart." Although they might claim to support female emancipation, freethinkers had the misconceived notion of wanting "to 'perfect' us so that we would be worthy of them . . . [rather than] perfecting *themselves* so that they *would be worthy of us.*" With reference to education, she took pleasure in quoting the educational reformer Paul Bert, a "great feminist freethinker," who had said: "It is curious that whenever the subject of girls' education is raised, no one ever invokes *their right* to this instruction and this culture, nor the *personal* and *direct* advantages they could derive from it . . . but only the necessity of making agreeable spouses and enlightened mothers of them, while the rationale for educating the other sex is completely different, and one never sees at the door of boys' schools: Here good fathers of families and companions for wives are trained."[84]

Roussel's address received long applause, and it was summarized and published all over France. However, not a word about it appeared in the journal whose directors were the principle organizers of the Congress, because it had caused so much controversy among them. Many feminists strongly protested this omission, but to no avail, which led them to conclude that a "schism must have occurred over this subject" within the freethinking League of the Rights of Man.[85]

Roussel's criticism of freethinkers and the publicity it received had lasting echoes in the press. One took the form of a two-month long polemic with Henri

Duchmann in *Le Libertaire*, an anarchist and Dreyfusard periodical. This exchange was a harbinger of future opposition to Roussel from the Left. It also contains some of the logic behind the enduring ideological conflict between feminism and socialism. Duchmann launched a systematic, often emotional attack against Roussel and feminists in general, believing that their motivations for participating in politics were personal, and that they ignored larger issues of social injustice wrought by capitalism. He even compared feminism to anti-Semitism, because it was "hostile to a certain category of individuals."[86]

The concept of "patriarchy" that acknowledged unequal gender relations as inherent in all social institutions—routinely employed by feminists today, though still controversial in its definition—had not entered the feminist lexicon in Roussel's time. But without using the word, she focused her argument on the notion that inequality between men and women went far deeper than the capitalist system of production. She thus responded to Duchmann in the subsequent issue of *Le Libertaire* by insisting that feminists did not oppose individual men but rather "the monstrous social organization," and she reiterated the points she had made in previous lectures about motherhood as a choice and women's need for economic independence.[87] Duchmann retorted that Zola's novel *Fécundité*—which revealed the decadence of bourgeois women who avoided motherhood—had taught him about women's fate. He then embarked on yet another way feminists were transgressing their natural roles in an attack on one of Roussel's colleagues in the UFF: "When [Roussel] defends herself by seeing in Feminism nothing more than a declaration of war against institutions and social organization, is she ignorant that Mme Kauffmann, for example, proposes that women practice muscular exercises in order to be able to impose force on men?"[88] Kauffmann's proposition provoked a contradictory response from Duchmann. On the one hand, he presumed women wanted to use violence against men in an apolitical, personal context. On the other hand, he also argued that women could not be true revolutionaries because they had neither the intellectual nor the emotional predisposition to engage in violence. "Would Mme Nelly Roussel," he asked, "like to make revolution without breaking windows?" And he concluded, "What Mme Nelly Roussel demands *now*, we other revolutionaries only envision *afterward*."

Female physical education had, indeed, grown popular since the 1880s. Feminists such as Caroline Kauffmann and Madeleine Pelletier advocated physical strength among women, as did nonfeminist women, such as Colette, who exhibited a new "feminine ideal" of physical health. Physical strength had also become a part of the public school curriculum for girls.[89] Duchmann saw in female muscular strength a threat to the whole gender system: it violated the most important mark of "natural" difference between men and women, as well as the very difference that undergirded male honor codes. Physical force in defense of one's honor lay at the heart of masculine identity, and it served as a real and symbolic basis for excluding women from the public sphere of politics and journalistic debate. With the explosion in the number of periodicals in the Third Republic, journalism had become an important arena for contesting the "truth" and defending honor, particularly during periods of intense conflict, such as the Dreyfus Affair. Insults and libels in newspapers often resulted in the need to defend honor with a duel between men who did not wish to bother with the court system, because it was ineffective in such matters.[90] Like the detractor in their neighborhood newspaper, Duchmann used ridicule and insult to attack Roussel, questioning her truthfulness, knowing that she would not back herself up "like a man" by challenging him to a duel. Duchmann was not the first, nor was he the last, to challenge Roussel in this manner. As though to affirm that his wife could not defend her own honor, Henri Godet entered the polemic the following week. He accused Duchmann of usurping the "revolution" and revolutionary tradition for anarchists of his ilk, and said the feminist question would endure as long as women remained unequal to men.[91]

At the heart of Duchmann's attack is what has come to be known as "French universalism," the notion that any demand for rights must apply to everyone. When feminists demanded rights for women, they were doing so, according to this logic, on behalf of a special group whose special interests would undermine the rights of others. "Others" implicitly meant males.[92] Duchmann persisted doggedly for several more weeks. He accused feminists of drawing their knowledge exclusively from their bourgeois boarding-school experience and from reading novels, rather than from having to earn a living. He began by casting the issue in capitalist terms: "It is not in the wordlets [*parolettes*] of *La Fronde* or Mme Marguerite Durand's salon that the results of social antagonisms are manifest," he wrote, but outside, among the unsheltered women of the people, prostitutes, and working mothers separated all day from their children, who were degradingly forced to compete with their husbands, thus causing the latter's salaries to fall. "That is where salaries drop in proportions unknown to the sculptor Godet and Mme Nelly-Roussel." Duchmann then shifted his argument from class to gender. If women were to obtain the right to vote and seek public office, he charged, female candidates would "tear themselves apart" with the same ardor that they manifested in their religious devotion. He believed, like the followers of Rousseau in 1793, that the political sphere would unleash in women some uncontrollable libidinal quality: "We shall see them entangled in 'last-minute [sexual] manipulations' [in the electoral mire] with the spirit that we know of them, without even hiking up their skirts. This cold obstinacy in wanting to taste the political cake reveals the feminist soul in all its ugliness and conceit." Evoking Eve's apple in the "political cake," Duchmann believed that in transferring their inborn senti- mental devotion from the Church to politics, women would unleash a sexual and political promiscuity that their religious devotion had otherwise kept intact.[93]

Roussel offered one last response to Duchmann, stating that she did not want to stoop to his level, where mockery and insult were substituted for argument. As though rising to his accusation that women could not engage in violence, she claimed that her feminism was a "declaration of war" against the social organiza- tion, and that along with socialists, she considered capitalism was one of the worst enemies of women—but so too were the men who "violently" blocked women's path to liberty. Duchmann could not allow her the last word. In an article entitled "Ne touchez pas à la Reine" (Do Not Touch the Queen), he complained that he had never received an adequate response from Roussel and accused both her and Godet of "willful incoherence." He argued that the "strike of wombs" had not in practice achieved the social effects neo-Malthusians had expected. Working-class women could not pay for bare necessities, let alone afford contraceptives or even Paul Robin's brochures. Only bourgeois women would have access to "control over nature," allowing them greater individual pleasure that would do nothing for the social good.[94]

The polemic even extended to the United States when an American sent his hearty congratulations to Duchmann for his journalistic courage. The radical feminist Cleyre Yvelin, also in America, then came to Roussel's defense in the last article of this debate published in *Le Libertaire*. She affirmed feminists' con- cerns about their unfortunate sisters. In their defense, she said with a telling logic and choice of words:

> These [feminists] are fortunately gifted, [and] neither ugly nor ridiculous . . . and
> that is what indisposes the mockers, who stand on their hind legs to applaud fail-
> ures! . . . these generous thoughts have caused a sensation overseas! . . . intrepid
> women speak in public; a few of them are endowed with talent, applauded, ad-
> mired. . . . This brave [Roussel] is neither old nor ugly, nor a deserted wife! Happily
> married and a mother, that is what disconcerts the critics."[95]

Duchmann's polemic reflected one continuous thread of left-wing thinking about gender from 1793 through the nineteenth century, which manifested it- self both in intellectuals such as Jules Michelet and anarchists such as Pierre Proudhon. It sustained the notion of an eternal feminine in which women could only be "housewives or harlots." As much as the Left detested the Church, it also feared what women would become without religion, as Roussel would continue to discover.[96] Though ironic, it is also understandable that this polemic would thus end with a feminist praising Roussel for her femininity, wifehood, and motherhood, as though these qualities would lend legitimacy to her otherwise revolutionary message.

Roussel would eventually learn the strategic importance of such labels. But what was she thinking as she read Yvelin's article and clipped it for her scrapbook?

Renewed Martyrdom

The body of the ideas Roussel articulated through 1903 served as the core of one of her most popular and frequently delivered lectures entitled "La Liberté de maternité." Literally translated as "freedom of motherhood," it might less awkwardly be translated as the nineteenth-century American concept of "voluntary motherhood," which also advocated women's control over the number of pregnancies they had. An essential difference in Roussel's concept, however, was the moral justification for contraceptive devices.[97] Moreover, implicit in the French syntax is the possible translation "freedom *in, for,* or *from* motherhood." She delivered it for the first time with this official title in Paris on April 9, 1904, almost two years after her son's death and—most ironically—at the very moment she learned about an unexpected third pregnancy. Recalling the terrible outcome of her previous experience, she wrote to her grandfather the same day as her lecture:

> In this ill state in which I find myself, your letter, I confess, rather pained me. It seems to me that you welcome very calmly the news to which everyone here refers as "my tragedy." You nonetheless are among those who witnessed intimately the lamentable condition in which my last childbirth put me. You know that the poor state of my health has no other cause; and that a new maternity is for me, *from every point of view*—physically, morally, financially—a veritable catastrophe.
>
> "Children," you say, "are a fatal consequence of marriage, you must resign yourself to them." If I die from them, would you say with the same philosophy: "Death is a fatal consequence of life; you must resign yourself to it"? Misfortune truly pursues me. Each time I begin to feel better a new "blow" falls on my head! . . . I shall have spent my youth suffering! Here I am again in the grip of this black and terrible depression from which I have had such difficulty freeing myself. And the prospect of beginning again the martyrdom that I endured for so many years panics and

exasperates me. [Henri and I] believed that the worst had passed; we were forcing ourselves to drive out the painful memories. Alas! They return incessantly! And if we do not succeed, Henri and I, if our profound affection does not sustain us a little in mutual consolation, I do not know how our life will be and how we shall be able to sustain it.[98]

She had, after all, spent a year publicizing the fact that a "strike [of wombs] had been declared within a small circle of those women" and that that circle would expand ceaselessly.[99] Yvelin's words must have struck Roussel with irony, and not only because they stressed that her own motherhood legitimized her message, but because she discovered herself pregnant again just as the polemic ended. As a member of the circle she was trying to expand, and indeed as its main apostle, this pregnancy made her both a strikebreaker and a heretic. It also threw her into a state of renewed depression.

Given her mission to publicize the need to prevent such unplanned pregnancies, and even more important, her profound desire not to have more children, how could she and Henri have been so careless? Did they lose themselves in a moment of passion? Did neither one of them use protection? Did the protection not work? A letter Roussel wrote two months later to Marguerite Durand provides some clues: "I really believed that I was sheltered from these formidable ordeals that so profoundly undermine my health. And I was hoping to provide an example of the "strike" [of wombs] that I advocate. Alas! Despite all the progress of Science and conscience, poor humanity is not yet completely mistress of its own destiny; we have not definitively conquered Fate!"[100] It seems, then, that she had taken "scientific" precautions that failed her. Henri must have felt profound remorse, which perhaps explains the zeal with which he made sacrifices to build her career, as the next chapter will begin to elaborate.

CHAPTER THREE

The Making and Marketing of a Spectacular Apostle

And this will not be an ordinary spectacle, the phenomenon
exhibiting her barnum!!

Nelly Roussel to Henri Godet (May 19, 1905)

Roussel's activities from the fall of 1902 through the spring of 1904 suggest that she had fully recovered both her mental and physical health. In addition to lecturing, writing, and performing *Par la révolte*, she contributed articles to *La Fronde*, *L'Action*, *Régénération*, and other newspapers. By the spring of 1904, she had taken up myriad other activities: on Mondays, she attended a course at the Franklin Institute. Tuesdays were her "reception day," when she welcomed family members, friends, and acquaintances, including Paul Robin and the feminists Marguerite Durand, Gabrielle Petit, Marbel, and Caroline Kauffmann. On Thursdays, she gave diction lessons at her home, and on Fridays, she attended a course by Paul Mounet at the Comédie-Française.[1]

Roussel began giving diction lessons in February because of "great demand," and her course included training in pronunciation, the art of declamation, and reading. She charged ten francs per month, and subscribers of *L'Action* or *La Fronde* received a 20 percent discount. In addition, she served on the Executive Commission of the National Association of Free Thinkers. In between these activities, she squeezed in sessions with Henri in his workshop, where she posed for a bust he was sculpting of her and Mireille. Now four and a half, Mireille lived with Nelly's mother and stepfather in the house Nelly had grown up in at 73 avenue de Saint-Mandé, around the corner from the Roussel-Godet residence on rue Michel Bizot. This living arrangement may have begun during Roussel's illness in 1902; it is unclear when it became permanent. Nelly and Henri saw Mireille daily. They often had meals at the Montupet home, especially on Sundays, when the extended family gathered there for lunch and then took a long and leisurely walk in the Bois de Vincennes. Mireille would "return to the paternal home" when the Montupets were away from Paris.[2]

Nelly felt the shock of her third pregnancy all more profoundly, not only because, as she told her grandfather, she had worked so hard to fight off the consequences of her last one, but because she was just beginning to taste the fruits of her nascent fame. The address she had given at the International Congress of Freethinkers and the Duchmann polemic that ensued had spread her name throughout France. One figure whose attention she captivated—and whose admiration began to play a role in her career—was Émile Darnaud (1826–1914), a former army captain, officer of the Legion of Honor and of Public Instruction, and mayor of Roquefixade (Ariège), a village of 400 inhabitants. Darnaud exemplifies the difficulty of pigeon-holing individuals into stable political identities; he also demonstrates the ease with which Nelly Roussel could fulfill individual fantasies. An ardent freethinker since he had been "in his mother's womb," he said, Darnaud was also an anarchist sympathizer. His abiding fondness for the opposite sex made him into a "feminist." Despite his left-wing politics, he was also a social Darwinist and believed in the superiority of the white race. As an officer, he had been seriously wounded in the Franco-Prussian war, but his experience and intellectual beliefs led him to accept war as "inevitable." Like others in his era, he also viewed war as a means toward progress. Darnaud was married to a woman twenty-two years his junior. She shared neither his freethinking nor his feminism, but she gave him "enormous leeway," and they enjoyed a stable marriage, living "parallel lives."[3]

In his late seventies, Darnaud attracted young unmarried women—most often schoolteachers who had been trained in the École normale of Foix, where he resided. They viewed him as an "indulgent *bon-papa*" in whom they could confide. If they were freethinkers or feminists, they would seek him out; or he would seek out local schoolteachers to try to convert them to freethinking and feminism. He devoted his time to collecting as many newspapers as he could get his hands on across the political spectrum (including the ardently Catholic *La Croix* and the feminist *La Fronde*), though he focused mostly on those devoted to free thought. He read them, took notes, contemplated, and each day wrote ten to twelve lengthy letters to friends and to strangers whose politics attracted his attention.[4] Darnaud's ruminations offer a wealth of information about Roussel's impact, as well as about her own self-construction as a public figure. Though he wrote copious self-confessional letters to her about his public and private life, she responded with letters revealing only her public self.

Roussel first came to Darnaud's attention in January 1903, when Paul Robin—whom he knew from the political circles they shared—sent him a copy of *Régénération*. Darnaud had known of Robin's educational work, but he had no taste for neo-Malthusianism. In fact, at that time, he agreed with Jacques Bertillon's assessment of the population problem; in his view, "in our terrible period of transition, when everything, absolutely everything is thrown into question, transformed, metamorphosed, we must allow evolution to operate."[5] But Roussel's article "L'Amour fécond, l'amour stérile" (Fertile Love, Sterile Love) in this issue of Robin's paper, caught his attention, and henceforth he studied her ideas by reading her articles and summaries of her lectures in *La Fronde* and *L'Action*. In the early months of 1904, he began corresponding with Nelly. That spring, he formed a "Feminist Committee of Roquefixade" and became its secretary. The group consisted of sixteen young women, most of whom were schoolteachers. When articles by Roussel appeared in *L'Action*, Darnaud bought every copy of that issue in Roquefixade, and he also purchased copies of *Par la révolte* to distribute to the local feminists.[6] Thus began a prolific and nearly obsessive ten-year correspondence with the object of his intense admiration. A frequent contributor to the local newspaper, *Les Annales de l'Ariège*, Darnaud spread Roussel's reputation with his own articles and established further contacts for her.[7] Many of the women with whom he put her in touch began writing to her; he became a regional publicist on her behalf just as her public speaking career was beginning to take off. Until his death in 1914, Darnaud both supported Roussel and acted as a foil in shaping her ideas and influencing her self-presentation to the public.

Roussel's collaboration with *L'Action* and freethinkers also began to pay off mightily. Although she had expressed bitter disappointment at Marguerite Durand's abandonment of *La Fronde* (still being published at this point), *L'Action* lived up to its promise to include articles on feminism and reached audiences that otherwise would not have heard or read the feminist message.[8] *L'Action* provided a national platform for networking freethinkers across France, and Roussel's visibility in the paper began to make her known among freethinkers in the provinces. Soon she was receiving invitations to speak from several freethinking groups in the Midi affiliated with the association Ni dieu ni maître (Neither God nor Master).

Fruits of Success: The Tour of 1904

On April 14, 1904, just five days after writing to her grandfather about her three-month-old pregnancy, Roussel embarked on her first speaking tour, departing alone from Paris for a twenty-hour train trip to Béziers (Hérault), near the Mediterranean. Over the course of the next five and a half weeks, she delivered eight two-hour lectures in the south of France (see map 3). In all but one case, after each lecture, she performed a 30-minute dramatic reading of her "symbolic scene," *Par la révolte,* after which she sold copies of the play. The newly federated freethinking societies sponsored most of the tour, which meant that she went to those areas where such societies were most prominent. Depending on the locale and its resources, she was paid a fee as high as 50 francs. Socialist municipalities could offer venues at no charge, which reduced expenses; but elsewhere the organizers had to pay for theaters, which meant that her fees depended more on receipts. Sometimes, however, she spoke gratis, accepting only reimbursement for her expenses. The organizers usually charged .50–1.50 francs entry, according to whether the audience was mainly working-class or more bourgeois; and often women were admitted free of charge in order to encourage their attendance, or—perhaps to assure control over the female audience—the organizers promoted free entry for any woman accompanied by a man.[9]

The freethinkers' associations brought Roussel to audiences who would never otherwise have heard her: industrial workers, minor functionaries, schoolteachers, café keepers, wine growers, craftsmen, agricultural workers, and peasants. The spring of 1904 was, moreover, a propitious time for her to spread her message. That year, there were 1,026 strikes, involving 271,097 industrial workers, with local work stoppages igniting strikes throughout France. The wave of strikes peaked in 1906, with 438,500 strikers, but strikes continued through 1907. Strikers made their protest highly visible, pouring into the streets carrying flags and singing the "Internationale" and other revolutionary songs. The fear and concern they fueled among conservatives eventually resulted in a brutal backlash. Because many of these striking workers also belonged to associations of freethinkers, Roussel's affiliation with the latter connected her more directly to the foundations of working-class material and political life. The Duchmann polemic and other left-wing criticism of feminists and neo-Malthusianists had also sensitized her to working-class issues and helped hone her rhetoric. Roussel's willingness to address workers starkly distinguished her from the vast majority of Paris feminists, especially Marguerite Durand and others associated with *La Fronde.* She was the first feminist to venture into the provinces and to begin to "decentralize" feminism.[10]

Nelly left Henri behind to work on the local elections and to finish sculpting the mother-daughter bust; she also left him to his own dark thoughts about her tragic suffering from childbirth the previous year and his worries over her physi-

cal and mental health. But Nelly took pleasure in her journey, traveling alone by
train, for the very first time, in an era when it was still uncommon for women to
do so. Despite her discomfort and fatigue, she felt joy in viewing the mountain-
ous landscape in the light of dawn. She thoroughly enjoyed her independence.
Upon her arrival in Béziers, a "dozen 'brothers' and 'comrades'"—Freemasons
and freethinkers—met her on the quay, and one of them drove her to her hotel,
where she settled in, dined, and slept for twelve hours. Although she complained
that bedbugs awakened her repeatedly, Nelly was quite content with her "pretty
room, large, comfortable and gay, with many mirrors and a balcony looking out
on the promenade below." It was only in retrospect a year later that she confessed
to having felt sad and lonely on her first night there.[11]

Upon her arrival Nelly received an emotional letter from her grandfather, responding to her own anguished letter five days earlier:

> The news of your future maternity made me sorry for you. I have not forgotten
> the distressing repercussions that your last childbirth had on your health, but it
> seems to me that my role in this circumstance was more to have you envision a
> future without fear. . . . Rest assured that I was wishing with all my heart that my
> intervention would make you realize that your new child will restore to your health
> what the preceding one destroyed. This occurs rather frequently, and it is my most
> ardent desire.[12]

The letter focused not on the baby that might somehow replace her lost son, but
on the restoration of Nelly's health. It reinforced what previous silences suggest:
that the loss of her health—mental at least as much as physical—hurt Nelly more
than the loss of her son, though it would be mistaken to think the two could be
separated. Perhaps her grandfather's letter helped her sustain the lightness of
heart she expressed at the onset of her journey. Her second letter to Henri glee-
fully recounted how four of the "gentlemen" looking after her had picked her up at
the hotel for a drive in a "very chic" automobile. "The owner is a young widower,
a rich wine wholesaler (the first in Béziers), whose mission is to entertain lectur-
ers. . . . He drove us to the seaside . . . to an immense and magnificent beach of
sand, where we breathed the invigorating, salty fresh air with delight ."[13]

Few wives would be so candid about the attentions from men their husbands
did not know; few husbands would feel comfortable having their wives be so dependent on the hospitality of men they had never met. Even little Mireille found
her mother's travels odd; while dining with Henri at her grandparents', she suddenly stopped eating and burst out: "So, papa, why did mommy leave all alone?"
Her father replied, "So, tell me why it should have been otherwise?" "Because,"

Mireille said, "when ladies travel it's always with their husbands, and gentlemen with their wives." Henri silenced his daughter by pointing out that "Pépé" (Montupet) had traveled to Lille alone two days earlier and would be going to Bordeaux alone the next day. "This silence," Henri recounted to Nelly, "meant that Pépé was not a woman, which, moreover, I did not contest."[14]

Henri was bemused by his daughter's observations and expressed no concern whatsoever about his wife traveling alone and being escorted by unknown "comrades." Indeed, he shared Nelly's excitement, and he seems to have been unworried by the attentions she received from men.[15] She recounted her first full day in Béziers to him: after they returned from the seashore, the gentlemen had dined with her in the hotel. They then went "to the theater (a real theater, you know, like those in Paris), where I harangued a crowd of 1,200 to 1,500 people, who came above all, I think, out of curiosity. Think about it! A woman lecturer! . . . what a strange beast! . . . The 'phenomenon' did not displease, and was strongly, warmly received. Oh! If you only could have been there, my poor dear 'barnum.'" From this point on, Roussel and Godet referred to one another respectively as "the phenomenon" and "Barnum"—the latter because of Godet's role in managing her as a "spectacle."[16]

Roussel owed her large turnout to effective advertising. Her appearance in Béziers had been billed as a lecture on feminism by an eminent former actress of the Comédie-Française. The *Depêche* of Toulouse had advertised her as a freethinker with "vigorous oratory talent, elevated even more by the grace of a woman and the diction of an artist" and strongly encouraged women to attend. Seven regional newspapers summarized her lecture and described audience reaction. She spoke for two hours about "The Social Question and Feminism," addressed many of the issues that Duchmann had raised, and "refuted the sophisms used to combat feminism." The summary of her lecture included all the elements essential to female emancipation; she made only oblique reference to the "liberty of motherhood," and made no direct mention of neo-Malthuisanism.

The *Pétit Méridional* reported that the hall had been "overflowing," and that Roussel "took over her audience with the first words she spoke." She delivered "an erudite, well-documented, extremely interesting lecture in both form and substance. . . . After having been many times applauded during her long talk, the audience gave her a warm ovation at the end. . . . At the exit, we heard ladies saying to men, 'Well, you had your hides tanned!' They were completely enlivened."[17]

"Numerous women attended, adding to and heightening the brilliance of this demonstration, which will surely bear fruit. The sustained attention and the frenetic applause . . . [may] permit us to hope so," the *Union républicaine* wrote, noting that Roussel's reading of *Par la révolte*, "with a truly remarkable diction and a grace of incomparable gestures," also met with enthusiastic applause.[18] Nelly sold half of the one hundred copies of the play that she had brought with her, and she and her sponsors celebrated with champagne, drinking to Godet's and Mireille's health.[19]

The ability to captivate such a large audience for two hours, followed by a reading of her play, testifies to Roussel's charisma. She also profited from coverage in the local press, which projected her voice well beyond the audiences at her talks. The *Dépêche* reached about 150,000 readers of the "popular milieu" in Toulouse and its surrounding region; similarly, the *Pétit Méridional* of Montpellier enjoyed circulation throughout the Mediterranean region of Languedoc.[20] Such publicity had its intended effect. To her surprise, a thousand people, most of them women, attended her next lecture, in nearby Cazouls-les-Béziers, where she had not expected a large audience. Nelly reported her "luminous success" to Henri: the audience, "composed above all of agricultural workers" crowded into a "rustic and bizarre . . . hall." The director of the local school and her four assistants expressed enthusiastic delight. Nelly thought that if all schoolteachers responded this way, her ideas would spread rapidly.[21]

By her fourth day, Nelly wrote that her stay in the Midi "would really be agreeable if, on the one hand, I did not miss you, my poor dear abandoned one! And if, on the other hand, I felt completely alert and in good health." With oblique reference to her pregnancy, she said, "The thousand little inconveniences inherent in my state somewhat spoil my pleasure. Nonetheless, I'm doing as well as possible. I don't need to tell you that we speak about you often, and I think about you constantly. Despite my distractions and activities, I am already finding the time long, and sometimes get bored being alone this way." She told him she had been paid 250 francs and apologized for the "telegraphic" tone of her letter, which she closed with "thousands and thousands of kisses."[22]

Before departing definitively from Béziers, Roussel's escorts took her by automobile to two other nearby towns, Agde and Murviel-les-Béziers. She reported enormous audiences, larger than had ever attended lectures there, but she found them "less intelligent, less open, less attentive." Nonetheless, she thought her performances went well and was particularly gratified by her success in "enchanting schoolteachers" everywhere she went. "I planted the first marker, I sowed the first seeds, and leveled the road for others to follow me. Now there is a job that is fairly noble and fruitful, about which I have no regrets." She was also pleased that she had made such a strong impression on the organizers, for she thought she had rid them of their old prejudices about a female lecturer and dispelled their fears of a "militant feminist."[23]

Roussel next lectured in Vallauris, also on the invitation of local freethinkers. The secretary of their association took her to his home for lunch. She described her hosts as "a nice family of workers, very simple and affable people." She noted approvingly that the daughter was about to have a civil wedding, and that she was very impressed with the son, a young worker of barely twenty, who had feminist ideas and admired her for her diction. The family informed her that they "assiduously" read *L'Action* and *La Fronde*, where they had enjoyed both her and her husband's articles. Her host was a potter, and he took her to his workshop to show her how vases were made. She then delivered her lecture in the garden of a café to an audience of 2,000, which included many women. Here the publicity had worked especially well, for women in this region, she was told, rarely attended public meetings. The audience consisted mostly of workers and petit bourgeois but included even nationalists and clericals, who were "attracted by the desire to see the 'feminist lecturer,' this unknown animal that they imagined so bizarre." Once again she was very satisfied about her success.[24]

Press coverage in *La Vérité* (Cannes) noted that the master of ceremonies had "opened the meeting in correct and courteous language" and (suggesting that working-class rowdiness had been anticipated) that the audience had listened to Roussel's lecture with "profound reverence." She not only spoke about feminism but also discussed motherhood, casting it in terms with which she thought workers could identify, particularly given the climate of social unrest. She spoke of oppressed workers' right to strike, and emphasized that no one should be forced to accept anything against his or her will. "It is only by revolt, that is, in refusing to be subjected to what is unjust that one will succeed in throwing off the yokes that weigh on the proletariat and that particularly grip the feminine sex." She stopped short of calling for a "strike of wombs."[25] She proceeded to Nice, and then Vienne, where she found the audience "very mediocre."

The pinnacle of Roussel's achievement on this tour came in Lyon, where she derived special satisfaction, because the Lyonnais "are, as they say, very cold and very distrustful. I hardly noticed it; and nowhere (except in Paris, of course) have I had an audience so attentive, so intelligent and so warm." But her talk in Lyon had more significance than its success alone, for it resonated more deeply and disruptively in the political culture of the period. Unlike at her other venues, a group of feminists sponsored this lecture; thus much of her audience consisted of the already converted. Moreover, members of the Lyonnais section of the League of Human Regeneration also attended. With this audience, she had both the courage to address her subject in bolder terms and a more pressing need to do so. She spoke about the liberty of motherhood and the "strike of wombs" to "enthusiastic bravos." The League of Human Regeneration was so pleased with her performance that its members immediately invited her to return to give another lecture on freedom of motherhood.

Because she had spoken more explicitly about reproductive rights, Roussel's performance in Lyon incurred vicious attacks in the conservative press. Her impact also had to do with the constellation of national and local, feminist and socialist politics. Key to the controversy here (and elsewhere) was the attraction feminism held for schoolteachers, and the central place teachers held in the future of French schoolchildren. Odette Laguerre, a contributor to *La Fronde,* with whom Roussel now began a lifelong close friendship and collaboration, was the primary organizer of the Lyon event. Laguerre had moved to Lyon to organize a group called L'Éducation et action féministe (Feminist Education and Action), which included schoolteachers, workers, and freethinkers. It advertised itself as "frankly anticlerical, anti-militarist, and socialist" and warned women workers against "certain philanthropic enterprises of worldly ladies who, in appearing to be interested in the people, only dream in reality of serving the Church and the interests of reaction."[26] Among such "enterprises" loomed Léonie Talsans's philanthropic ladies' society in the working-class city of Saint-Étienne. Talsans felt intense rivalry with the Lyonnais group, and she was particularly incensed that it received the support of Mme Desparmet-Ruello, the first female director of a girls' secondary school in France. At the core of this rivalry lay bitter competition for the hearts and minds of women workers and schoolteachers.

In response to Roussel's lecture in Lyon, Talsans wrote a long article in the organ of her philanthropic society, *Le Travail de la femme et de la jeune fille* (The Work of the Woman and Young Girl).[27] The article gained importance because the associated Catholic press reprinted excerpts of it in newspapers throughout France—and it represents the stakes in the struggle between clericals and freethinkers. By her own unapologetic admission, Talsans did not even attend Roussel's lecture but only heard "echoes" of it; her absence did not, however, deter her from vividly describing what the audience had seen and heard. She began with a biting critique of the reversed gender roles in the staging of the event, with the women in the center, flanked by "a certain number of representatives of the strong sex [who] decorated the ends of the stage." Describing the content of Roussel's lecture posed more difficulty for Talsans than its staging, because "to reproduce her talk exactly, without offending the legitimate modesty of her female readers, she would have to resort to Latin," she said, which, unfortunately, she did not know well enough. Talsans therefore proceeded to summarize the talk without explicit mention of these "brutal" doctrines. Roussel's ability to make "outrageously scabrous remarks . . . for an hour without batting an eyelid" proved that she was devoid of scruples, Talsans proclaimed. Roussel's "prodigious gestures, exhibiting muscular force, attest that she cedes nothing to the masculine portion of humanity," Talsans said, and her "strong voice" was unsettling all by itself (even though Talsans had not heard it), being devoid of "the natural softness of the feminine inflection."

What Talsans found most scandalous about Roussel's feminism was the means she advocated for women to emancipate themselves. The first method would be coeducation, "the extraordinary and edifying results of which," the author added in sarcastic reference to the Cempuis scandal, "M. Robin has given an admirable example." This education would "naturally" lead to free unions that would replace marriage. Talsans said that even in a free union, which she claimed Roussel advocated, "women's particular nature and particular constitution would charge her with the responsibility of childbearing." But instead, "the woman will be a mother only if she wants to be, when she judges it convenient and useful. The League of Human Regeneration, of which Mme Nelly Roussel is the apostle . . . openly preaches, Malthusianism . . . monstrous theories that are today accepted without protest in certain milieux, and little by little they make their way. Only a few years ago, one would have booed or sent to the padded cell of an insane asylum a woman so bereft of the most elementary modesty or so deprived of good sense as to utter such insanities."[28]

Talsans's critique operates on two levels. First, as with the profound discomfort Duchmann had expressed at the "muscularization" of Caroline Kauffmann, Talsans—in most respects Duchmann's opposite—also "saw" in Roussel's very presence on stage, and "heard" in the strength of her voice, a similarly threatening masculinization of womanhood. Second, excusing herself from explicating Roussel's doctrine gave her greater leeway to misrepresent it. Although Robin's educational experiments actually did have "edifying results," she used his unproven misdeeds in the Cempuis affair as the logic on which she based a bizarre cause-and-effect relationship: coeducation would readily lead to cohabitation in the form of free unions, and these free unions would be all the more degenerate in their barrenness. Roussel never advocated free unions. Privately, as a matter of principle, she opposed marriage, but she did not think free unions would advance women's status.[29]

Talsans made another interesting and paradoxical point in her description of the audience reaction she had not witnessed. Reflecting the prevailing ideas about the psychological behavior of crowds, widely popularized by Gustave Le Bon, she claimed that the audience, composed mostly of young people of both sexes, had become an "unconscious crowd" at the end of Roussel's lecture and had "frenetically applauded" like a "band of swooning lunatics in contortions," uttering "incoherent declamations." At the same time, however, the audience's complete composure during the lecture itself, despite its lascivious content, proved to Talsans that Roussel had put it under a spell.[30]

Over the next two months, owing to the organized network of Catholic press agencies, Talsans's interpretation of Roussel's Lyon lecture found its way into newspapers in other towns and cities, each reproducing portions of her article word for word, usually without attribution, sometimes with further embellishment. For example, in *L'Éclair comtois*, Jules Burty of Besançon (Doubs) wrote that Roussel implied that boys and girls might as well share dormitories, "in a touching promiscuity." And if Roussel had her way, parents would want to rid themselves of their "litters" like "tomcats." One of the most menacing aspects of Roussel's presentation, according to Burty, was that the director of the public girls' school had organized it, proving the absence of morality in the government's administration of female instruction.[31]

These reactionary responses touched on the destabilization of boundaries between girls and boys, men and women, youths and adults, and human beings and animals. They also used religious metaphor in describing Roussel as an "apostle on a mission with a gospel," sensing and fearing the messianic appeal of her message. Indeed, Roussel's words resonated so deeply in the Catholic press because she spoke them in the midst of an acute crisis in Catholic education. On becoming prime minister in 1902, Émile Combes, a fanatically anticlerical Freemason, immediately implemented measures against the Church, using the 1901 law on associations to evict or disband most religious orders. On July 5, 1904, less than two months after Roussel's tour, the National Assembly passed a law that prohibited all congregations from teaching. Roussel's demands for educational reform, and the fact that teachers were so receptive to her ideas, touched Catholic nerves. Jules Burty asserted that the students being trained as teachers at the *écoles normales* shared Roussel's views, and "by the suppression of congregations and of the freedom of instruction, M. Combes does not hide his intention of subjecting all our young girls to this intellectual and moral discipline in the *lycées*. . . . Mme Roussel just preached this morality to us in all its cynicism. . . . she suppresses conjugal love, maternal love, filial piety, which sink into the ignominies of debauchery . . . human morality will forcibly lead to these bestial consequences when they are not invigorated by the spirit of God."[32]

Overall, Roussel's tour was a great success in terms of the publicity she received, her large audiences, and the sale of *Par la révolte*. A conservative estimate of her collective audience is more than 6,000; her talks were summarized or otherwise commented upon in at least thirteen regional newspapers; she sold several hundred copies of her play.[33] Once news of her success spread, requests poured in for repeat performances. Astruc, the organizer of the first lecture of her tour, wanted her to return to Béziers immediately, and Eugène Humbert, now leading the neo-Malthusian movement, asked her to extend her tour and to do another with Paul Robin. But her advancing pregnancy made any further lectures impossible, although admitting this caused her intense embarrassment. Without mentioning her pregnancy, Roussel wrote back to Humbert to say that she would not be able to accompany Robin on another tour because she would be too tired. But she assured him that she would return the following year to address "liberty of motherhood," because "there is almost a complete ignorance of it in the Midi." Henri meanwhile took upon himself the task of telling Humbert the real reason for his wife's response, also specifying "what he could say and what he must not say," assuring Nelly, "I left it to him to understand your situation—and you can rest assured that he received it well; this guy is not an imbecile."[34]

In the meantime, Godet was busy with his own life, as well as with their daughter. "Mirelle continues to be a love," he wrote. "Yesterday, as I was taking her to your mother's, I said to her, 'Do you think about your mother sometimes?' And with a volubility such that she almost swallowed her words, she screamed her response, 'When you write to her you must tell her that I always think about her, and that I received my toys from Vallauris [small items the potter had made for her] and that I wanted to write her a postcard.'" Godet wrote articles for *L'Action*, showed his sculptures, and presided over the voting section in their arrondissement, a "wretched burden that I thought I must accept, like other burdens." Nelly offered sympathy and concern for his health, as well as contempt for the "vile electoral crowd." She told him to rest, and "leave these dirty politics aside." She added in parentheses, "I am becoming an anarchist." She shared Duchmann's anarchist disdain for electoral politics because women did not have the vote.[35]

Godet continued sculpting the bust of Nelly and Mireille, a virtual celebration of mother and daughter, and he sent her a photo of the nearly finished product. Nelly expressed pleasure at how Mireille appeared, but her own likeness displeased her. He had rendered Nelly's eyes cast downward, no doubt gazing at her daughter adoringly, like mothers in other sculptures of his (figs. 5 and 6). She demanded that Henri "open the eyes," suggesting that she preferred instead to be shown facing away from her daughter, gazing outward to her public, just as she was doing in her actual life. He complied with her request, and completed the bust prior to her return. He exhibited it at the Salon des artistes français, where it attracted "great notice and the most flattering comments," according to a newspaper account. Henri said that "everyone recognized her."[36] The irony in his portrayal of Mireille as attached to her mother (fig. 9), during yet another of the latter's prolonged absences, is inescapable, especially since Nelly does not seem to have missed Mireille when she was away for nearly six weeks. Though she occasionally expresses homesickness and yearning for Henri, she rarely mentions Mireille in her letters. She did, however, write to her daughter separately.[37]

By the end of April, about two weeks into her trip and four months into her pregnancy, Nelly's physical condition became more burdensome. From Monaco, where she had gone to visit her grandfather and gamble, she wrote, "I am feeling very heavy, very weary, and already I am having difficulty walking. I hardly go to the Casino—the atmosphere turns my head and deafens me; nonetheless I won ten francs the day before yesterday!" By the end of her tour, she complained of her weight, having already put on about twenty pounds.[38] She also became acutely aware of the maternal burdens that others suffered. When she visited her friend Honorine in Beaucaire, Nelly noted how "her children really filled the house." Honorine's little girl was recovering from bronchitis, "and the last, Jules, one month old, is breast-fed by his mother," which Nelly found remarkable. She envied her friend her quick recovery from childbirth, but also empathized with the suffering Honorine had previously endured. Similarly, when she visited her recently married and very close friend Juliette Supply, she commented: "Juliette finds me looking excellent [for being pregnant]; but unfortunately, I cannot pay her the same compliment." And with reference to her friend's unintended pregnancy, added "she is very tired and thin . . . for, let's admit it, stepmother Nature has played what can be called a dirty trick on her as well [as on me]. . . . It is so unfortunate that she is feeling sick during the first months of her marriage."[39] Thus even while on her speaking tour, Roussel observed in other women the very burdens about which she spoke publicly, and from which, on this particular tour, she suffered herself.

Roussel received many compliments from her friends about how well she looked, on the other hand, which pleased her immensely—not because of her pregnancy—but as proof that she could defy her condition. But the passage of time did nothing to reconcile her to her future child. She learned in May, during a second visit with her grandfather, that her sister Andrée had just had a miscarriage. In reaction to this news, she wrote Henri, "I am impatient to have the details; and I really hope to receive a letter soon . . . what a stupid thing all the same! Why couldn't this have happened to me two months ago?"[40]

Two highlights particularly stand out in Roussel's five-and-a-half week trip. Her grandfather attended the lecture she gave in Nice, and congratulated her warmly, "declaring that he was really astonished." He had had no expectations, but he told her that "he had never before heard a speaker who had given him so much pleasure." Thomas Nel's pride in Nelly must have meant more to her than anyone else's, perhaps even Henri's, whose praise she could take for granted. A second event, an unscheduled "lecture," also thrilled her. While in Toulon, she saw her cousin Jules Nel, an officer in the navy, and his wife, Ninie. Ninie took her aboard a destroyer under the command of one of Jules's friends. They chatted with three officers, one of whom inquired about Roussel's trip. She recounted to Henri:

> I explained that I was doing a lecture tour . . . first amazement. They asked on what subject; Ninie responded: on feminism; . . . second and more profound amazement! Then we chatted, and never before have the walls of a destroyer heard such things! Imagine me expounding my theories in front of three navy officers! Reactionary and clerical like almost all their colleagues but—equally like almost all their colleagues—distinguished, friendly, and courteous. Ninie found this very funny. She said to me afterward, "You are astonishing! You didn't get flustered!" These gentlemen had the wind knocked out of them, I would say in the language of a sculptor. They didn't expect anything like that, and never has your "phenomenon" produced such an impression. The commander spoke of organizing a lecture for the squadron, which, he said, had great need of it! . . . And then he promised from now on to read newspapers that address issues of feminism.[41]

Even this non-lecture resonated in the press. Godet wrote an article for *L'Action* about the success of Roussel's scheduled lecture in Nice, and then added the story about her visit on the destroyer. The widely circulating conservative paper *Le Figaro* picked up the latter story, taking advantage of Roussel's conversation on the warship to attack the anticlerical, antimilitary navy minister, Camille Pelletan, against whom it was waging a long-term battle. The article described her as a "particularly zealous collaborator" of Robin, who "distinguished himself at Cempuis, and now directs a league for the propagation of 'The Art of Making Angels' [abortion]." It referred to Pelletan—who had had absolutely nothing to do with Roussel's appearance on board the destroyer—as an "educator," as though he had organized a formal lecture by her. "By this fact," the article continued sarcastically, "it appears that M. Pelletan is preoccupied with adorning the minds of French sailors with new and healthy ideas."[42]

Roussel discovered new dimensions of herself on this tour. Although she loved the sense of independence travel gave her, she also had to endure long periods of solitude and loneliness, not to mention the practicalities that often challenged her. She reveled in her ability to "conquer" the less sophisticated provincial audiences, and in the praise and the attention she received from the lecture organizers; she cherished time spent with her friends and her grandfather, and she loved being at the Mediterranean. Most remarkably, Roussel learned that she could market herself, her doctrines, and her published "playlet" to a wide variety of audiences. Although she delivered every lecture on this tour under the same title, the content varied, for she always spoke about her well-rehearsed subject without a written text. This allowed her to calibrate the content according to whether her listeners were working-class, urban, rural, freethinkers, feminists, neo-Malthusians, or simply seekers of spectacle. She also conquered her body, in that she was able to perform to her utmost despite the increasing burdens of her pregnancy.

Roussel's large audiences and success resulted in part from the rise in the status of public intellectuals and in the popularity of public lectures during the Belle Époque. She also owed her success to support from the federated network of freethinking associations. The pending fusion of *La Fronde* and *L'Action* was intended to promote an alliance between freethinkers and feminists. The collaboration was both logical and symbiotic. Freethinking provided both a philosophical and structural basis for promoting feminism, as Roussel's tour demonstrated. The Association of Freethinkers was also a more "legitimate" organ for the dissemination of her ideas than either feminist organizations or the neo-Malthusian movement, both of which also sponsored her lectures. At the same time, Roussel and her feminist doctrine helped promote free thought, and her entire tour was an advertisement for *L'Action*. Freethinkers also benefited, because they had in Roussel a dynamic speaker who could spread the message of anticlericalism to provincial audiences who might otherwise have been unreceptive. Peasants, workers, shopkeepers—people of all classes and both genders in the countryside—flocked to hear her, not only because of her dramatic talent as a speaker, but because she was a female public speaker, something uncommon even in Paris, and spectacular entertainment in the provinces.[43]

Roussel's other main support was her husband, particularly in respect to publicity. The large size of her audiences shows that they had been well advertised. Provincials experienced few of the newer entertainments current in Paris, but they certainly knew such phenomena as vaudeville and traveling circuses. Roussel was quite correct in perceiving that she drew crowds, not because of the nature of her message, but because what she had to offer was "spectacular," in the sense that she was out of the ordinary, almost a circus figure. By 1900, French provincials had been well exposed to spectacle and its power to lift them out of the commonplace. Advertisement of such entertainment also became a spectacle unto itself: Buffalo Bill's Wild West show used gigantic posters that covered walls throughout towns and cities, and in 1889, it even succeeded in competing with the Exposition universelle in Paris. Barnum and Bailey achieved a new level of the extraordinary with their five-year European tour at the turn of the century. The press spread word of its colossal grandeur to those who had not witnessed it and interpreted it for those who had. Godet had personally witnessed the impact of such publicity in Châlons, a much smaller town, where he encountered the Barnum and Bailey circus. He marveled at walls "covered as though by magic with multicolored posters . . . and this only for a day."[44]

Although Henri described this display somewhat disdainfully, he had begun to think of his wife's performance in terms of marketing and of himself as her "Barnum," the publicist of "the phenomenon" that she now proclaimed herself to be.[45] While she was on tour, he made certain her lectures were advertised through posters and the local press and covered in *L'Action*. But he also managed the smallest details of her life: he told her how much to pay in tips and sent her copies of *Par la révolte* to sell as her supplies of it became depleted with each performance. He answered much of her correspondence, and he advised her about what to say in letters she had to write herself regarding future lecture tours and other practical matters. In answer to her complaints that *L'Action* had not written about her lectures in the Midi, Henri insisted that she write summaries herself, taking advantage of her time vacationing in Monaco to do so. He advised her particularly to emphasize the enthusiasm she aroused among schoolteachers. He also told her to send an article to *La Fronde,* and then to the other freethinking newspapers, listing four of them. After her lecture in Vallauris, he chastised her for not announcing her forthcoming lectures in the nationally circulating Paris newspapers. In short, he had to encourage and guide her in her publicity, and her success depended on his unflagging support.[46]

Redemption from Pain

Roussel returned to Paris on May 21, after a thirty-eight-day absence. Now visibly pregnant, she informed friends and colleagues of her condition, including Paul Robin. She was obliged to continue to turn down invitations. Marguerite

Durand asked her to accompany her to Berlin, all expenses paid by Durand, to attend the important International Council on Women. Nelly sent her regrets: "You will easily understand my abstention [from accompanying you on your trip] when you know why. Know thus, my dear Madam, that I am expecting another child in September! This will no doubt astonish you. But no one can be more astonished than myself." She then went on to say that she had thought she was "sheltered from these formidable ordeals," and that she had hoped to provide an example of "wombs on strike." She continued:

> Here I am thus condemned to complete rest for several months; and I shall not be able to pick up my active life before the end of the year. My lecture tour, which I did not want to give up, and which, moreover, was salutary for my morale in distracting me from my sad thoughts, also made me excessively tired and I now have to spend time recovering. This time I don't want to overlook anything, to avoid the disastrous consequences of my previous pregnancy. You will certainly understand, dear Madam, why I wish that the news of this event spread as little as possible. Adversaries of the theories that are so dear to me will doubtlessly see in [my pregnancy] a subject of mockery and triumph.[47]

Roussel's pregnancy and fears of the future continued to weigh on her, but the memory of her tour renewed and sustained her sense of self. Two weeks after her return, she wrote exuberantly about her experiences in *L'Action*. Her portrayal reveals how she saw herself and how she wished to be viewed by others: as a Christlike missionary bringing the "truth" that would set women free to backward regions of France. She found the women of the Midi more oppressed than in any other part of the country and simultaneously felt "pride and a sadness that no one had yet gone there to make the cry [of revolt] heard." The farther south one went, she wrote, the more "oriental" the mores:

> the antiquated and pernicious separation of the sexes is practiced on a vast scale, with deplorable obstinacy. Women are relegated to the home, closed in a narrow and dreary circle of domestic occupations. The men pass almost every hour of their leisure at cafés; and the few who, on Sundays, prefer to go out with their families instead of drinking, expose themselves to the mockery and reproach of the others. Rare are the households where there is a communion of spirit—a moral intimacy, a mutual and profound trust, a warm and enveloping tenderness—which provides valiant support for life's hardest burdens.

The local freethinkers, Roussel continued, complained about their wives' churchgoing, not understanding that the Church offered women their only source of sociability, since they had no access to other public spaces. (Realizing the importance of this point, she incorporated it into subsequent lectures and later wrote a play about the subject.) She was proud of being a confessor to the women she met and exclaimed: "if all these husbands knew all the secrets and complaints I received. Everywhere, I had the profound joy of seeing the faces of these unhappy women, resigned [to their condition], light up when for the first time in their lives they heard a voice rise to defend and glorify them."[48]

Roussel wrote ten more articles on feminism that summer, the last of which appeared the day she went into labor. She published most of them in *L'Action,* but she also wrote for Gabrielle Petit's feminist-socialist newspaper *La Femme affranchie* and for the newspaper to which Darnaud contributed, *Les Annales de l'Ariège.* One of the articles she wrote for *L'Action* praised Darnaud's Feminist Committee of Roquefixade for its efforts at self-education, combating clericalism, and educating peasants, as well as for being both "vast" and practical in its goals. She hoped that such groups would multiply throughout France and inform *L'Action* of their existence.[49] Darnaud, meanwhile, having read accounts of her performances during her tour was quite beside himself with admiration, and he wrote to her saying that she was "the youngest and most eloquent of French feminists," an "apostle" who "electrified" both her auditors and readers. He said that although he had long considered himself a feminist, he had had doubts about the "delicate question of *liberté de maternité*," but that her article "Aux femmes" in *La Femme affranchie* (August 1904) had changed his mind.[50]

Roussel devoted much of the summer to leisure; she spent afternoons with her mother and Mireille in their garden, took walks in the forest of Vincennes, and received visits from friends and family. She also undertook careful preparations for the birth of her baby. In early June, she went with her mother on her first visit to Dr. Lucas in his "Anesthesiology Establishment" in Passy, in the wealthy sixteenth arrondissement of Paris, and she made at least four subsequent visits in the company of her mother and Henri. Nelly had chosen Dr. Lucas with great deliberation, for he had made a medical discovery that was supposed to significantly reduce the pain of childbirth and its damaging effects. She also prepared for her baby's postpartum care. At the end of August, Nelly, her mother, and Henri visited the *pouponnière* of Porchefontaine in Versailles.[51] Unlike a *crèche,* or day nursery, a *pouponnière* was a "home" for children under three years of age, where they lived both day and night.

At 9:30 a.m. on September 9, 1904, Nelly arrived with her mother at the Anesthesiology Establishment, and her sister Andreé arrived later to spend the afternoon with her. The following day, her mother and Henri visited. Regular and "serious" labor pains began at 4:00 p.m. Dr. Lucas arrived at 7:00, and Nelly entered the delivery room at 8:00. Marcel was born at 10:00 p.m. This time, Nelly was spared the experiences of her previous two deliveries. Inspired by the former Sorbonne professor of physiology, freethinker, and minister of education Paul Bert (1833–1886), Dr. Lucas had learned to produce "all the degrees of anesthesia, from the light intoxication analogous to champagne to the complete sleep that resembles death," using a mixture of compressed air and nitrous oxide. Because its strength, and thus its side effects, could be regulated so easily, this mixture resolved the previously insoluble problem of possible paralysis. Rather than constraining the natural labor of parturition—the danger of other anesthetics—it actually accelerated it.[52] In fact, the use of nitrous oxide was not new, though perhaps Lucas's particular mixture was. Nitrous oxide numbered among several gases and combinations of gases that had been in use to ease the pain of childbirth since about the middle of the nineteenth century. But the French medical profession as a whole frowned on the use of anesthesia in childbirth and so did not train physicians to use it in that manner; those who did wish to use it were left, as was Dr. Lucas, to their own experimentation. An enigmatic statement six years later suggests that these methods were not entirely safe: "Yes, it really is our Dr. Lucas who died," Henri said after reading the newspaper, "after having killed many women, it seems."[53]

But in 1904, Dr. Lucas, mercifully, killed only Nelly's pain and rescued her from her fears of childbirth; neither mother nor son suffered any ill effects from the procedure. The day after Marcel was born, Nelly received visits from friends and family, including Mireille. Yet it took more than a week for her to get out of bed to eat, and she remained in the establishment for two weeks after the birth. Dr. Lucas did not charge Nelly for his services, because of her "financial situation," which was not the best, since Henri had not succeeded in selling his sculptures. Instead of a monetary payment, he asked that Roussel publicize his method, which she did by writing an article about it a month later.[54]

The day following Marcel's birth, Henri, accompanied by their maid Louise, took him to the Pouponnière de Porchefontaine. Seven weeks passed before Nelly first visited her son. Such behavior might shock modern sensibilities, but in fact Roussel was only doing what had been common in her mother's generation, when women of all social classes put their children out to wet nurses. Working-class women sent their infants to wet nurses in the countryside, where they had no contact with them for a year or two, while bourgeois women hired wet nurses to come into their homes. By the end of the nineteenth century, however, only about 10 percent of mothers—primarily of the working classes—sent their children out to nurse. Wet-nursing was declining in part because pasteurization had made bottle-feeding more sanitary, and hence safer.[55] Indeed, the *pouponnière* was an institutionalized replacement of traditional wet-nursing, a "social work" dedicated to lowering infant mortality. The *pouponnière* served the double purpose of instructing mothers in "order and devotion" and in raising infants. One supporter claimed that the infant mortality rate in the *pouponnière* of Porchefontaine was below 4 percent, while the general rate was 14 percent. This institution also instructed unmarried mothers about how to feed their children and how to be housewives, so that they would be marriageable.[56] Roussel, of course, did not receive instruction in motherhood and housekeeping, but at least she was assured that Marcel would receive good care and be spared the fate of her previous son.

The medical profession as a whole increasingly insisted on the benefits of maternal breast-feeding to reduce infant mortality. Anne-Marie Sohn concludes on the basis of judicial records that, by the end of the nineteenth century, public opinion had begun "to associate breast-feeding and love, castigating the mother who was heartless enough to escape this natural function."[57] As already noted, maternal breast-feeding became an issue among feminists as well. For many of the contributors to *La Fronde,* and for many other "maternalist" feminists as well, breast-feeding was an integral part of a mother's duties.[58] But as Rachel Fuchs has pointed out, complex factors determined parents' choices regarding infant care. Placing babies outside the home did not necessarily indicate lack of maternal affection. Some mothers relied on wet nurses because they had to work, but others did so for reasons of maternal and infant health. Even in this period, some doctors still advised patients to send children out to nurse for the sake of both mother and infant, and Roussel may have been advised accordingly. Given her sensibilities, it is unlikely that she had breast-fed Mireille, and her own poor health had surely prevented her from breast-feeding the ill-fated André. Despite public opinion and the persistent propaganda about breast-feeding, private, practical concerns prevailed among a critical mass of women. Bottle-feeding "triumphed" in the first five years of the twentieth century, but wet-nursing continued in France until World War I.[59] Sending Marcel to the *pouponnière* probably did not shock Roussel's contemporaries, and no evidence indicates that anyone in her family or circle of friends was in the least concerned about it. That Louise Nel and Henri accompanied Nelly on preliminary visits to Porchefontaine suggests that her family fully supported her as well, particularly given their awareness of the suffering she had endured with André.

Despite Roussel's long stay in Dr. Lucas's Anesthesiology Establishment, she resumed work in no time; she contributed an article to *L'Action* just five days after

Marcel's birth. Less than a month later, *L'Action* published her article about the unnamed Dr. Lucas, "Un Bienfaiteur de l'humanité" (A Benefactor of Humanity), fulfilling her debt to him. She gave no hint that she herself had experienced this doctor's method; she only said that "we" had visited his establishment, which allowed her to describe it in detail. She explained that his anesthetic not only eliminated pain but would do away with "the terrible apprehension of future births in the mother who had already been subjected to the indescribable torture [of childbirth]." She hoped that "proletarian mothers, poor workers, abandoned girls, all women who were . . . victims of nature's cruelties as well as Society's injustices," could benefit from this method. She then suggested a reason beyond modesty for this young doctor to conceal his identity: he had no illusions about those who would oppose him, the "blind defenders of dogmas . . . the fanatics who saw in Motherhood the fatal and necessary chastening for this stain of profane love, those faithful to the Bible, which said to woman, 'You will give birth in pain.'" She reiterated her attack on freethinkers for whom nature had become a "divinity" and ended her article with an invocation of Robin's doctrines.[60] Dr. Lucas's insistence on anonymity in Roussel's article, the facts that he did not charge them for his services and that his method did not spread, and Godet's later comment that Lucas had "killed many women" suggest that his anesthetic was experimental and dangerous.

Roussel's positive experience gave her another platform on which to militate against female pain. Nonetheless, it caused further embarrassment in a particularly ironic manner. In September 1904, just after Marcel was born, Roussel's fervent admirer Émile Darnaud—still not having met her in person—wrote an article that he intended to publish in the *Annales de l'Ariège*, entitled "Maternity." He began with a description of Godet's recently completed mother-daughter bust: "The head of the little girl is graciously tilted on the shoulder of the young mama, whose face is of a sculptural beauty." But then Darnaud continued into sensitive and compromising terrain, demonstrating not only his persistent reluctance to embrace Roussel's "freedom of motherhood" doctrine but his ignorance of her true situation:

> Madam Nelly Roussel, not content to have her Mireille, desired a big boy, who arrived on September 10. And he was already well on the way on May 15, when she gave a most eloquent lecture on freedom of motherhood in Lyon. [Was it not her right, when] she was going to have a second child, without herself, dreading misery, to cry out: Woman must only be a mother when she wants to be, and she must only want it with circumspection.

But if it is just and good that a woman abstain from bringing children into the world who are inevitably doomed to unhappiness, should not we fear that she will abuse the freedom of motherhood solely to avoid the pains of childbirth? To this question, science responds by suppressing the pain.[61]

Darnaud then described the process Roussel had undergone with Dr. Lucas, summarizing the article she had just published on the subject. His message was that the "science" Roussel advocated in the birthing process would abolish the fear of childbirth, as well as the reason women might have for not wanting children, thereby making birth control unnecessary. Not only did he completely miss the broader context of Roussel's discourse about reproductive rights, but he imputed to her an attitude about her own pregnancy exactly the opposite of what she felt, with regard both to the dread of having another child and the political shame she felt over her compromised position. Fortunately, Darnaud sent her the manuscript prior to its publication, and Roussel reacted quickly and firmly by insisting that he pull it from the newspaper.

But Darnaud had not waited to receive Roussel's response before giving his article to the *Annales de l'Ariège*, which in turn had already sent it to the printer. Roussel took this matter so seriously that Darnaud, in Roquefixade at the time, had to prevail upon a worker to rush a letter to Foix instructing the printer to suppress the article. Mistaken as he was about Roussel, she carefully avoided revealing her true self to Darnaud. She told him that he had erred in saying that she wanted a "second" child, because in fact Marcel was her third; she allowed him to believe that she wanted the article withdrawn because of that mistake. Darnaud apologized, "The error which you attribute to [the reference to] the *second* child, instead of the *third*, had the merit of proving that the article was spontaneously written by a stranger to your family," and obviously, to Roussel herself.[62] Of course, he could interpret her pain over the loss of the second child as he wished, but he would never understand her embarrassment at having become pregnant with a very much unwanted third child and, to be sure, her desire to escape childbearing, regardless of its pains, just as he feared women might want to do.

By the middle of October, Roussel resumed holding her "reception day," giving diction lessons, and attending meetings of the Union fraternelle des femmes, where she collaborated in writing a "feminist almanac," whose purpose was to introduce feminism to those who knew nothing about it, in the form of small, inexpensive brochures.[63] She contributed numerous articles to *L'Action* and other newspapers. On October 29, the day before she saw her seven-week-old son for the first time since his birth, Roussel delivered her first lecture since the previous

May. She spoke about an issue of profound importance for feminists—the Napoleonic Code—whose one-hundredth anniversary was being celebrated. Before an audience of a thousand at the lecture hall of the Sociétés savantes, she joined Marguerite Durand, Odette Laguerre, Gabrielle Petit, and Alexandra Myrial in condemning the Code and its centenary celebrations. Roussel in particular targeted article 213 of the Code, which stipulated that a woman must obey her husband. This meeting was summarized in several newspapers, and the summaries were in turn reproduced in several others. *L'Action* also published Roussel's speech.[64] During the five subsequent months, she delivered eight public speeches, including an address at the annual *Noël humaine* sponsored by *L'Action*, the secular version of a Christmas banquet celebrated by freethinkers. She also spoke at the funeral of her heroine Louise Michel and for the first time delivered her most comprehensive lecture, "L'Éternelle sacrifiée" ("She Who is Always Sacrificed") in Paris, on January 18, 1905, to the League of the Rights of Man, and again to an audience of 2,000 in Châlons (Marne) in early March.[65]

This lecture, her longest and most general, combined all the subjects on which Roussel had previously spoken and that she believed to be central to feminism: women's place in the capitalist economy, the Napoleonic Code, motherhood, marriage, education, and the hypocrisy of freethinkers and Freemasons for chastising women's religious devotion while they denied them the very associations that could offer an alternative to the Church. The title itself provided the unifying theme of her feminism: the pain and humiliation to which nature and, more important, its accomplices, society and the Church, subjected women. She delivered this lecture thirty-five times in 1905. Her presentations in Paris and Châlons rehearsed the provincial tour she would begin in April.

Cultivating the "Wastelands": The Spring Tour, 1905

On April 7, 1905, Roussel took the train from Paris to the somber working-class town of Firminy (Loire) in the highly industrialized Stephanois Valley. It was a less aesthetically pleasing start to her tour than the previous one, with cold, humid weather and a small, primitive, dimly lit hotel room. But she proudly wrote to Henri that the *camarades* who met her at the train station, "say 'Nelly' the way they say 'Louise' [Michel] and 'Sébastian' [Faure]," thus comparing herself with two revolutionaries far more famous than she was. At the end of this letter, she added a revealing personal note: her pen, running out of ink, was, she said, "almost as dry as the heart of physician 'torturers,'" who believed that pain and sacrifice were natural to womanhood. In ink that is even more difficult to decipher today, Nelly added at the end: "here is a precious hand-written letter, which will fade quickly, I fear; and will be missing from the 'Intimate correspondence of Nelly Roussel' published after my death."[66]

Despite her self-conscious celebrity, Roussel seems to have been less self-absorbed on this tour than on the previous one, more accustomed to being in the limelight in unfamiliar places, and less fazed by the vagaries of audiences. Although the weather remained very bad throughout most of her tour, she keenly took in the details of her changing environments, both geographical and human, and became ever more convinced of, and dedicated to, the need to bring her message to the "ignorant masses." She did, however, continue to be acutely concerned about her success—or lack thereof. Her lecture at Firminy, in her view, was a "fiasco," for only a hundred people attended. The young and inexperienced organizers were "stupefied" and deeply apologetic, attributing the small attendance to poor publicity and late preparation. She was nonetheless satisfied with her own performance, and they paid her more than the going rate for her lecture and begged her to return.[67]

The next talk was scheduled for Le Puy, a town in the hills above the Stéphanois valley. So reactionary was this area that the organizers—"The Lay and Republican Youth of Velay"—felt that they could not even display posters advertising her talk. Nor did it calm her nerves to be told that she would be the first woman speaker ever to appear there, and that audiences in Le Puy sometimes emitted "animal cries." But even in these circumstances, she was a success: the hall overflowed with more than a thousand people, and *L'Action républicaine* of the Haute-Loire reported that during the two hours of her lecture "the entire audience hung on her every word." When she stopped, she became "almost timid while the electrified hall gave her an unforgettable ovation." She then "tirelessly mounted the stage again, and there the magnificent, tragic, radiance of a superhuman beauty began to perform for us the magnificent . . . *Par la révolte,* with a voice into which she put her entire heart and soul."[68] Roussel then went to the textile town of Bourg-Argental (Loire) in the Vivarais mountains, where she again learned that her lecture had been poorly advertised because of the conservative political climate. But once again she drew a huge working-class crowd that spilled into the hallways. *La Tribune* of Saint-Étienne noted how pleased the audience was, and especially the women, whose large numbers were unprecedented. They, especially, "went home very moved and strongly impressed."[69]

Roussel had reason to take pride in her courage in traveling alone into provincial France and establishing meaningful contact with working-class men and women. Her devotion to the cause made it easier for her to repress many of her bourgeois sensibilities, to stay in uncomfortable hotels, and to spend much of her time with men, and to a far lesser extent women, who came from backgrounds distinctly different from her own. They spoke a "rougher" language, suffered material conditions unfamiliar to her, and were immersed in local cultures she could only have imagined with great difficulty prior to encountering them. Whereas in Béziers it had been "gentlemen" who had orchestrated her tour, in St. Vallier (Drôme), they were "comrades," among whom she found some really "worth knowing" and "quite amusing" but others quite "vulgar." There she stayed in a village inn, where she had a "primitive little room, cold and dark" and the weather was "ugly, humid and gray, which has nothing joyful." "Ah!" she remarked to Henri, " It is necessary to suffer for the Idea." In Olarques, high in the mountains of the Hérault, Roussel spoke in a "shed," and the locals asked how a woman could ever have gotten the idea of coming to their village to lecture. She recounted to Henri, "You can imagine how I disrupted this savage population. . . . Oh, my friend! It is in traveling thus that one understands the immensity of the work to be accomplished . . . that this terrain is still an absolute wasteland and needs to be cultivated! . . . but what is consoling and admirable is that in the most remote and most primitive corners, one finds active and courageous militants who try to shake the apathy and indifference of these ignorant crowds."[70]

After Bourg-Argental, Roussel traveled on to Grigny and Oullins (Rhône), and then finally Lyon, where she felt quite happy spending four days in a "civilized" place with a hotel room that even had electric lighting, a not so common luxury. From there she traveled on to twenty-four other villages, towns, and cities across eleven departments—the Isère, Drôme, Vaucluse, Alpes-Maritimes, Hérault, Ariège, Gironde, Charente, Maine-et-Loire, Indre-et-Loire, and Loir-et-Cher (map 2). She looked forward with some nervousness to her return to Béziers, her first venue the previous year, because she wondered whether she could live up to the reputation she had already created. Her lecture there took place in another unusual setting, the seat of a local wine cooperative, an immense, poorly lit warehouse lined with wine barrels, in which 1,000 to 1,200 peasants—half the population—"squeezed together, standing, sitting, clambering on top of the enormous barrels." This "unsophisticated" audience, which included many children, was easily distracted; but as usual the teaching personnel seemed very interested.[71]

One highlight of this tour, at least for Émile Darnaud, is that after much doubt on his part, he had been able to arrange a lecture in his hometown of Foix and, alas, he finally met Nelly. His observations about her lecture and reactions to it lend an important perspective to her impact on audiences. In the months prior to the tour, Darnaud fretted endlessly over finding a venue, as well as an organizer, an effort that was fraught with tensions associated with both local politics and his own domestic relations. Looking forward to "intimate conversations" with Nelly and Henri (who was with her for this portion of the trip), he was chagrined to learn that his wife, who while tolerating his freethinking politics, nonetheless "silently condemned them." She would not permit him to receive Roussel and Godet "under her roof." Perhaps she was also tired of her husband's attentions to younger women. Darnaud worried as well about Roussel presenting the same lecture that she had given in Nice, and asked her not to speak about freedom of motherhood, because he thought the population of Foix would have no "taste" for it.

To Darnaud's great relief, all went smoothly and her presentation of "L'Éternelle Sacrifiée"—in which she did indeed discuss freedom of motherhood—was an enormous success. The next day he shared three observations, inspired by his knowledge of Gustave Le Bon's theory of crowd behavior: (1) the audience, composed of "disparate elements," had been "transformed into one, hypnotized by the orator, so that it constituted 'a crowd,' applauding the ideas suggested to it"; (2) Roussel was able to accomplish this feat because of her prestige and because she possessed the rare faculty of fascinating her audiences; and (3) she won over her audience, not because of her eloquent delivery or what was physically, morally, and intellectually "seductive" about her, but because her convictions were so sincere that she "sacrifices her entire being in order to propagate them." Darnaud's reading of Le Bon led him to think that her impact would be ephemeral, and that the day after her lecture, members of the audience would return to their individual habits of thought and their individual, inconsequential interpretations of Nelly Roussel—and they would then soon forget her.[72]

But three weeks later, Darnaud wrote to Nelly again in a state of disbelief over the growing—rather than diminishing—effects of her lecture; it was "increasingly the subject of every conversation." What surprised him most was the impact she had had on "young ladies," who now, he said, constantly alluded to freedom of motherhood. He apologized for having tried to divert her from the topic. Even his wife, having heard her lecture "celebrated" so much by friends she respected, would eventually, he thought, accept Roussel's ideas. "*Régénération* doesn't produce any effect, even on women. It requires your dignity, your conviction, your delicateness, all your talent, as gracious and pleasing as it is ardent and logical, to speak effectively about the *liberté de maternite*."[73]

Despite the hardship and fatigue, Nelly thoroughly enjoyed this tour and had success with every lecture, selling somewhere between three and four hundred copies of *Par la révolte*. On only two or three occasions did she express disappointment at a poor turnout, resulting from the ineptness of the local organizers, from which she again learned the importance of timely advertising with prominent posters.[74] Otherwise, she relished her good health and loved being in the limelight. She missed Henri, and her letters are filled with deep affection for him; unlike the previous year, she mentioned Mireille more frequently and with greater affection, often ending her letters with instructions to kiss her. She only mentioned Marcel once after having received news of him: she expressed happiness at his weight gain and asked Henri whether he would be visiting the baby again soon. Henri, on the other hand, mentioned the children in almost every letter, even though he saw little of Marcel, and Mireille continued to live with Louise Nel and Antonin Montupet.

Visits with family and friends provided a welcome respite during Roussel's tour. She stayed with Odette Laguerre in her house outside of Lyon, and at Henri's suggestion, her mother (*petite mère*), Montupet, and Mireille spent a Sunday with Nelly in Valence. Mireille, to whom Nelly referred as her "little cabbage," "little wild rose," and "little queen," blushed with excitement when she saw her mother at the train station, and Nelly took pride in showing her off to the owner of the café-hotel in which she was staying. She once again visited with her grandfather in his elegant villa apartment in Monaco. He attended her lecture in Nice, where she delivered "Liberté de maternité," and again delighted Nelly with his enthusiastic reaction: the "scientific side of the question above all seduced him," and he found her performance superior even to that of the previous year.[75] But what she looked forward to most was Henri's visit, and with each day, her impatience grew as his itinerary and timing remained unclear. Henri went to Marseilles to try, most unsuccessfully, to sell his sculptures. From Béziers, she wrote that her hotel room, the same one she had had the previous year, looked "even prettier because she would be receiving him there." She was rejoicing, not just in the prospect of seeing him, but in showing him off to her friends there. "And this will not be an ordinary spectacle," she wrote: "the phenomenon exhibiting her barnum!!"[76]

Roussel had much to be grateful to Henri for: as during her first tour, throughout this trip, he provided numerous support services, again performing as her "Barnum," only more so, because the 1905 tour had a longer and more complicated itinerary and posed more challenges with regard to publicity. The details of her lectures—time, place, and who would preside—often fell into place only at the last minute, but he made posters to advertise her talks and sent them to the appropriate destinations so that they could be put up in advance. He also advised her about which lecture to give at each location.[77] Both he and Nelly exercised a firm hand in the publicity for her talks, insisting that the announcements in newspapers, posters, and leaflets describe her talent. Meanwhile, at Godet's constant prompting, *L'Action* published summaries of her lectures and glowing accounts of their success. They also published her speaking schedule and invited other groups to take advantage of Roussel's passage through the region by inviting her to give a lecture, further complicating Henri's task.[78]

Just as Nelly was self-consciously shaping her image as a talented public speaker, Henri and others began to create a counterimage that stressed her role as wife and mother, casting her feminism as "relational." When Odette Laguerre introduced her lectures in Grigny, Oullins, and in Lyon, she presented Roussel as the wife of Henri Godet and mother of Mireille, and told stories about Mireille (which Roussel found charming). The secretary of the Free Thinking group of Grigny wrote to *L'Action* that Odette Laguerre "presented the citizenness Nelly Roussel to us as the model of feminine moral perfection."[79] An article about her Lyon lecture by "Marianne" in *L'Idée socialiste de Lyon,* made a point of talking about her husband as a socialist and feminist who would accompany his wife on the second part of her tour: "Nothing is more charming than this young household, unified by a complete community of ideas." As a family they evoked "better times, a future time, when the woman, at last emancipated . . . will really become the companion of the man and his associate in the work of human progress."[80] Émile Darnaud contributed to this image in his prolific letter-writing; he constantly viewed Roussel in relation to her children and her husband and extolled her motherhood—even though he never witnessed it firsthand.

The importance of Roussel's image as a "legitimate" woman became clearer to her in Montpellier, where her hostess, Mlle Ruben (a friend of Henri's) told everyone who asked that Nelly was married to "the most charming man in the world." Mlle Ruben did so because the Montpelliérains were very worried about Roussel's morality and wanted to know if she was an "honest woman." "They are astonished," Nelly said, "that an 'honest woman' can say things that are so brazen." Emmanuel Lévy, a distinguished law professor at the University of Lyon, known as a champion of the proletariat, chaired the meeting at which her lecture took place, but he was "dreadfully scared." Prior to her performance, he begged her "not to go too far, not to compromise him, not to risk the critiques of adversaries." His pleas did not deter her, however, and Roussel's lecture received the usual lively applause from the audience of 1,200. Afterward, Levy congratulated her, but he also confessed that he did not share her ideas and had to disengage himself from any responsibility for the evening's event.[81]

From this point on, Roussel and Godet would make motherhood a more prominent part of her public image. Having escaped from motherhood and its pains, she learned, especially on this tour, that with many audiences it would be strategically advantageous to incorporate a maternal image into her public persona, because doing so gave her more appeal and legitimacy. She also more clearly grasped the disruptive power of her doctrine. If working-class audiences flocked to her lectures in order to see the spectacle of a woman speaking publicly, they departed as changed individuals. Her lectures provoked not only debates in the press but debates between local men and women of all social classes. It is not surprising, then, that opposition to her came from all directions and grew more serious.

CHAPTER FOUR

The Public and Private Politics of Female Self-Sacrifice

Audience Reception

And I shall see you again today, Nelly Roussel, your uncanny face in the shadow of your large hat, flapping like the wings of a bird taking flight—you invoke for me the superb "Strong Virgin" and the almighty "Loose Woman," the integrated, and suggestive, and energetic, and nonetheless gentle "Future Eve."

Lucien Ledont, "Une Conférence de Nelly Roussel au cirque" (1905)

On a Saturday evening, January 20, 1906, 400 people crammed into the overflowing Maison du Peuple hall in Caen (Calvados). The city's residents had never before seen a female speaker, let alone heard a lecture on feminism. Nelly Roussel was supposed to appear at 8:30 p.m., but she walked in forty-five minutes late, which proved to at least one observer that "even as a feminist, she remained a woman." He considered her timing "charming coquettishness" that lent more force to her argument. When she finally entered the hall, the crowd burst into applause. Draped in a velvet black dress that accentuated her pale skin and jet-black hair, the speaker looked small and frail (fig. 10). But as she boldly mounted the stage, Roussel suddenly became larger than life. From the shadow of her broad-brimmed hat emerged a face whose pallor was compared with the "white petal of a camellia." Self-composed before her restless listeners, she began in a soft voice, measured and articulate, that brought her audience to complete silence: "Gentlemen, Ladies, dear Comrades: if there is a universal question par excellence, a question that interests . . . not only all women of all classes and of all countries, but all human beings . . . it is the question we are going to discuss tonight—equality between the sexes." As she continued, her voice grew louder and her gestures more dramatic; her entire body trembled with the conviction of her message. Her black eyes appeared as "sparks bursting forth from a fireplace burning with thought." Like the thick black velvet atop her translucent skin, Roussel embodied contrast, if not contradiction. Her voice filled huge rooms with the timbre of "vibrating crystal." Her feminine toying with the gold chain around her delicate throat nonetheless seemed to clash with the logical rigor of her words and the "male vigor" with which she spoke them. Defying categorization, Roussel always evoked opposites—logic/poetry, reason/passion, frailty/strength, paleness/flame, charm/audacity, beauty/virago.[1] Lucien Ledont, who saw Roussel as a new Eve who combined the qualities of Jean d'Arc (saint) and sinner, needed those opposites to define her. Much taken with her lecture, this assistant master at a private high school in Châlons said that thanks to her, feminist theories would no longer cause smiles or mockery from "imbeciles."

Roussel did not provoke very much mockery, but she did evoke considerable reaction everywhere she went. Journalists' amazement at the conviction with which she spoke reflected their presumption that publicly defending one's word was incompatible with femininity; for in the eyes of many, women were by nature dissimulating and could not be held accountable for what they said.[2] The charm of her personality, her anticipation of objections, her deft responses, and her artful wit left even those who opposed her uncertain about whether they should consider themselves her enemies or her seduced admirers. "If the arrows that she directs . . . at our politicians in particular and at men in general are often very sharp and very hard, they are launched with such tact, so much art, and such good grace that we, those of us of the strong sex, can only applaud, and applaud with both hands," one journalist wrote, expressing a sentiment that was repeated by numerous others.[3]

Men and women flocked to Roussel's lectures because—as a dynamic female speaker—she provided spectacular entertainment. She even earned an entry under the category "amusements" in a popular American travel book, *A Woman's Guide to Paris,* which urged its readers to make a point of attending one of her lectures.[4] But beyond the impact Nelly Roussel had as a visual spectacle and auditory marvel, what did those who heard or read her words understand? Audience reception is exceedingly difficult to gage. This chapter analyzes more closely the positive and negative reactions among both her public and private audiences. As noted in Chapter 3, recipients of Roussel's message were highly diverse, both in Paris and in the provinces. In the former, depending on the venue and organizers, her audiences consisted of bourgeois feminists, freethinkers, neo-Malthusians, anarchists, and syndicalists. The provinces yielded audiences of working-class and lower-middle-class men and women. Schoolteachers especially sought her out. Because freethinkers sponsored most of her talks, they likewise attended her lectures and read her articles in the nationally distributed *L'Action*.

Although Roussel honed each lecture according to the composition of her audience, the underlying goal in all of them was to uproot the deeply embedded cultural assumption that pain constituted a natural element of womanhood, a religious notion that was undergoing a secular rebirth in the Third Republic. The concept of womanhood among most men of the Left, especially in the provinces, differed little from that of the Church: nature, rather than God, had created women's unchanging essence, which included irrationality and self-sacrifice. The concept of self-sacrifice became the foundation for literary "ideal types" and "intuitive abstractions" that survived through the twentieth century.[5] At this, the apex of her career, Roussel brought her battle against assumptions about female pain to the forefront in "L'Éternelle sacrifiée" (She Who Is Always Sacrificed). The title itself drew on the image already lodged in the French imaginary of self-sacrificing womanhood. Here *sacrifiée* substituted for the *féminin* in *l'éternel féminin*, placing female sacrifice itself above historical change. Eve's sin condemned women to perpetual *self*-sacrifice. Unlike men, who redeemed themselves through action, women had no choice about the sacrifice they would make; they were born to endure pain as the passive receptacles of reproductive labor. Reactions to Roussel's efforts to break down these ideal types reveal how entrenched they were in both Catholic and secular imaginations.

Roussel delivered "L'Éternelle sacrifiée" on sixty-four occasions between 1905 and 1908. She also presented "Liberté de maternite" (Freedom of Motherhood) and the closely related "Beaucoup d'enfants?" (Many Children?) fourteen times, and "La Femme et la libre pensée" (Woman and Freethinking) twenty-nine times. Other lecture titles during this period included "Amour et maternité" (Love and Motherhood), "Amour fécond, amour stérile" (Fertile Love, Sterile Love), "Le Suffrage des femmes" (Women's Suffrage) and "Créons la citoyenne" (Let's Create the Female Citizen). Altogether during these four years, she delivered 122 lectures, 74 of which were in the provinces, and 57 of the latter were followed by a dramatic reading of her short play *Par la révolte*. She also delivered lectures in Switzerland, Belgium, and Hungary. As already noted, she sold from 25 to 150 copies of her play after each performance, providing another mode for spreading her message to those who did not see her. The play went through five editions and sold 3,964 copies from 1905 through 1907. When she first performed it at one of the popular universities in Paris in 1903, it was an immediate success.[6] But her twenty-minute reading of it following her lectures in the provinces particularly enhanced the power of her message among these entertainment-deprived and less educated audiences.

The single most important performance of *Par la révolte,* which took place in September, 1905 in conjunction with the International Congress of Freethinkers, offers a good starting point for systematically examining the reactions she provoked. As noted in Chapter 2, this play is an allegory, in which "Eve," enslaved and chained, faces her oppressors, "Society" and "The Church," and then succeeds in liberating herself when inspired by "Revolt." On this occasion, Henry Bérenger and his newspaper *L'Action* sponsored the play and staged it in the luxurious Sara Bernhardt theater. The International Congress of Freethinkers had drawn 20,000 participants from Europe and the United States, and 2,000 of them nearly filled the theater. Roussel played the role of Eve, accompanied by actresses from the Comédie-Française (fig. 7). Her audience included local and national dignitaries as municipal councilors and left-wing members of the Chamber of Deputies, as well as feminists, Freemasons, and freethinkers.

This gala production, and Roussel in particular, received the usual acclaim. A. B. de Liptay, having witnessed the performance, also read her "little masterpiece" with "the same joy that I reread Victor Hugo or Lamartine . . . the beauty of *Par la révolte* resides in the force of sentiment as well as in the grace of expression." Also having read it after witnessing the performance, Isabelle Gatti de Gamond felt herself "penetrated by the symbolism and the color." Roussel received requests, which she granted, to have the play translated into Russian and Portuguese. Victor Ragosine, writing to her in October 1905, had already translated it into Russian. Looking forward to the fall of "the Russian autocracy, the principal rampart of European reaction," he considered that her play would contribute to that effort, given the startling energy with which Russian women had just battled for the freedom and rights "of man and citizen" in their recent revolution. Three Portuguese wrote to request permission for translation, one of whom had witnessed Roussel's performance at the Sarah Bernhardt theater; she recounted how it had "fortified in me such a strong sentiment of indignation, it moved me to notice the cruelty, the bad faith, the indignity of the society in which women are always the victims." She believed that having a Portuguese translation of *Par la révolte* would make a difference, especially because it would make this important message accessible "to the four out of five million" in Portugal who could not read. Indeed, the play did touch the hearts of less educated women everywhere, including Paris, as shown by the letters Roussel received requesting more performances.[7]

Audiences found Roussel's lectures as compelling and entertaining as her play. Local newspaper reports convey important details, not only in the summaries they provide, but in descriptions of audience reaction—they often, for example, note points at which applause interrupted her. Roussel received just the sort of favorable responses for which she had hoped at the time when she had first envisioned her career: they came from women who felt voiceless and isolated. Her words appealed to schoolteachers who wanted to escape the Church's control; to women who felt physical and emotional pain as a result of motherhood, but had neither words to describe that pain nor an audience; to impoverished working-class mothers and, in particular, those who had been seduced and abandoned. Although some feminist organizations concerned themselves with women's work, none focused on issues of gender relations in private life the way Roussel did. She publicly articulated the private thoughts of "everywoman."

Liberating the Eternally Sacrificed Woman

In her effort to reach provincial working-class audiences, whose backgrounds were so unlike hers, Roussel manipulated language in three ways: she used familiar religious terms, symbols, and metaphors, even in an anticlerical message; she used the language of working-class militancy, casting women's plight in the familiar labor movement terms of justice and dignity; and she described women's universal experience of childbirth and the female body. She used familiar language to dislodge abstract assumptions in the public imagination.

Having once been devout herself, religious memories continued to influence Roussel even in her anticlerical, antireligious adulthood.[8] We have already seen her use of religious allegory and symbolism in *Par la révolte;* she and others construed her entire campaign in religious terms, with frequent use of words such as "apostle" and "mission." The use of Christian vocabulary—even Christian-like ritual—often appeared in the cultural practices even of those starkly opposed to the Church. Freethinkers followed the Christian calendar by acknowledging religious holidays irreverently, such as in eating pork on Good Friday and celebrating the *Noël humaine* on December 25, which even included its own kind of "communion." Such practices had deep roots in French culture. Christian eschatology created a "messianism" and the vision of a "Promised Land" among nineteenth-century workers.[9] Roussel's invocation of religious imagery similarly drew from a Christian eschatology that offered the promise of a new society, as well as shameful judgment on those who "sacrificed" women. In "Liberté de maternité," she said that motherhood should have the status of a priesthood and compared its stages—pregnancy, childbirth, convalescence, then "slavery" to an infant's ceaseless demands—to Christ's torture: "these are the painful, sometimes murderous stages, these are steps of Calvary that must be climbed slowly"—only to lead women into more self-sacrifice.[10]

Some of Roussel's listeners regarded her as a Christlike figure. After hearing "L'Eternelle sacrifiée" in Le Puy (Haute-Loire), a schoolteacher from a nearby village wrote to her: "I hung on your lips, I drank your words [as she might have drunk wine in the celebration of mass], worthy Apostle of feminism. Oh yes, 'apostle' is the word!—you have revealed an unknown landscape, such as those who preached the Christian Doctrine must have done. This flame, this sincere faith, your ardent facial expressions . . . bring new adherents to feminism." As one would have said of Christ, and of the mission at hand, she continued: "Oh, how good you are! . . . because you must possess an immense treasure of love for us [because you] courageously dare to affront a public that has always been hostile to our most worthy demands. Believe, Dear Citizenness, the ideas that you have developed with such great clarity have made a profound impression on me, which gives me the courage to take them up and propagate them." She then went on to complain of the "clerical ulcer, whose roots are so deep in the women" of her region.[11]

Roussel sought to reach beyond provincial schoolteachers. Few French feminists came from or ventured into the provinces, let alone spoke to workers. Most of them were urban and bourgeois. Roussel distinguished herself by making working-class women a priority in the effort to spread her message. It was among these women, especially in the provinces, that the birthrate remained high. She went out of her way to study working-class women's material conditions. In her spring 1905 tour, for example, she visited one of the factories in the textile town of Bourg-Argental (Loire), and she later recounted: "These factories employ almost only women; the work demands little muscular strength, but [it requires] close attention, meticulousness, and extraordinary vigilance; and the intolerable noise must make this job very painful for beginners. At this moment an entire enterprise is on strike. Many of the workers are, it seems, abandoned single mothers."[12] On another tour two years later, she visited a spinning mill in St. Hippoyte-du-Fort (Gard), where prior to her evening lecture, she saw her female audience at work. "The labor seems much less difficult than that of the weavers; but it is also much less lucrative. What man would consent to work twelve hours a day for only thirty-two sous?" She noted the warm, humid atmosphere of the mill, which, in the long run, she believed, would make the women "anemic." That same night she attended meetings of both the workers' syndicate and freethinkers, where her host, using a mill-related metaphor, introduced her as "unwinding the cocoon of her thought across France." From 1,200 to 1,500 people attended her lecture, and 200 had to stand outside without seats. It was the biggest crowd ever gathered in St. Hippolyte, "despite the efforts of clericals, Catholics and Protestants" to discourage attendance. And though the acoustics were terrible and her audience distracted, she was "appreciated, if not understood."[13]

The religious references in "L'Eternelle sacrifiée" appealed to provincial working-class women; just as significantly, Roussel addressed the issues of their material lives in a language of labor militancy already familiar to them, using a vocabulary that had helped fuel revolutionary movements in 1848 and 1871, as well as the syndicalist movement of her own epoch. During the nineteenth century, male workers had collectively made progress in establishing some dignity on the basis of their productive labor with regard to the rights to associate, to work, to bargain for higher wages, to strike, and to consume. Even unorganized workers demanded dignity in labor.[14] But since reproductive labor was private and unpaid, motherhood could not form any basis for association that could seek justice. Roussel applied the language of production to women's reproductive labor. In "L'Éternelle sacrifiée," she argued that maternal labor,

> just like any other form of labor, even more than other labor, [should] assure independence and well-being to those who accomplish it, but instead this work has never been anything but a cause of slavery and inferiority. Of all the social functions, the first, the most magnificent, the most laborious, is the only one that has never earned a salary! . . . The poorly paid worker refuses to work; the right to strike is no longer contested today. And we—*we women, we mothers—are the most poorly paid of all workers;* and there would be no *strike* more legitimate than ours.[15]

Roussel also emphasized the legal and personal power that motherhood denied women in their private lives, for they did not even have rights over their own children: "Married, your child will remain the *property of his father* . . . whose entire task is limited . . . to a few moments of pleasure." Like a proletarian, the woman had no right to the product of her labor. The civil code legally "alienated" her from her child by granting parental rights only to the father; and she, the mother, owed obedience to the father, her husband: "in marriage, annihilated as a woman, you are also annihilated as a *mother,*" she hammered into her audiences.[16] Single mothers, who suffered legal and economic situations far worse than those of their married sisters, composed a significant portion of her spectators. Addressing them with the familiar *tu,* as though she were one of them, Roussel said: "As an unwed mother . . . you alone will support the weight of what bourgeois hypocrisies contemptuously call your 'sin.'" Even the economic burden of supporting a child alone did not offer sufficient atonement: the single mother had to suffer the "physical torture of childbirth" as a "ransom for love," alone in her attic apartment, without help, without consolation.

Society only further chastised the unmarried mother in the form of abandonment, contempt, misery, and—perhaps most important of all—the "impossibility of rebuilding [for herself] a happy and free life,"—a goal some lower-class provincial women were beginning to envision and pursue.[17] Many single mothers were forced to make the "sad choice between *suicide* or *prostitution!*" Then there was infanticide. Roussel offered her empathy for this worst choice: "And if then, frantic, hopeless, weary of suffering, you do away with this little being whom you would have wanted so much to be able to love . . . [society] will find judges to send you to finish your miserable existence as a pariah on the straw mat of the prison cell." Thunderous applause interrupted her lecture at this point.[18]

Roussel began to deliver this lecture in the provinces during the spring of 1905 amid a wave of strikes that had begun the previous year. As labor disputes persisted in subsequent years, she presented it in many hard-hit departments, including the Loire, the Rhône, and the Isère (map 2). The number of strikes peaked in 1906, the year of a gas explosion in the mines of Courrières (Pas-de-Calais) that killed 1,300 miners. That April, she offered the proceeds from one of her lectures to the victims of that catastrophe. She also repeatedly visited the "proletarian peasants" of the Midi, who entered the working-class battles with unprecedented combativeness in 1907.[19]

Unlike schoolteachers, who had the writing skills and confidence, workers seldom wrote in response to her lectures. But they did speak to her afterward, and sometimes they sought her out in her hotel to seek "practical and precise" information about birth control.[20] When she delivered "L'Éternelle sacrifiée" in the working-class textile town of Bourg-Argental (Loire), which employed large concentrations of women, she recorded their reactions: "Everybody was talking about me [the day after the lecture], all the women in the region, especially in the silk-weaving factories. [These factories] are numerous and employ only women. All those who had not dared attend the lecture were terribly sorry and asked if "this lady" would come again another time. Even the women who support clericalism regretted their absence. And I am told that *Par la révolte* circulated from hand to hand." The male listeners, Roussel said, told her that when she had looked them in the eye during her lecture, they "felt ashamed and wished they could sink into the ground [*auraient voulu rentrer sous terre*]." Some of the women had cried, and "their seducers, also present, admitted responsibility for their actions."[21]

Roussel also used a language reflecting the experience of all women, regardless of class distinctions or religious belief. In "Liberté de maternité," as in "L'Éternelle

sacrifiée," she graphically described the ways in which repeated pregnancies ravaged women's bodies and marginalized them into real and metaphorical "attics"
of society. "Several times a mother," she said, identifying with her audience, "I
believe I am in a good position to speak logically about [the so-called 'joys' of
motherhood]. I must add that I do not rank among those who deserve the most
pity . . . I cannot recall the pain with which my joys were paid, without thinking
of all those who have even more pain, but infinitely less joy." She quoted a letter
from a woman who had responded to a prominent daily newspaper conducting a survey of its readers' opinions about large families. The correspondent's
mother had borne twelve children, and each birth had been horribly painful. But
that pain hardly marked the end of this mother's suffering. Of the twelve whom
she bore, four died as infants, and a fifth was killed in the Franco-Prussian War;
another "expired in his mother's arms at age thirty-three," invoking for some the
image of the Pietà. This mother, the letter continued, "following the fatigues of
labor and breast-feeding, saw her stomach degenerate; then rheumatism set in,
and she could not rest for atrocious neuralgia. Finally, she developed breast cancer—that horrible nursling—in the breast that had fed eight children. . . . After
a life of inexpressible physical martyrdom, and moral tortures that were even
more cruel . . . the death agony began, slowly and implacably," and she suffered
horribly until the very end.[22]

This letter offered Roussel's audiences graphic, authentic testimony about the
fecund motherhood that pronatalists wished to force upon Frenchwomen. She
noted that this particular woman could have come from any social class; but if
she were also impoverished, then (again invoking religious imagery) "there is
no Inquisition that could invent a more cruel torture for her punishment, nor
a religion that could imagine a worse hell, than this mother's existence! . . . the
chapter on maternal pain is endless."[23] Several women and men wrote to Roussel that this and other lectures provoked tears, even among the Paris elite. "Your
lecture made hearts beat," Blanche Cremnitz (a.k.a. Parrhisia), an associate of
Marguerite Durand's and member of the UFF, wrote. "You caused tears to fall,
at the same time pity for the victims you portrayed." They also noted the delicacy
with which she addressed these "forbidden" topics of private life.[24]

Regardless of her audience, whether Parisian or provincial, bourgeois or peasant, Roussel articulated pains with which women were intimately familiar, but
about which no one had ever spoken publicly. A recurrent theme in the letters
and reviews women wrote in response to her lectures was how she exposed what
"we mothers, we women have lived and suffered." Provincial women in particular
wrote that Roussel expressed "natural sentiments" that "all women feel," senti-

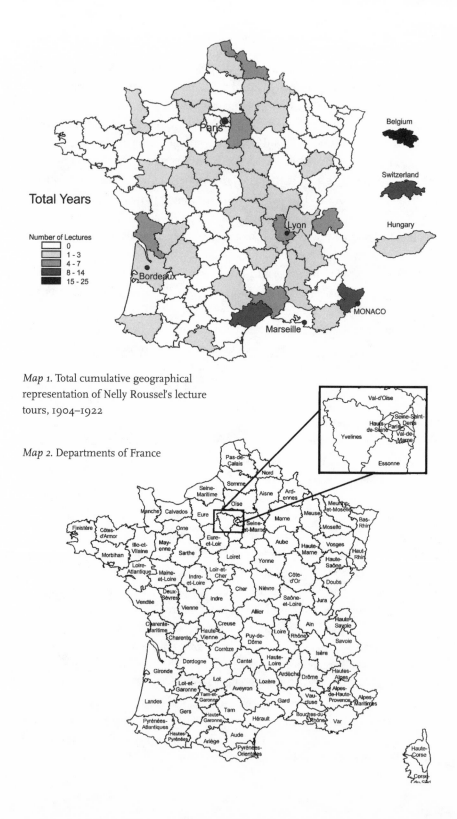

Map 1. Total cumulative geographical representation of Nelly Roussel's lecture tours, 1904–1922

Map 2. Departments of France

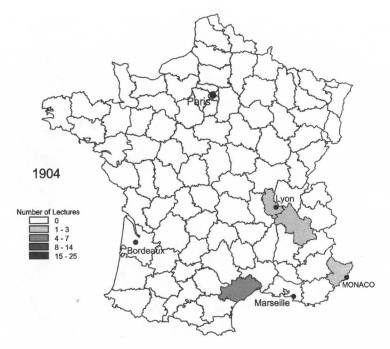

1904

Number of Lectures
- [ ] 0
- [ ] 1 - 3
- [ ] 4 - 7
- [ ] 8 - 14
- [ ] 15 - 25

Map 3. Geographical representation of
Nelly Roussel's lecture tour, 1904

Map 4. Cumulative geographical
representation Nelly Roussel's
lecture tours, 1904–1908

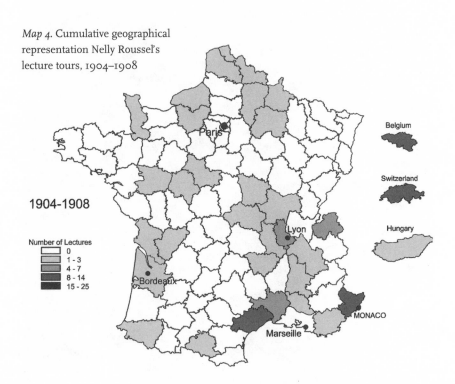

1904-1908

Number of Lectures
- [ ] 0
- [ ] 1 - 3
- [ ] 4 - 7
- [ ] 8 - 14
- [ ] 15 - 25

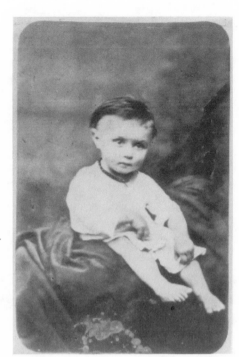

Figure 1. Nelly Roussel c. 1880.
Mairie de Paris–Bibliothèque
Marguerite Durand.

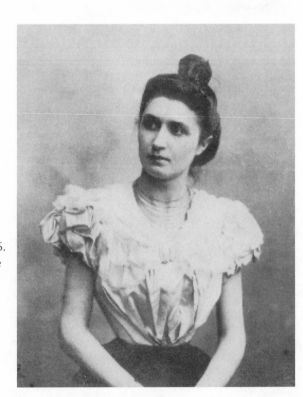

Figure 2. Nelly Roussel c. 1896.
Mairie de Paris–Bibliothèque
Marguerite Durand.

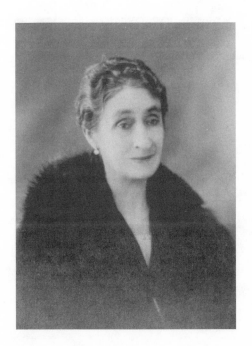

Figure 3. Nelly Roussel's mother,
Louise Nel. Mairie de Paris–
Bibliothèque Marguerite Durand.

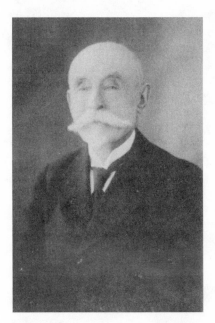

Figure 4. Nelly Roussel's stepfather,
Antonin Montupet. Mairie de Paris–
Bibliothèque Marguerite Durand.

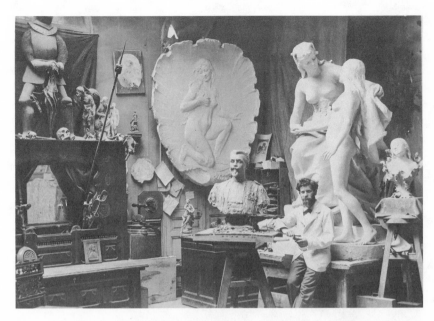

Figure 5. Henri Godet in his workshop c. 1904. Musée d'Orsay.

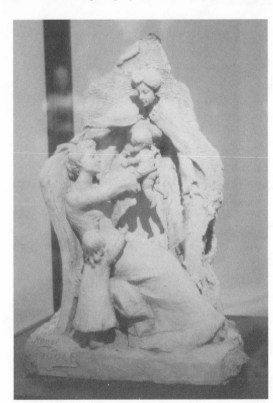

Figure 6. La Maternité by Henri Godet. Courtesy of Christiane Demeulenaere-Douyère.

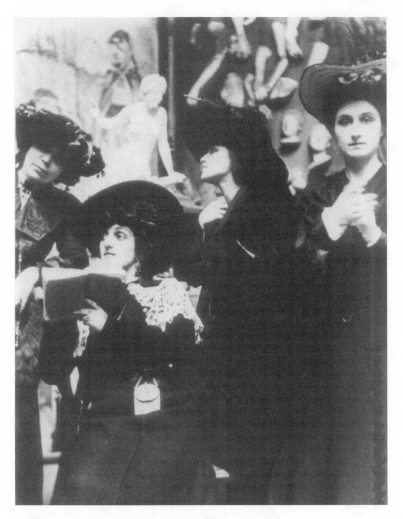

Figure 7. Actresses in *Par la révolte*. Mairie de Paris–
Bibliothèque Marguerite Durand.

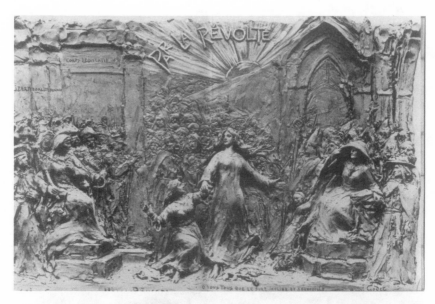

Figure 8. Bas-relief by Henri Godet illustrating Nelly Roussel's *Par la révolte,* inscribed: "All of you whose destiny is to be bowed down and kneeling, it is I alone who can break your chains." Mairie de Paris–Bibliothèque Marguerite Durand.

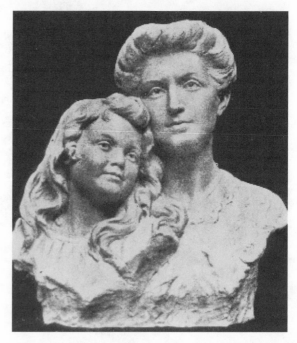

Figure 9. Bust of Nelly Roussel and her daughter Mireille Godet by Henri Godet, 1904. Mairie de Paris– Bibliothèque Marguerite Durand.

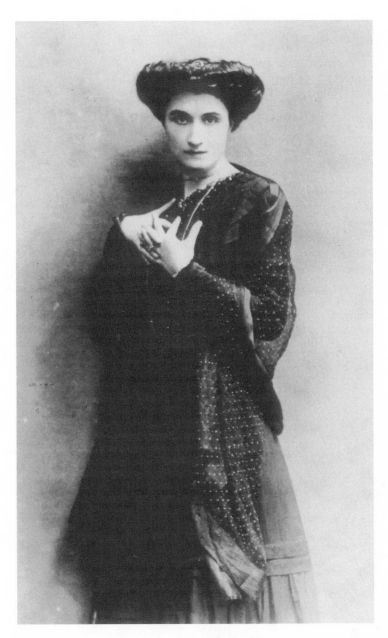

Figure 10. Nelly Roussel as a public lecturer, 1908. Mairie de Paris–Bibliothèque Marguerite Durand.

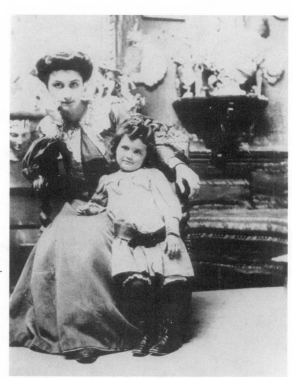

Figure 11. Nelly Roussel and her daughter Mireille Godet in Henri Godet's workshop, c. 1905. Mairie de Paris–Bibliothèque Marguerite Durand.

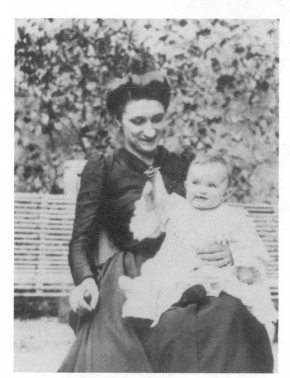

Figure 12. Nelly Roussel visiting her son Marcel Godet at the *pouponnière*, c. 1905. Mairie de Paris–Bibliothèque Marguerite Durand.

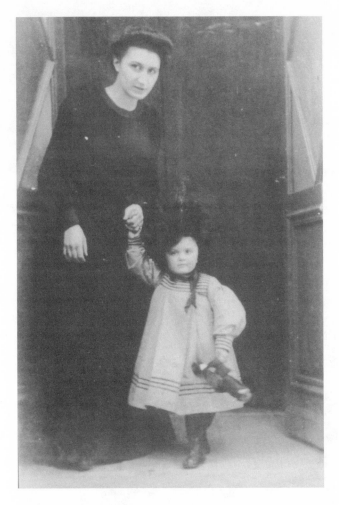

Figure 13. Nelly Roussel and her son Marcel Godet, possibly on
the occasion of his homecoming from the *pouponnière*,
c. 1906. Mairie de Paris–Bibliothèque Marguerite Durand.

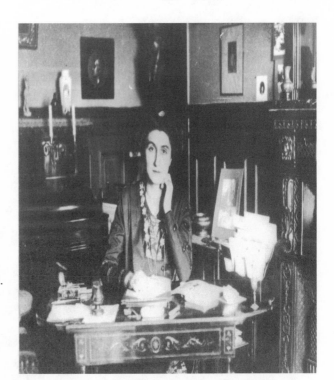

Figure 14. Nelly Roussel in her study, c. 1909. Mairie de Paris– Bibliothèque Marguerite Durand.

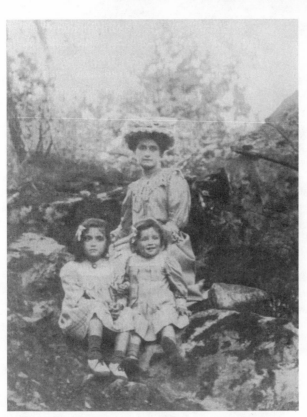

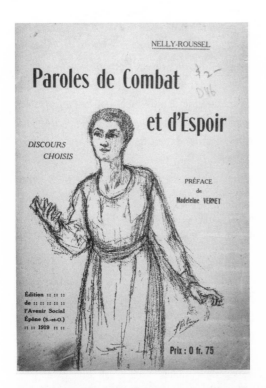

Figure 16. Front cover of Nelly Roussel's *Paroles de combat et d'espoir.*

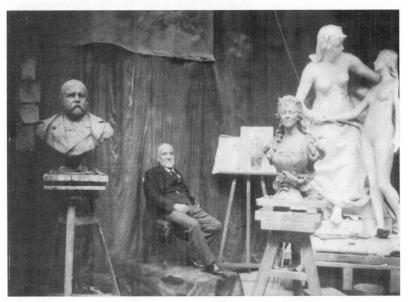

Figure 17. Henri Godet in his workshop in the 1930s. Musée d'Orsay.

Figure 15, opposite. Nelly Roussel, Mireille Godet, and Marcel Godet in the forest of Fontainebleau, 1906. Mairie de Paris–Bibliotheque Marguerite Durand.

ments that "should need no awakening." Roussel was the first publicly to discuss "everywoman's" private pain. She had helped them escape their "moral isolation," correspondents told her.[25] Even if the women in her audiences had not themselves experienced the pain of childbirth, suffered from unwanted pregnancies, been seduced and abandoned, or witnessed the deaths of their own infants and children, they knew someone who had and whose fate they feared for themselves.

Even women who had only heard about her lecture by word of mouth came out of their mental attics to tell her what she meant to them. One such twenty-year old woman, who lived in a village of 1,500 and proclaimed herself "illiterate," produced the following extraordinary letter, to which Roussel surely responded:

> I hate and despise clerics [*ensoutanés*]. This is to say to you that with such ideas I no longer have any religious status, and that it hardly bothers me to say that the church-goers [*calotins*] are hypocrites and sanctimonious bigots. According to the clericals . . . I am a demon vomited from hell, and many other things as well. It also requires a true courage for me to dare to hold my head up to these watermelon eaters. . . . I just content myself with shrugging my shoulders and complaining about these stupid people. But Madam, do you understand this rubbish? It is to ask you for advice that I bother you with my prose, to have encouragement, if I merit it, from a woman with heart and intelligence, like Nelly Roussel. . . . Madam, I only know how to write with my heart, and I think that suffices.[26]

In emphasizing its pains and indignities, Roussel in effect proclaimed that motherhood dehumanized women, and that repeated, unwanted pregnancies made them like animals.[27] She made this comparison when addressing pronatalist demographers in an article she wrote for *L'Action:*

> If these *messieurs les statisticiens* would take the pains to leave their numbers behind in order to look at life itself . . . if they gave any thought to the prolific females [*femelles pondeuses*] whom, drunk one night, a brutal male thoughtlessly fertilizes [*féconde*], [males] unconcerned right to the end about the heavy, aching bellies of the females, who struggle, "slaving away" for the whole family, serving the men, taking care of the brats [*marmots*]; and who, after having gone through labor on the straw mat of an attic room, without air in the summer, heat in the winter, . . . in three or four days, hurting all over, resume the job of the beast of burden, waiting in anguish for the next pregnancy.[28]

If thoughtless motherhood turned women into animals, civilized society had the responsibility, through science, to control nature and allow women to be fully human. Because freethinkers prized science as a source of human liberation,

Roussel thought they offered a path for female emancipation. She continued to discover deep-seated prejudices in them as well, particularly with regard to their conception of "Nature" in whose name they condemned "caution in procreation" as immoral. She pointed out that the "cult of the goddess Nature" did not prevent them from using science to fight disease and destroy germs that nature had also created. "How could man's conquest over the forces of reproduction," she asked, "be more immoral than surgical operations or medical treatments . . . [or] the canalization of rivers" and other measures that all "go against, transform, tame and master nature?"[29]

Roussel continued her attack on freethinkers in her lecture "La Femme et la libre pensée," which she delivered 39 times between 1906 and 1910. Building on her original address to the National Congress of Free Thought in 1903, she incorporated criticism from anarchists such as Henri Duchmann and her friend Émile Darnaud to further her critique of left-wing men who opposed political rights for women because of their supposed domination by the Church. She began her lecture with an attack on Catholic dogma, especially the notion of the immaculate conception, which made chastity the dominant virtue, treated "love" (sex) as a "stain," and reduced women to objects of reproduction who had to obey and suffer. Women had difficulty extricating themselves from Church doctrine, not because it was in their nature to be religious, but because they had no other respectable place to go, especially while men spent all their free time in cabarets. In her tours through the provinces, she had witnessed the pattern, even among freethinkers, in which men and women inhabited starkly separate spaces. This division reinforced the very problem—women's relationship to the Church—that both she and freethinkers wished to tackle.[30]

If churchgoing women were not mature enough for liberty, cabaret drunkards were no more so. To shouts of "Bravo!" Roussel said, "While you seek to eliminate the Church from our morals, think about eliminating the cabaret from yours." Men demonstrated no moral superiority to women; moreover, freethinkers humiliated their wives and daughters by hypocritically behaving as lords and masters in their families, thus violating their own injunction "neither God nor master." Women sought out the Church as a refuge from their own suffering, even though the Church itself reinforced the ideology and institutions that made them creatures of self-sacrifice. Roussel challenged freethinkers to give women an alternative to churchgoing and demanded their right to "integral happiness." If freethinkers admitted equality between the sexes, religions would cease to attract suffering women, and all of humanity could be intellectually emancipated.[31]

Opposition

Roussel's written and spoken words drew opposition from men and women across the political spectrum. Conservatives not surprisingly labeled her lectures immoral, imprudent, and shocking, and proclaimed that the French people would never dream of a woman abandoning the home for occupations that were not the prerogative of her sex. They reminded their readers that religion "emancipates" the woman from her "natural propensity to sin" and "fixes her place in the home; it defines her role as a young girl, a wife and a mother, granting her a beautiful and noble part." Protestant women, of whom she encountered many in Switzerland, stressed that it was only the Catholic Church that treated women badly and urged her to come into the Protestant fold.[32]

Several feminists publicly or privately opposed her. Pauline Kergomard, a contributor to *La Fronde* who promoted infant-care education for girls, "bitterly reproached" Roussel for giving neo-Malthusian lectures—even though she had never attended one—and refused Roussel's offer of a preferred seat so that she might attend.[33] Augusta Moll-Weiss not only opposed her views but, like so many others, feared the power Roussel exercised over "crowds" and claimed she was usurping the "feminist flag." After seeing her present "Fertile Love, Sterile Love," she wrote that the audience was "carried away in spite of itself," as it listened to Roussel proclaim "the merits of sterile love, of today's joy without tomorrow's pain, of ecstasy without remorse." Before this assembly of feminists, Roussel uttered "blasphemies"; because her voice was so "captivating," not a single mother was able to respond to this "superb and paradoxical" speaker. The feminists, Moll-Weiss declared, "extraordinarily, remained women—fearful of a public debate, blushing over being unveiled in front of everyone," and too hesitant to protest their own defilement as women, "too upset to dream of defending their dear feminist flag, violently torn from the heights where they had planted it in the name of the woman who came to speak."

Moll-Weiss said that, from a feminist standpoint, Roussel was unleashing the "fiercest, most formidable enemy." Her promises of intellectual superiority would only make woman more egotistical than man, and turn her into "a courtesan incapable of will." And attacking the point most central to Roussel's thinking, she said: "It's not in pleasure and joy that character is forged; it is through pain." Pain, she claimed, was what gave women a greater capacity for compassion. Evoking Christ's sacrifice, she concluded, "Our superiority is in a crown of thorns; in tearing it away from us, Madam, you should fear that instead of pushing us toward a supreme achievement, you will push us toward an abyss."[34]

Others attacked Roussel for not being radical enough—or out of petty jealousy. Aria Ly, a feminist who advocated celibacy, and who also had not attended any of her lectures, complained to Caroline Kauffmann (Nelly's close collaborator in the UFF) that Roussel never advocated *"equality* between the sexes but only *equivalence!* Which is not at all the same!" Ly further questioned the authenticity of Roussel's talent, claiming her lectures were full of clichés taken from the classics; "the sacred torture of mothers," Ly asserted, was "pinched" from Victor Hugo. Roussel's association with *La Française* meant that she could not possibly be revolutionary. Ly concluded she was a "fake who thinks she is much better than she really is!"

Not long after Ly wrote this letter, Roussel contacted her with a very friendly overture about matters relating to the UFF. Ly by that time had read her lectures and confessed admiration for Roussel. However, Ly also emphasized their point of diversion: the only reason to have sex at all, this advocate of permanent virginity declared, was to have children.[35]

Roussel's most intractable opposition, however, came from men on the Left. Freethinkers, socialists, and anarchists attempted to counter her arguments with "theory" that differed little from that of the religious right-wing. Both sides held remarkably similar views about women's nature, and especially their propensity for "sin." Men of the Left particularly feared women's vulnerability to the "seductions" of priests. On the occasion of her 1906 northern tour through the departments of Calvados, Manche, Seine-Maritime, Nord, and Ardennes, one contributor to a local paper insisted that Roussel's feminist social theories were "inadmissible" for anticlerical thinkers, because "giving rights to women amounts to giving rights to the priests who penetrate their conscience and audaciously exert power over them." Women did not flock to the Church simply out of moral or physical distress; even "rich and happy" women expressed ardent devotion. "Who would ever believe that a woman emancipated in her own household would distance herself from the enveloping, tempter priest, who mediates access to paradise in the afterlife?"[36] The writer insisted that men and women must first be liberated through science, a bizarre reaction given Roussel's outspoken support for scientific progress—especially as it related to women—and her claim that churches would empty when women became emancipated.

As in other tours, this one produced considerable journalistic debate throughout the region. The audience in St. Lô had never seen a female speaker, and some among them—even freethinkers—found "L'Éternelle sacrifiée" risqué and unsettling. Her single lecture in Caen generated political debate in five long newspaper articles that even engaged some who had not attended it.[37] At issue in these debates was not just women's presumed domination by priests, but their inescapable physiology that predisposed them to both spiritual and physical seduction. For example, when *L'Action* began publishing Roussel's articles, Camille Guesmere complained privately to the editor, Henry Bérenger, that he was among "a certain number of readers" who opposed the "invasion" of feminists. Nature had denied women the moral strength "distributed to a man by his physical structure," he argued, and he facetiously suggested that women would require mental therapy and medication if they were to participate in the public sphere. Like so many others across the political spectrum and gender divide, Guesmere located female morality and intelligence in the prison of an unchanging body, rather than in a mind that could reason and evolve. Invoking the Revolution to emphasize that any public presence of women would undermine republican ideals, he spoke of women's "rage for *servilisme*," a rarely used term for feudal servility that had been current during the First Republic. "Unconsciously," he said, "woman needs to have masters . . . she [only] feigns to want to emancipate herself." Women had been accomplices of the clergy since 1793 (the year the Terror began), and they threatened to "return us to the lovely days of absolute power [of the monarchy]." Guesmere closed his letter by asking Henry Bérenger "to ban *l'éternel féminin*" from *L'Action*.[38]

Between 1904 and 1907, Guesmere wrote several long letters directly to Roussel. Although she never wrote or spoke specifically about contraceptives, he accused her of giving a "little course on practical gynecology" and advocating "conjugal cheating" in *L'Action*. He sarcastically suggested she consider the infallible method of abstinence instead, for "nothing is easier, especially for feminists." He recommended yet another method he presumed familiar to "the league against masculine tyranny": the "practice dear to the divine Sappho" (lesbianism).[39] Even as a self-proclaimed anarchist, Guesmere resorted to the biblical source of morality when he said, "Woman shows her fall from grace, man hides it," suggesting that a woman should not be able to avoid the consequences of her sexuality—that is, hide her sin—through birth control. No statement could have more adeptly cut to the issue at hand: the power that female sexuality would have if it were separated from reproduction—and religion. Guesmere was hardly unique in defining woman's "eternal" nature as located in the body. Jean-Jacques Rousseau had made a similar argument in *Émile*, saying that whereas man's reason allowed him to control his passions, woman's "boundless passions" could only be restrained by modesty.[40]

The physiological component of the "eternal feminine" manifested itself in other reactions, even among apparent supporters, such as that of an M. Celérier who wrote to her a "few minutes" after having been "under the charm of her word." After complimenting her, he presented his argument against her: women could never be the equals of men, or even persons in their own right, because the heterosexual relationship subjugated them and turned them into passive receptacles. When a man "has" a woman (in sex), he argued, the woman loses all moral initiative. The will of a woman annihilates itself "when she submits to a stronger will." "Isn't consented love a voluntary [and irrevocable] servitude [of the woman]? This—if I am not mistaken—is the conclusion of 'La Rébelle.'" With this last comment, Celérier further revealed his predisposition by wrongly calling *Par la révolte* "The Woman Rebel." He thereby lent the play a meaning different from what Roussel intended by associating it with female sexual liberation that would subject women anew. "Language offers us a verification of this inferiority of the feminine will," he continued, using a very postmodern argument. "A woman 'gives herself,' a man 'takes'; these are not just simple words; they translate a physiological and moral fact. The will of the person who abandons herself is inferior . . . to the will of one who behaves in some way actively." This question, he thought, merited a "physiological, psychological, psycho-physiological analysis."[41]

Such an analysis indeed took place. Consciously or not, Celérier attributed to the sexual act the same significance it possessed in classical Athens, where it was an "action performed by one person upon another"; sex polarized individuals and created a hierarchy. What David M. Halperin writes of this society could be applied to Celérier's statement here: "The extraordinary polarization of sexual roles . . . merely reflects the marked division in the Athenian polity between this socially superordinate group, composed of citizens, and various subordinate groups . . . composed respectively of women, foreigners, slaves, and children (the latter three groups comprising persons of both sexes)." In early twentieth-century French society, only girls and women permanently lacked full civil rights. Feminists of that era (Aria Ly), as well as recently (Catharine MacKinnon), have used the same logic to argue against heterosexuality.[42]

Like Guesmere, Moll-Weiss, and so many others, Celérier believed that the ability to avoid pregnancy would not change women's nature but instead bring out the worst in it. He was not, moreover, alone in misinterpreting the meaning of "revolt" in Roussel's popular play. After the 1905 Paris production, she was forced by the reactions of certain individuals to write an article clarifying her true intent. With "Society's" statement that Eve was made "to give, not to receive," she captured the meaning of the eternally sacrificed woman; and her solution to Eve's plight was "revolt" through the refusal to bear children. Several men who wrote to her personally or who published newspaper articles thought that "closing one's flanks" meant refusing to have sex with men, thus missing her whole point about freedom to love without bearing children. Flammèche, a contributor to *L'Action,* compared the play with Aristophanes' *Lysistrata,* in which women refuse to sleep with their husbands until they stop war. Roussel responded, "Reassure yourself, dear colleague Flammèche, it is not the strike of *lovers* I want, but the strike of *mothers.*" She explained, moreover, that by "revolt," she meant "the legitimate re-fusal to suffer, the fight against injustice, the resistance to oppression," and that similar to the orderly strikes of workers, the "best" revolts were calm.[43]

The Right Not to Suffer Legally Denied

Attention from Roussel's opponents on the Right intensified by the end of 1905, when she appeared not just with anarchists such as Sébastian Faure, but with respectable politicians such as the Paris municipal councilor Eugène Fournière, director of the *Revue socialiste.* A lecture she delivered on November 20, 1905, became the focus of particular alarm, resulting in a long-term contro-versy that revealed the subversive and unsettling impact her words had on public discourse. The mere announcement of the lecture in *Régénération* and on large posters placarded throughout Paris provoked the popular right-wing newspaper *L'Eclair* to publish an article whose title dubbed the League of Human Regen-eration the "Ligue pour la Dépopulation" (League for Depopulation). In citing the grave danger neo-Malthusianism posed for France, it specifically mentioned Roussel's scheduled lecture and listed the other modes by which the group dis-tributed its sinister message and contraceptive methods: medical "recipes," ad-vertised products, bibliographies, lists of "practitioners," and suggestive post-cards. The meetings and lectures they sponsored and advertised, such as those of Roussel, gave "the impression of a movement much more active than had been previously supposed. . . . It is the duty of each man concerned with the future of the race to see what happens from this side. The extension of this doctrine, which will be preached all over Paris in a few days, is a symptom. . . . It would be a social crime to ignore it willfully." The article was published in three other provincial newspapers, helping both to spread the "warning" and to advertise the lecture itself.[44]

The next day *Le Matin* joined in the attack on the "League for Depopulation" with the same criticisms and reported that it had asked the opinion of Senator Edmé Piot. Piot had just published another book with even more dire statistics, showing that France was "more dead" than the previous year because of a lower birthrate and higher death rate. The senator responded that he did not think the actual events of this propaganda were too important, and that the neo-Malthusians had failed so far. He did, however, deeply regret that Eugène Fournière had lent his support to their efforts. Fournière was, after all, not just an editor, but a government functionary who taught at the École polytechnique. The government had banned all religious instruction from schools, the *Avenir de la Vienne* lamented, yet "apostles" of the modern Malthus could preach from within. The debate about the neo-Malthusian threat—generated by *Régénération*'s mere announcement of Roussel's lecture—spilled over into provincial newspapers. A presumably female contributor to *Le Petit Provençal* of Marseille warned that "mocking nature" would cause "women to burn from within," and that it had become necessary "to tell all women . . . that they are built to have children."[45]

Fournière presided at the meeting of November 20 before an audience of 500 to 600 people. Roussel spoke for two hours under the title "Beaucoup d'enfants?" After covering all the points about maternal pain, religion, nature, and science articulated in "Liberty of Motherhood," she ended her lecture by saying, "We have a right to love." Her attentive audience interrupted her numerous times with applause.[46] Although Roussel had already lectured on these topics in Paris and the provinces, this event constituted a particularly controversial turning point, because—from the perspective of its critics—neo-Malthusianism seemed on the brink of becoming a mainstream movement. But the lecture also evoked more strident reaction from populationists. Immediately following her presentation, *L'Éclair* again interviewed Senator Piot, whose stance about the neo-Malthusian threat had dramatically changed in just four days. Roussel's lecture, he said, obliged him to ask the government to take measures against the neo-Malthusians.[47]

The following January, Guy de Cassagnac, director of the conservative newspaper *L'Autorité*, published an article in which he decried the "scourge" of depopulation, lambasted the neo-Malthusian movement as "anti-physiological madness," and protested the public silence with which such outrages were met. He then cited Roussel's lecture of November 20 ("Beaucoup d'enfants?") as an example of the sort of propaganda that should be outlawed. He ranked her among "these sorts of viragos, unsexed women who saturate literature and modern politics," and who "mount their pens the way they would mount a broom to go to a midnight orgy. Sterile or scorned, they avenge their disgrace by insulting Nature." But where other female revolutionaries had been placed in mental institutions or prisons for having transgressed their sex, such as Théroigne de Méricourt (Revolution of 1789) and Louise Michel (Paris Commune), "the delicate Nelly Roussel travels across France with impunity behind the banner of her skirt," suggesting that her feminine appearance protected her from persecution.[48]

Not one to ignore personal attacks, Roussel wrote Cassagnac a letter in order to rebut his views on neo-Malthusianism and to defend her honor. In response to being called a "virago," "unsexed," "sterile," and "scorned," she sent the legal proof of her "true womanhood," a document signed by the bailiff at the Tribunal of the Seine, indicating that she was married and had two children. Cassagnac sarcastically mocked her "proof." He withdrew the words "sterile" and "scorned," but not "unsexed" or "virago." He refused, moreover, to publish her letter in its entirety because he wanted to "protect his female readers" from her explication of neo-Malthusian theory.[49]

Cassagnac's refusal to publish the whole of Roussel's letter provoked her to sue him. Her case rested on a law that obligated a newspaper to publish in its entirety any letter of response from anyone named or designated in the same newspaper. Exceptions could be made only for letters containing a "direct provocation to debauchery" by "exposing an immoral and antisocial doctrine" that was "contrary to laws and good morals." *L'Authorité* regarded the court proceedings as an opportunity to humiliate and ridicule Roussel and her female supporters. The paper described these women as "the fine flower of the League of Regeneration: one of them, in order to show that she is truly liberated from the masculine yoke, is unafraid to let her mustache grow, [which] she wore with particular grace." Unable to label Roussel herself as "unfeminine," it described her "whole being as shaken by a slight trembling, which would appear to be the sign of habitual neuropathology."[50] In fact, as numerous descriptions of her "performances" indicate, Roussel spoke in public with such intensity that her body often did tremble, lending a decidedly dramatic effect.

The court decided in favor of Guy de Cassagnac and his newspaper, because it found the suggestions in Roussel's letter to be "a direct provocation to voluntary sterility of women" and a "violation of the maternal and moral law of procreation." Her words encouraged debauchery, because they sought to persuade women that they had the right, as well as easy access to, "obstacles to conception," which would cause them to forget their duty to bear children. The judicial wording naturalized motherhood and woman's obligation. It equated a woman's desire to have fewer children through contraception with willingness to have an abortion or commit infanticide; it thereby implied that the desire itself was immoral, unnatural, and murderous. Contraception, abortion, and infanticide had in common the elimination of the "sign" of the sexual act. This legal opinion reflected the belief, as Camille Guesmere had expressed it, that women's "fall from grace" had to be visible. The court also decided that Cassagnac had the right to suppress the part of Roussel's letter that made "an appeal to his female readers."[51]

The court also dismissed Roussel's accusations of slander but found Cassagnac and the editor of *L'Autorité* guilty of the lesser charge of "injurious insult" for calling her an "unsexed virago"; the fines were 25 francs each, and 100 francs for damaging her interests. Cassagnac ended his own account of these proceedings by conceding that "to have doubted the sex of this lady would have been worth five gold pieces. I would have willingly given her more if she had asked me nicely."[52] Bridling at this final patronizing insult, Roussel refused to surrender her case. But at another hearing the following spring, the Paris Court of Appeal again decided in Cassagnac's favor. It recognized women's right to protect their bodies through chastity but blatantly denied their right to engage in sexual activity *"without fear of suffering"* (my emphasis).[53] What is significant about this appellate court decision is not its anticipated condemnation of birth control but its intolerance of any desire to avoid pregnancy in order to escape physical, psychological, or emotional pain.

Originally of religious origin, this moral precept regarding female pain continued to inform and determine secular justice in the anticlerical Third Republic. Indeed, it is important to keep in mind that the French were already well acquainted with birth control in its traditional forms—withdrawal, condoms, abortion—so that, on a private level, the issue was one of method rather than morality, at least for a large portion of the population. The problem Roussel and the League of Human Regeneration posed was their loud and visible attempt to place reproductive control in women's bodies rather than in men's, promoting not only their capacity for sexual pleasure, but their potential for sexual independence.

Neo-Malthusians, however, were not of a single mind, and some among them—especially those who were eugenicists—opposed Roussel. Several years after the Cassagnac affair, in reaction to a particularly successful lecture Roussel had just delivered, a correspondent to the neo-Malthusian newspaper *Rénovation* declared that those who suffered from inheritable defects and those made unhealthy by the ravages of capitalism should have the means to avoid conceiving children. But the writer noted that the bourgeoisie already practiced birth control, which "deprives humanity of a considerable number of healthy individuals." This writer concluded that for Roussel to demand "absolute liberty even for the rich and robust woman not to procreate—[just because] it pleases her not to [is] . . . criminal."[54]

Somewhat more surprising, however, was the opposition from Roussel's loyal friend Émile Darnaud, a freethinker and self-proclaimed feminist. Darnaud sincerely believed that the instructions to use contraceptive devices would provide too graphic an anatomical education, one that would "overexcite" female readers.

Just as a certain instinct had been bred into hunting dogs, he claimed, female prudery and chastity had been handed down through generations to girls—a Lamarckian notion of the evolutionary process common among the French. Knowledge of physiology would destroy those qualities. If young girls read these neo-Malthusian newspapers, they would "deliver themselves to profligacy with impunity." He agreed that abstinence would be impossible among married couples, but nonetheless he thought it would be "humiliating for the wife to serve her husband *without purpose*."[55] Seeing the wife—or at least wanting to see her—as only serving her husband rather than engaging in mutual pleasure, implies that Darnaud shared the widely held public opinion—and that of the court in the Cassagnac affair—that female sexuality had no purpose other than reproduction.

The Political as Personal

How could Roussel consider Darnaud one of her staunchest supporters if he held the very assumptions against which she fervently spoke? Through the height of her career and until his death in 1914, Darnaud engaged Roussel and Godet on numerous issues that concerned her career and her private life. He admired Roussel's independence (even when she disagreed with him), her militancy, her logic, and her speaking ability—talents he found so rare in women of his era. He constantly expressed his adoration of Roussel from every viewpoint; his age gave him license to feel and express his "paternal" affection for her. He referred to himself as "the disciple of Nelly Roussel," whom he cherished not only as a "prodigious militant" and female public speaker, but also because she was "still woman in her physical beauty." But most important to him was her role as a mother, for which he offered incessant praise: "And now let me use my octogenarian rights, beyond all sociology; feminism, free thinking, et cetera, to say to you that it is not only 'Our Nelly' with whom I am taken [*épris*], but also Madame Henri Godet, mama of Mireille, of Marcel." It was her status as wife and mother in private life that legitimized her—a lesson Roussel began to learn well. He urged her to emphasize in her lectures that feminism was perfectly compatible with motherhood and family.[56]

Roussel and Godet hardly dismissed Darnaud as the eccentric octogenarian that he appears to be in his letters. He was a good advertisement for her, and she regretted "not having a Darnaud in every department."[57] He corresponded with many people about her, recommended that they see her speak, and copied his correspondents' reactions to her talks and sent them to her, thus providing another source of audience reaction, as well as publicity. But she also took his own reactions and opinions very seriously, for he was a foil against which she could either sharpen or temper her own arguments. His correspondence reveals an epistemology that reflected the contradictions and complexities of modernity— the rise of mass democracy, nation-states, theories of race and evolution, war, and human rights. If his beloved Nelly Roussel was, as he called her admiringly, a woman of the future, he was a man of the present who embodied a political culture of his era that he shared with many: a culture desperate to preserve a hard-fought-for republic, whose origins dated back to a revolution that had very consciously excluded women from politics. Like other men of the Left who disagreed with Roussel, Darnaud's thinking about women in general exemplified the influence of earlier democratic thinkers, particularly that of Pierre-Joseph Proudhon and Jean-Jacques Rousseau. He admitted that, to a degree, he accepted Proudhon's highly criticized maxim that women were either "housewives or harlots," particularly with regard to bourgeois women, who "rarely desired to be housewives." Most were not literally harlots, he conceded, but they lived "exactly like *cocottes*," and he wondered whether such behavior contributed to the rise in divorces.[58]

Though Darnaud was not a misogynist, he disdained and distrusted certain aspects of femininity. As had Rousseau, he appreciated beauty, but hated the manner in which women used artifice—he especially hated unhealthy corsets— to make themselves conform to sick, superficial standards of fashion. Roussel inspired passionate devotion in Darnaud because in his mind—despite her corset, for which he relentlessly scolded her—she embodied the ideal woman in her integration of physical beauty, acute intelligence, logic, and independence. As a freethinker, Darnaud supported feminism, because unlike many of his freethinking colleagues, he thought that one day women could be emancipated from the tight grip of the priests. He thought they should be granted more civil rights, but like other freethinkers, he believed they should not have the vote until they had lay educations. On these grounds, he was far more conservative than Roussel. But at the same time, his brutal critique of the conservative "feminine" feminists with whom she maintained contact is telling. He said Jane Misme and the contributors to her newspaper *La Française* gave secondary importance to feminism, even though they supported suffrage. Misme herself was a "coquette," a kept woman. She and one of her associates, the aristocratic and Catholic duchesse d'Uzès, were just the sort of females whose votes one would not be able to trust.[59]

Darnaud's letters to Roussel produced a degree of candor not found in newspapers or other correspondence. Just after Cassagnac initiated his attacks on Roussel in the winter of 1906, Darnaud wrote, "your writings and your talks on conscious motherhood make me your disciple. That does not prevent me from finding that Paul Robin goes too far. When I ordered for myself the 4th edition of *Par la révolte*, out of curiosity I asked for various publications from the offices of *Régénération;* and, after having read them, I burned them . . . I go as far as you go, but not beyond that." But in fact he knew Roussel did go "beyond that" in her beliefs, as well as in her words. He thus repeatedly expressed his revulsion at the neo-Malthusian "accessories" advertised in their newspapers and shared the opinions of others who found such methods disgusting.[60]

For his part, Godet, who must have felt personally dishonored by Cassagnac's attacks, also continued to try to steer his wife away from her association with neo-Malthusianism. For example, in April of 1906, he urged her to talk about suffrage—a topic of secondary importance to her—because the upcoming elections made it relevant. He thought a good summary of her lecture on this subject would then provoke debate in other newspapers, and she would receive more recognition for it. It would also allow her to "avoid going in the same circle," reference to the issues raised in the ongoing Cassagnac affair. But Nelly continued to defend Robin and her association with him, pointing out that her lecture in Chaux-de-Fonds (Switzerland) had been well organized because Robin had contacts there and had told them about her. "And all this proves that this good Robin is for me a sort of Darnaud."[61]

Cassignac, Darnaud, and Henri did, however, influence the self-image Roussel henceforth presented to her public—for somewhat suddenly, motherhood became a more visible part of it. During her tour in the spring of 1906, ever aware of the importance of publicity for her lectures, she instructed Henri to send her "many copies" of a photograph of the mother-daughter bust he had sculpted (fig. 9). She wanted it published in the newspapers and displayed at the Palais de Gelée, where she would be speaking.[62] Friendly press coverage of her lectures and testimony from her supporters increasingly emphasized her identity as a wife and mother. For these sympathetic commentators, she offered living proof that a feminist could have a loving relationship with a man; they portrayed her marriage as a model of companionship. In this manner, Roussel differed significantly from other feminist birth control advocates, such as Gabrielle Petit, who was not bourgeois and "lacked culture," or Madeleine Pelletier, whose celibacy, disgust for sexuality of any kind, and lack of femininity many found off-putting.[63]

Private Life

And what of Roussel's actual motherhood? The sculpture of Mireille emanating from her mother's chest belied the physical distance between the two of them. Mireille, six years old at the time of the 1906 lecture tour, continued to reside and travel with her grandparents. Marcel, who was never included in the publicity, remained in the *pouponnière* for the first two years of his life. To a large degree, Roussel escaped her own "natural" maternal responsibilities while she ardently pursued her career. But it appears as well that she did not harbor maternal proclivities, at least as regards the care of infants and small children.

When she turned twenty-eight in January 1906—happily married, enjoying good health and a widespread reputation—Roussel was on the point of reaching the apogee of her speaking career. Her peak coincided with heightened working-class unrest, renewed tensions with Germany over competing interests in North Africa, and the final separation of Church and state in France—national issues that provided a backdrop for her message, but whose unfolding events would later contribute to its suppression. From 1905 to 1908, she spent close to a third of her time on lecture tours, going to many different departments (map 4). Her speaking fees and the sale of her brochures earned an impressive income—10,014 francs from 1905 through 1908, more than an average of 2,500 per year—and paid for her trainfare and sometimes her hotels; if she arrived home with a profit, she kept it for future trips and did not contribute it to the household. She appeared at peace and at ease with herself during her extensive travels away from home and family. She also continued to derive great pleasure from her successes and from the visual effect of her black velvet dress. Though her detractors sometimes upset her, she thrived on controversy.

Family and friends also recognized her achievements. When in Nice during her 1906 tour, her grandfather heard her speak for a third time, and other family members were present as well. Their reaction thrilled her. Thomas Nel showed how seriously he took her ideas when, the following day, he insisted on talking about feminism with a guest who came to lunch. One of the family friends who had attended the lecture told Nelly's mother that even though she found the ideas "daring," she had "unreserved admiration" for her daughter. This reaction pleased Godet, because both Louise Nel and Antonin Montupet held right-wing political views, and up to that point, they had never attended any of the lectures. Soon they and the rest of the family and many of their friends began attending Roussel's lectures in Paris.[64]

Roussel's lecture tours offered more than the ability to display her talents; they gave her the freedom to exert her irrepressible and unusual (for the era) independence. On her 1906 tour, for example, she decided to stop in Clermont-Ferrand (Puy-de-Dôme) for a couple of days because tentative plans for a lecture elsewhere had been cancelled. Henri fretted over how alone and isolated she would feel, and he urged her either to go directly to Le Puy, where people would receive her, or to Vichy for a rest cure in the mineral waters. But Nelly ignored his advice, and instead took the opportunity to hike alone in the Auvergne mountains. She sent Henri an exuberant description of the clean air, the melting snow, and the extraordinary vista of the Cévennes.[65]

Roussel also took advantage of her travels to sightsee and otherwise amuse herself with lecture organizers, usually young men. While in Le Puy, they took her to see the huge statue of the Virgin Mary, made from melted cannon taken from Sebastopol after the Crimean War, meant to "dominate and protect" the city. They irreverently subverted this religious iconography by placing neo-Malthusian stickers "in all the holy places," on churches and cross pedestals, in addition to the Virgin and other statues. The League of Human Regeneration had produced twenty-four versions these stickers, an example of which read "Abortion is dangerous / Prevention of pregnancy / is easy and without danger / Let's have few children."[66]

Roussel relished vacation time while on tours, especially in the Midi. She met her sister Andrée in Monaco, and from there they went to lunch with friends in Cannes, sailed to the island of Ste. Marguerite, and visited with their cousin Jules's wife, Ninie, in Toulon. Nelly wrote to Henri from atop the hills of Nice, on the terrace of the château of her friend Georges Danjou (whom she had met through Darnaud) "installed under the mimosa," as though to underscore the difference in their respective situations. She described the exquisite view of the sea and said how content she had been with her day. She added, "In almost all your letters you speak to me of sadness, lack of spirit, drunkenness. I am sorry about that. Despite the charm of my holiday, thinking about taking the first rapid train home to break your ennui makes me crazy with desire to see you. Poor dear friend! We would be so happy here, the two of us." She then imagined that they would spend all their time embracing and looking at the sea. "But let's leave that subject. I don't want to augment your regrets, and mine." Henri, in response, complained that she seemed to have "lost the habit" of writing to him.[67]

Henri fared far less well than his wife during her tours. He occasionally wrote of suffering from hangovers, and many of his letters appear to have been scrawled in a drunken state, late at night. They are full of rambling free association about his activities, complaints about the problems of daily life, and incoherent non sequiturs. Meanwhile, Godet persisted in trying to sell his sculptures and also engaged in the business of selling blocks of uncut marble, not for art, but for the building industry. On one occasion, he solicited Nelly's marketing help in Clermont-Ferrand, even though he urged her not to stop there; and when she went to

Marseille, he facetiously and not very subtly suggested that she separate herself from politics for a brief moment to help with the business—he asked her to visit clients on his behalf without shouting "long-live socialism" or singing the "Internationale."[68] Henri otherwise filled his time with freethinking artists' meetings and feminist and left-wing lectures. He revised the statutes of the International Federation of Freethinkers, replacing the word "nature" with "matter." Electoral politics also consumed his attention; deprived of the vote, Nelly did not share his passion, which irritated him. He complained of time spent on mundane household chores. He also had to assume the less trivial responsibility—on Nelly's orders—of firing their domestic, with whom he was not on speaking terms.

Godet's "Barnum" activities multiplied as Roussel's fame grew. He opened the increasing amount of mail sent to her and then decided which pieces to answer himself and which to forward, often advising her on how to respond. Roussel's early tours had taught them both the importance of skilled publicity and tight organization; but working such details out as she traveled was never easy. With a twenty-four- to forty-eight-hour turnaround in the mail, they were always rushing to finish their respective letters in time for the mail; the whole organization of her lecture tours depended on frequent and reliable trains and mail pickups and deliveries. The inevitable gaps sometimes caused tension between them. Henri often complained that she did not write frequently enough and failed to provide him with sufficient information about her schedule in time for him to be able to make posters, send brochures, and advertise her lectures in the nationally circulating *L'Action*. Sometimes he did not know when she would reach a particular destination, or how long she would stay there. Consequently, many of his letters had to be forwarded from one location to the next one, resulting in his frustrated complaint that he needed a more precise idea of her plans so that his letters would not "remain *en panne* [broken down] like vulgar automobiles."[69]

Deeply political in his sensibilities as well as his activities, Henri genuinely believed in his wife's mission and took it very seriously. He gave her continuous encouragement and support, and even addressed the envelopes of his letters "Madame Nelly-Roussel, World Champion of Pure Eloquence"; "Madame Nelly-Roussel, Celebrated Orator"; or "Madame Nelly-Roussel, Illustrious Lecturer," while she addressed him affectionately as her "stone breaker," the pen name he used as an art critic. Godet was convinced that a broadsheet distributed by the infamous right-wing nationalist Paul Déroulède made allusion to Nelly, proving that her propaganda influenced elections. In his effort to promote her, he suggested at one point that she write to the Socialist Party leader Jean Jaurès, who was trying to rescue his newspaper, *L'Humanité*, from the brink of bankruptcy.

Nelly, he thought, should offer to raise money for the newspaper by lecturing and contributing articles on feminism and socialism. Roussel responded to his "humanitarian idea" by saying it would have little chance of success. Henri's genuine desire to help Jaurès—*L'Humanité* was indeed on the verge of bankruptcy—was also an opportunity to launch his wife into the high elite of Socialist Party circles, where she would be assured yet more publicity, even though her more radical feminist, not to mention neo-Malthusian, views would have had to be tempered, if not suppressed.[70]

Roussel's independence, love of travel, devotion to her career, and minimal contact with her children for months at a time do not fit Darnaud's image of her as a devoted wife and mother. Despite her long periods away from home and occasionally overt attentions from other men, her devotion to Henri was steadfast. She saw little of Marcel, who was still living in the *pouponnière,* and often did not see Mireille for two months at a time. They did, however, spend vacations together. It was typical of urban French bourgeois families (and still is) for the women and children to spend the summer months in vacation residences, while the men remained in the cities and visited their families on weekends. The Roussel-Godet family was no exception to this summer habit. For example, on July 22, 1906, Nelly departed for St. Quay on the Normandy coast, along with her daughter, her sister Andrée, and their mother, where they remained for six weeks. Her letters to Henri express frank and profound affection for Mireille. She spent everyday at the beach walking, hiking, climbing rocks, either alone or with the others. Ever conscious of herself as a public figure in these private circumstances, she wrote to Henri: "Madame Nelly Roussel, the distinguished lecturer, her skirt raised to her knees, climbed [on the rocks] and splashed in scandalous fashion."[71]

Belying this leisured vacation were financial difficulties that increasingly plagued Henri and Nelly. After dismissing their domestic servant, they did not hire another, a telling aberration for people of their social class. Instead, they relied on the meals prepared by Andrée's domestic. But Nelly's sister offered more. In August, she suggested they move in with her and her husband Paul Nel. Their apartment was large, and owned by Montupet's company, for which Paul worked. Nelly and Henri would only have to pay the cost of the water, coal, and gas that they consumed.[72] They certainly needed more space than their own apartment afforded, because they planned, finally, to retrieve Marcel from the *pouponnière* that September.

In the two years since his birth, Nelly had visited Marcel only every few weeks. As she and Godet prepared to bring him home, an exchange took place between them that reveals much about their respective sensibilities as parents. The previous May, 1906, when Nelly was on tour, Henri had written, "Marcel must be doing well—he must even be getting old. I have not been to see him once in order that he not develop, to your detriment, a passion for me. This cost me a lot, I assure you." While Nelly and Mireille were in St. Quay that July, Henri wrote to the director of the *pouponnière* to say "I can no longer live without my son." But he also told her that she had to keep him until September 10, his second birthday. Since it was too "bothersome" to go to Versailles alone to see Marcel, Henri instead telephoned to get news of him. Meanwhile, still in St. Quay, Nelly implied through her planning for the following fall that the return of her two-year-old son would make little difference to her schedule. She accepted an invitation to speak in Toulon on September 23. By that time, she figured, they would be settled in their new domicile, and Andrée had offered to take care of the *mioche* (kid). She also thought she would then take another "dozen days" to go from Toulon to Switzerland to give a few lectures.[73]

Shortly after returning from the Normandy coast, Nelly and Henri took a full week to move from their apartment on 109 rue Michel Bizot into Paul and Andrée's apartment, number 254 on the same street. Mireille joined them in her aunt's apartment for two weeks. Nelly did not, after all, leave for a tour to Toulon on September 23, as she had planned, but instead departed in mid October for a two-week stint in Switzerland.[74]

The new household arrangement was not what Nelly had imagined it would be. The mercurial and unpredictably moody Andrée "whined" about Marcel distracting the maids and the care he demanded. Paul complained as well that Andrée spent too much time with Marcel, which in turn forced Henri to insist to Andrée that he was not *her* child. He assured his in-laws that henceforth he and Nelly would care for their toddler in a manner that would allow Andrée to be "tranquil with her maids." But until Nelly returned from Switzerland, Henri had his hands full. Although Mireille continued to live with her grandmother, Henri took care of her part of the day, and both children had colds. Marcel developed a "little eruption" on his backside; unable to recognize a diaper rash, Henri called a doctor. "Ah! Children! With or without boiled milk!" he complained. But worse were Marcel's "dirty tricks" and "diabolitries," which provoked Andrée to declare that she would not permit him to be left alone in any room. Like any normal two-year old, Marcel "climbed all over everything." Henri obligingly offered to remove objects from the toddler's reach by placing shelves higher. He assured his sister-in-law that he would repair the resulting damage to the walls, but she snapped back that she didn't want her house to look like a "stable." She ended up swearing at him, he vowed to dine elsewhere that weekend, and wished he could find "another social position." Henri resolved the issue by making a "stall" for Marcel in the attic. Whenever he left the apartment, he shut his son in the bathroom, having removed all accessible items. Even that strategy was not foolproof, because on one occasion Marcel managed to have a spoon (engraved with Nelly's name) with him and proceeded to eat sand from the bathroom spittoon, pretending it was soup. Finally, Henri proclaimed that they had "discovered" that his name was "Nono" (as in *Non! Non!*), a nickname that persisted for many years, ultimately to Marcel's deep chagrin and humiliation.[75]

Public Image and Private Behavior

The most glaring contradiction in Nelly Roussel's life lay in the difference between the maternal image she projected to the public and her actual behavior as a mother. Nelly showered affection and pet names on Mireille, saw her several times a week when not traveling, and spent some summer vacations with her. Mireille slept at her parents' apartment when her grandmother was ill or out of town. Marcel, as we have seen, came from the *pouponnière* to the home of a couple who fought loudly and incessantly. Henri's loving but incompetent care during Nelly's absences only fueled household tensions. This living situation, which lasted for two years, facilitated Nelly's continued extended absences from Paris.

Roussel's absences render all the more ironic her success at creating a public image of herself as a devoted mother. Her efforts to do so while on tour in the spring of 1907, moreover, provoked long-simmering tensions with Godet. Her travels at this particular time produced more than the normal frustrations in communication, because she had to make decisions from a distance about the publication of her first collection of speeches, *Quelques discours*. Henri gave his usual input, offering advice about which speeches should be included and how they should be edited. As important as the content, however, were the frontispiece and dedication, which would showcase the volume and, they hoped, sell it.

Henri grew frustrated because Nelly did not respond promptly enough to his queries about the title of the collection and the photograph she wanted him to use. Letters they each wrote on May 2 crossed in the mail. She told him she wanted her portrait on the cover, emphasizing "*you know which one.*" With regard to the photograph, he wrote on the same day, "zut, zut, Zut, zut, Zut, zut. I'll do what I want to all alone all alone all alone all alone. It's my own photograph that I'll put [on the cover] with Nono—who said yesterday without anyone asking him anything: 'Mommy is going to return to see Nono.'" Returning to see the two-

and-a-half-year-old Marcel was far from his mother's mind, as Henri was well aware. If his words about the photograph here were facetious, they also served as a reminder that he was the one "mothering" their son. The final choice for the frontispiece was a photograph of Roussel and Mireille in Godet's workshop, with his sculptures in the background (fig. 11). When she indicated that she wanted her own portrait to be used, she did not say "the one with Mireille," so this choice may have resulted from a compromise. In any case, it satisfactorily projected her maternal image.[76]

Henri knew that the way this volume was presented would reflect their marriage as well. He thus also had a hand in the dedication. In response to Nelly's first version, one unfortunately not saved for posterity, Henri protested:

> I just reread the dedication and permit myself some reflections: it has the fault of most dedications concerning women, [and] I would have preferred that it make clear that I opened this horizon of activity to you, [a horizon] you did not consider, that at least I had showed you the way, encouraged you to follow it. It's very difficult to explain what I mean to say—and I am tired, I am going to bed. I will add something Wednesday the 24th—that will perhaps be less idiotic.[77]

Nelly's original version had ignored Henri. His complaint about "dedications concerning women" must have referred to his sense that feminists acknowledged only the efforts of women and not those of men. While he could not justifiably claim the entire responsibility for her feminism, he had encouraged her to pursue public speaking, rather than a career in the theater, a path actually more difficult for women than acting, because it was rare and made them more vulnerable to ridicule. Moreover, he had become a partner in her career and had cared for their children in her absence. How could she have overlooked his contributions and his desire for public acknowledgement of them?

Roussel's response came four days later at the end of her letter, crammed into the margins almost as an afterthought: "I'm thinking of the dedication. It's upsetting that you don't like it . . . I was so happy with [it]! . . . it is necessary, above all, that you like it. We'll talk about it more." In her next letter, she offered him this revision: "To my husband, to my best friend; he who understood and encouraged my apostolate." But this version also left Godet frustrated and confused. On May 4, he wrote that he had "plunged his head in his hands" to try to figure out what it was that made this dedication so "farcical" to him:

> Why does your dedication resemble an epitaph? . . . it's because you speak in the past tense . . . here is what I propose, but the man proposes, the woman disposes

and even sometimes indisposes. "To my dear husband, who understands me and encourages me." It is less romantic, but you know, Victor [referring to their mutual hero Victor Hugo] is dead, and we must not raise the dead . . . in fact I don't know if one says it, but I suppose that many would find it bad—come on, I am saying a bunch of stupid things, it's the effect of the *tilleul* [lime-blossom tisane] that I just drank.[78]

Whatever Henri was drinking (probably not lime-blossom tea, given his sloppy hand, free association, and non sequiturs) did not afford him the courage to articulate his remaining thoughts. Did he not want to be referred to as his wife's "best friend"? Would he have preferred something more romantic, such as her "greatest love"? He wanted Roussel's readers to know that despite her feminism, despite her career, he remained the center of her life and they had a romantic marriage. But at this juncture, he felt helpless in their relationship. "The man proposes, the woman disposes . . ." (and in this case, also "indisposes"), was a popular twist on the proverb "Man proposes, God disposes," reflecting the view that the "eternal feminine" had ultimate power.

The final product had the desired results. Darnaud gave enthusiastic approval and expressed his particular pleasure at the dedication to Henri and the photo of Nelly with Mireille. Whatever the modern eye might make of the frontispiece photograph (fig. 11), in which Roussel leans away from her daughter and gazes outward, it made her into an "excellent mother" as indicated by one critic in *La Liberté* : "Madame Roussel has a severe eloquence. . . nonetheless, if we judge by the portrait that figures on the cover of the brochure, [she] is a young woman, very pretty, very elegant. A beautiful child leans against her: Mme Roussel is thus also an excellent mother. Bravo! All that is worth even more than revolutionary eloquence." Another reviewer noted, "Mme Nelly-Roussel has rendered herself almost notorious by her enthusiasm for preaching depopulation to the French. She is M. Robin of Cempuis, only more gracious. Do not believe, however, that [she] puts her theories into practice." The author then quoted the dedication to illustrate her wifely devotion, and continued, "the cover of the brochure presents a charming portrait of the orator, holding tightly against her a pleasant child. Mme. Nelly-Roussel, she's the modern matron, but she's still the Roman matron [with] her jewels." It is ironic that this reviewer admired Roussel all the more because he thought she did not practice what she preached. More noteworthy is that he failed even to see that she was not touching Mireille (with either arms or hands), let alone holding her tightly, which underscores the semiotic power this image had on predisposed viewers. Aria Ly also later reacted to this frontispiece photograph, writing to Roussel of how Mireille "leans against her dear and glorious mama in such an exquisite pose of adorable abandon and for which this feminist virgin can envy you despite her cult of purity."[79]

The introduction to the collection, authored by Roussel's feminist colleague in the UFF, Hellé (a.k.a Marguerite Dreyfus), also drew reviewers' attention for its treatment of Roussel's recurrent travels away from home, as well as Darnaud's hardy approval. "The spectacle is assuredly very rare of a happy woman, a happy spouse, a happy mother, leaving the warm shadow of the hearth in order to go off on great roads, free, uncertain roads, to serve a cause," Hellé wrote. "You abandon a soft quietude for the austere joy of speaking according to your heart and your faith, and you accept in advance the danger of being misinterpreted."[80] Hellé sought to reconcile Roussel's qualities as bourgeois wife and mother with her absence from the home by construing the latter under the typical rubric of female self-sacrifice, but in this case, sacrifice to a cause rather than to men and children. In fact, as we have seen, Roussel relished travel for its own sake, and she derived most of her identity and self-esteem from her career. During her absences, not once did she ever say she missed her children, and she rarely asked after them. She missed Henri and would often say that his absence marked the imperfection of an otherwise successful trip; she also sometimes felt herself to be a "martyr" in her travels as well. But her lecture tours provided far more of a basis for her self-esteem than self-sacrifice.[81]

The unusual strain, anger, and sarcasm in Roussel and Godet's correspondence in the spring of 1907 contradicts the image of conjugal harmony and happy motherhood they were at the same time creating for public consumption.[82] Nelly had already been absent for two weeks in February on a tour in Belgium, and had she been home for only just over a month before leaving on a two-month tour through Geneva, Lausanne, and the departments of the Haute-Savoie, Isère, Var, Gard, Ariège, Pyrénées-Atlantiques, Charente-Maritime, Maine-et-Loire, and Indre-et-Loire, where she gave eighteen lectures followed by dramatic readings of *Par la révolte*. Not only did Henri have to occupy himself with the usual affairs related to her speaking tours, but this one occurred just after the close of the Cassagnac affair, an experience perhaps more humiliating to him than to Nelly; it had, after all, given her and her cause more publicity and provoked gratifying public discourse, while he had been helpless in the battle to preserve her honor.

Meanwhile Henri's home life offered little solace. Paul and Andrée had serious marital problems, to which "Nono" contributed. Andrée attempted to find a nanny, but claimed she could not because Paul was too stingy to pay more than 30 francs per month. Despite their more than ample income from annuities,

Paul and Andrée incessantly bickered over money. Henri noted to Nelly the irony of their hosts' money battles, "while we, by my fault, moreover . . . are without a penny [but never fight]. Oh well, I would not change, if it were at the same time to mean inheriting this inveterate habit of fighting so stupidly."[83] But the lack of a nanny also meant that Henri had to occupy himself with Nono, a task that continued to challenge him, particularly around issues of toilet training. "Marcel went pipi on the floor and then dabbled in it, saying 'Nono is washing his hands.'" He also urinated on an issue of the conservative feminist *La Française* (an appropriate gesture, Godet thought) and ate his excrement. Nelly responded, "Horrible little Nono! Disgusting kid! Who always profits from my absence to do such things, because he knows that I am the only one who whips him conscientiously." Henri resorted to locking Marcel in an armoire on occasions when he became too obstreperous.[84]

During the long separation of the 1907 tour, Henri and Nelly had yet another reason to resent their son. They had planned to meet in Bayonne, because each of them would be en route to Bordeaux for the Congress of the League of the Rights of Man, and then slowly make their way back to Paris together, while she continued to give a few more lectures on the way. But all Henri's in-laws were leaving Paris, taking their servants with them, so no one was available to take care of Marcel over the long Pentecost weekend. Henri finally succeeded in finding a nanny—a fifteen-year-old girl from the provinces with "a look of stupidity"— pressed upon him by a neighbor who seemed eager to be rid of her. Henri hired the girl at the incredibly paltry rate of ten francs a month. Even Andrée thought Marcel should not be left alone with this domestic, which made Henri think he should shorten the trip. His doubts infuriated Nelly, who was desperate to be with her husband for as many days as possible. If Marcel was going to be left with the nanny at all, she queried, "what difference would five or six days make?" In fact, "Maria" turned out to be both incompetent (she "almost lost Nono") and "a small-time thief"; she lasted for only a couple of months, another failure in the family's recurring problems with domestics.[85]

We must not conclude from these exchanges that Nelly and Henri, preoccupied with one another and with their respective careers, did not feel love or affection for their son. Figure 12 of Nelly with Marcel on her lap at the *pouponnière*, suggests maternal warmth and tenderness; for once her gaze is on her child, rather than toward the camera and at the outside world. Figure 13 similarly conveys maternal affection in Roussel's body language, even though her gaze is on the camera.[86] Henri often wrote tenderly and lovingly about their son. In Nelly's absence he allowed Nono to get into bed with him in the mornings; he fretted over signs of the boy's sickness, and shared stories of his good deeds as well. He especially conveyed to Nelly how much Nono missed her and wanted her to return. But Henri was not beyond telling the child that his mother's return depended upon his good behavior, even though his behavior had nothing to do with her traveling schedule. Meanwhile, Mireille, the "chou en chocolat" (cabbage in chocolate), was a "perfect" child, content with her living arrangement, especially since she saw her parents frequently when they were in Paris. Nelly would often spend entire afternoons at her mother's, and she would always be at Mireille's bedside when she was sick. As Mireille grew older, Nelly took her to and from school and piano lessons. The extended family lunched every Sunday at the Montupets' home, after which they went on excursions in the Bois de Vincennes or elsewhere. Nelly, Henri, and the two children also socialized frequently with his extended family—especially Juliette and Fritz Robin, their son Maurice, and Fritz's mother, Louise Robin. Paul Robin, ill and increasingly reclusive, rarely joined them. The Godet, Robin, and Nel families shared a large multigenerational network of friends in Paris, Vincennes, Fontainebleau, and Monaco, mostly people associated with music, theater, and the arts, who often joined in family dinners and activities. All these people became an intricate part of the children's lives.[87]

By modern standards, Roussel appears to have been a bad mother. But by the standards of her day, she did not appear that way. After her initial memoir while pregnant with Mireille, she neither ever commented about her sense of self as a mother nor expressed anxiety, guilt, or second thoughts about herself in that role. No one else did either, including Henri. This was because motherhood (even according to pronatalists, as Roussel routinely pointed out) primarily meant bearing children, and—despite the growing sentiment that mothers should breast-feed—did not automatically mean nurturing them oneself. Roussel's behavior followed the pattern of the past, when mothers did not involve themselves much with their children. Those who had the means instead oversaw servants, nursemaids, and governesses who did. In Roussel's case, unable to keep a nanny for any length of time, let alone afford a team of servants, her family stepped in because doing so was normal. The transition from the preindustrial motherhood in which women integrated productive activity with maternal responsibilities—whether they were wage-earning workers, bourgeois business women, or aristocratic socialites—to modern motherhood was long and uneven, and not all women had the "instincts" that were supposed make it "natural" for them to devote themselves exclusively to the children they bore—exclusive in the sense of doing nothing but raising children, as well as in the sense of not caring for children other than their own.

Roussel's family and friends shared the assumption that childcare was not the exclusive responsibility of the mother and that other family members and friends should assume those tasks—and they did without question.[88]

Roussel and her contemporaries participated in a lifestyle that left little time for motherhood as the twentieth century came to define it, but that incorporated a collective care and concern for children. In addition to traveling, Nelly, her sister, and their friends filled their time with social visits, and in her case, political contacts.[89] Much of this social visiting, which excluded children, occurred within the upper-middle-class convention of hosting "reception days," a practice so regular that one's "day" was listed in the telephone book. Roussel received guests every other Tuesday, a day coordinated with those of Andrée and of their mother, so that family and mutual friends would not have to choose between them. On occasion, she might have as many as eight or ten visitors, most of whom were women, though men called on her as well. These occasions provided a space for female bonding, as mothers and adult daughters visited together. They also offered Roussel an obvious opportunity to talk about her own exploits and ideas. Some of these friends began attending her lectures, such as Mme Wolf and Germaine Lambert; even the frivolous Andrée began participating in the UFF.[90] It is not difficult to imagine that her reception days were informal "salons."

Roussel's career demanded—and acquired—another set of delicately balanced emotional relationships that appear contradictory. "Timorous" Louise Nel and Antonin Montupet were shocked by both the form and the content of Nelly's lectures. Louise Nel had raised her daughter as a strict Catholic, had ruled out formal education for her after she was fifteen, and had prevented her from pursuing an acting career. Moreover, Louise Nel and Antonin Montupet held political views that sharply contrasted with Nelly's. In 1907 Montupet, a ship-building engineer, began a prolonged stint as mayor of Fourchambault (Nièvre), where one of his factories was located, and where he had a residence. On one occasion, he intervened in a meeting of striking workers to explain that they needed to return to work for their own benefit, and that reduced hours or higher wages were not in their interests. After they expressed a few "timid observations" of their own about the social question, one that had become acute in 1906, Montupet asked his workers "who had put these ideas in their heads." One of them responded, "I became libertarian while listening to your stepdaughter." Louise Nel expressed her view that all the striking workers should be put in prison. Henri responded to her that during a time of strikes it might suit them, for most striking workers "would find a comfort [in prison] unknown to them in their own homes." He told Nelly that her mother had the reasoning of "an eight-year-old baby."[91]

Despite their political differences, Nelly remained extremely close to her mother. She saw her almost everyday when they were both in Paris, and she referred to her affectionately as "petite mère." And while Nelly toured Belgium in February 1907, her mother asked Henri to provide summaries of her lectures published in the local newspapers. Louise Nel then began attending her lectures in Paris, along with other family members.[92] Both Nelly and Henri, however, detested Montupet, not only for his political views, but because he lectured to them constantly. Their contempt for him did not, however, stop them from accepting his generosity in caring for Mireille. Nelly's and Henri's financial situation helped cement close family ties. The apartment they abandoned in September, 179 rue Michel Bizot, had cost 800–900 francs per year, but Godet also annually paid 1,200–1,500 francs for his workshop at 58 rue du Rendez-vous, a short distance from their home. Roussel's speaking fees afforded a small profit, but various signs—such as Godet's persistent complaints about his inability to sell sculptures or marble, and their not hiring a domestic at a time when they needed one more than ever—point to their increasingly precarious financial situation. They each nonetheless exhibited the mentality of people accustomed to a certain level of comfort. Godet at one point wrote in 1906, "These questions of money are so unworthy of our attention as millionaire apprentices that I am ashamed." Meanwhile, Roussel continued to purchase clothes frequently, most of which were tailor-made.[93]

Enjoying the peak of her career in 1907, Nelly Roussel had indeed risen above the fate she had so feared eight years earlier while pregnant with Mireille. What had tormented her then had been the "secret, voiceless and bitter revolt of all her instincts . . . against the destiny of Woman." Her experience with childbirth was worse than she had feared; then there was infant care, another pregnancy, another childbirth, which almost killed her, the loss of her infant son, and an unwanted pregnancy. She used her personal pain as a platform from which to launch a campaign, not just for herself and for all women, but for humanity. In the process, she generated opposition across the political spectrum, among friends, foes, family, and strangers. Responses to her demonstrate how deeply embedded the assumptions about female self-sacrifice were in French political culture. Undaunted, she intensified her campaign. In her private life, she enjoyed not only "freedom of motherhood" but freedom *from* maternal responsibilities. She had won, for herself at least, the right to pursue pleasure and avoid pain.

Roussel's audiences did not operate as a single-minded "crowd," despite the repeatedly expressed concern that she turned them into one. Like Émile Darnaud, her auditors filtered her words as individuals through their own needs, desires, and sexual, gender, class, and political identities. Almost everyone appreciated her speaking talent, even if they did not agree with or understand all that she said. If what she said or how she looked caused controversy, she was happy to disrupt assumptions and give voice to praise or protest. If the journalistic debates that her lectures so often provoked—especially in the provinces—constituted a measure of success, then she succeeded brilliantly. Still enjoying the peak of her career in 1908, however, Roussel would soon face a new source of pain—illness—that neither her rhetoric nor science could combat. Her precarious health, combined with the increasingly nationalistic and conservative political climate created insurmountable obstacles to the continuation of her career as she had known it.

CHAPTER FIVE

Pathologies and Persecutions

The evenings, obligatory exhaustion. And what is clearest of all is that I am in the process of losing again the little improvement I gained with such difficulty. I feel as bad as possible. And Nono only contributes too largely to this wonderful result. This child will kill me.

Nelly Roussel to Henri Godet (1909)

The government is resolved to clamp down on this destructive campaign against the French family. Let us think about what [U.S. President Theodore] Roosevelt has said: a nation whose men no longer want to make war, whose women no longer want to make children, is a nation stricken in the heart.

Deputy Gauthier de Clagny (Seine-et-Oise), quoted in L'Accord social,
December 12, 1909

After sifting through and cataloguing hundreds of letters written by French feminist women who were Roussel's contemporaries, Maïté Albistur wrote that the major event of their daily lives was their suffering bodies: "Their complaints, which run through all [social] classes and upset those in all conditions, fill their correspondence, transpire in each document"; their bodies, moreover, became a major handicap that weighed on them.[1] In the era prior to antibiotics, everyone suffered prolonged bouts of ill health, not just women. Bronchitis—to which Henri and Mireille were especially prone—could endure for weeks and be fatal. In the Roussel family correspondence, a nearly obsessive concern about the weather reflected the precariousness of daily health; it was believed that sudden changes in temperature, or excessive heat, cold, and dampness could cause serious illness. When Nelly traveled, especially on lecture tours, Henri cautioned her about her diet, overwork, and keeping her windows open at night to rid the air of menacing germs. From 1909 onward, from the time she was in her early thirties, these health concerns became more urgent and occupied more space in Roussel's diaries and correspondence. She suffered a series of disorders whose symptoms—insomnia, nervous anxiety, depression, digestive dysfunction, and eventually disabling menstrual periods—first appeared intermittently but later became more chronic.

Gauthier de Clagny's admonition (see chapter epigraph) captures the new political and international climate that coincided with the point at which Roussel's health began to decline, and within which she carried on her neo-Malthusian and feminist campaigns: a resurgence of nationalism and all its cultural trappings, which had implications for sexual politics. For the first time since 1870, rising international tensions fostered a widespread belief that war with Germany was imminent. In 1905, France took steps to gain control over Morocco in order to secure its position in the Mediterranean. Germany took this move as an insult, and Emperor Wilhelm II paid a visit to Tangier, where he declared that Germany wanted to protect Morocco's independence, bringing the two nations to the brink of war. An international conference of the major European powers averted armed conflict by affirming France's right to exert control over Morocco. In 1905, war against Germany would have been deeply unpopular in France; but this crisis introduced the idea of war into the minds of the French, and the political and diplomatic climate changed dramatically in subsequent years. Even Roussel's good friend Émile Darnaud expressed bellicose sentiments similar to those that later became fascist doctrine, writing in 1909: "Salute war! Would one know the value of man without war? Would one know the worth of peoples and races? Would we progress?" And with reference to the unexpected defeat of Russia by Japan five years earlier, he said: "Look at the Japanese! What were they! What have they become thanks to war?"[2]

Germany precipitated a second Moroccan crisis in the summer of 1911, after France had intervened in Moroccan internal affairs. Claiming to protect their commercial interests, the Germans sent a gunboat to the Moroccan port of Agadir. British-led negotiations averted war, but the effect of the crisis was to make Germany appear more threatening than ever. Moreover, in return for continued French domination in Morocco, Prime Minister Joseph Caillaux handed the Germans a large chunk of the French Congo. The Chamber of Deputies ratified Caillaux's move, but not gladly. In response to widespread anti-German feeling, it threw out Caillaux and his cabinet. His replacement, Raymond Poincaré, led a national revival between 1911 and 1914 that reflected increased fear and resentment about German behavior. As the nationalist Right became more bellicose, the internationalist, pacifist Left—including Roussel and the neo-Malthusian movement—became more antimilitarist. Nonetheless, patriotism infected moderates, radicals, and even some socialists. The new national mood converged with a Catholic revival in rejecting modernism, scientism, and secularism and helped produce the neoroyalist, antiparliamentarian Action française. Although this movement had little electoral influence, it inspired intellectuals, and its emergence coincided with a decline in the popularity of freethinking, one of Roussel's primary bases of support.[3]

Gauthier de Clagny's admonition further demonstrates how the neo-Malthusian movement fueled fears about German aggression, national degeneration, and unstable gender roles. One journalist wrote that men were being deprived of "the freedom to be fathers," which was the basis of honor and domestic happiness. Since 1905, the French had also become more acutely aware of how other nations perceived them; one journalist quoted a Japanese newspaper as saying that France "*is no longer what it was previously* . . . it is absolutely rotten in the heart; one can envy it for its refinements, its arts, its wealth, *but its vital energy is used up.*"[4] International tensions lent more gravity to French perceptions of national degeneration and infused pronatalist and repopulationist campaigns with more dogged purpose than ever before.

Thus, as of 1909, Roussel faced new personal and political challenges: her uphill battle on behalf of female dignity grew more difficult in the changing political climate. Did her health fail from a growing sense of defeat and demoralization? The persecution of neo-Malthusians most assuredly discouraged her, but her illness had other sources.

The Fraternal Union of Women and Neo-Malthusianism

In addition to her lecture tours, Roussel remained politically active in Paris circles, especially feminist ones. Despite her own radicalism, she readily reached out to and collaborated with those who were more conservative, as well as with the few feminists who were more radical than she, such as Madeleine Pelletier and Aria Ly. The Union fraternelle des Femmes (UFF) continued to be the primary group with which Roussel associated and in which she played a leadership role. The group remained small and focused on feminist issues of private as well as public life and provided a tolerant audience for her views on birth control. In addition to lecturing and distributing her publications, she invited others to speak on behalf of her cause, such as Dr. Lucas, who lectured on his method of reducing the pain of childbirth, and Dr. Danjou, a friend she had made through

Émile Darnaud, who lectured on female physical education. One of the important issues she advocated through the UFF was *recherche de la paternité,* the right of an unmarried woman to name the father of her child and seek support from him (though Roussel later advocated government support of single mothers so that they could be independent of their children's fathers). The UFF also took up the banner on behalf of women in the colonies, "where the abuses of white men without scruples lead to a considerable number of bastards."[5]

Feminists and neo-Malthusians inhabited distinctly different worlds, even though Roussel constituted a bridge between them in the UFF. Roussel played no organizational role in the neo-Malthusian movement; on her behalf, Godet had early on refused an invitation from Paul Robin to take on an administrative position. She did not generally socialize with the neo-Malthusians as a group, though she befriended and met with them individually, and continued to appear with them at major lectures. Through 1909, the movement enjoyed considerable success in its ability to spread birth control propaganda, both because and in spite of important structural changes. Unlike feminists, who organized themselves into an array of groups, neo-Malthusians were a motley collection of bohemian types who focused on propaganda, the sale of contraceptive devices, the sponsorship of lectures throughout France, and social activities such as banquets and picnics.[6] Many of them had working- or lower-middle-class backgrounds, and most were anarchists of one persuasion or another. Gradually, they won the support of a number of physicians, writers, journalists, politicians, and militants of the Left. More than ever, the movement addressed workers. Georges Yvetôt, the head of the General Confederation of Labor (CGT), was persuaded to take up the cause of family limitation and began giving speeches about it. Educational lectures on the subject were also organized in trade unions.

Although Paul Robin continued to consider himself the head of this movement, by 1905 or so, it owed its growing strength to a number of other key participants, especially Eugène Humbert, whose background and winning personality drew in more supporters. Robin did not have a winning personality, and he became increasingly cranky as his health declined. In March 1908, a major rupture occurred. Humbert, who had administered Robin's newspaper *Régénération* and managed the sale of brochures and contraceptive devices, resigned. Robin apparently accused him of pocketing profits from the sales he oversaw, but the breach also had to do with complex personal conflicts and rivalries, including sexual jealousies and betrayals within the group as a whole. Humbert then began publishing a biweekly, *Génération conscient,* and continued to sell contraceptive devices on his own. Robin planned to continue publishing *Régénération,* but he was seventy-two years old and ill, and he could not provide the necessary leadership for the new cooperative that formed after Humbert's departure. *Régénération* thus ceased publication in November 1908. A further schism occurred at that time, with Albert Gros (one of the editors of *Régénération*) breaking off and launching yet another newspaper, *Le Malthusien*.[7]

Upon returning from her spring tour that year, Roussel had repeated visits in quick succession from Humbert, Robin, Gabriel Giroud, and Albert Gros to secure her continued support as the movement splintered. Though she had regularly contributed articles to *Régénération*, Roussel had never been a member of the cooperatives that produced neo-Malthusian propaganda. She remained deeply loyal to Robin, but continued to collaborate with the schismatics and met frequently with Humbert, who solicited her articles and arranged lectures. With the reinvigoration that Humbert brought to the movement, Roussel henceforth published more of her articles in neo-Malthusian journals. She also continued to publish in feminist journals, but she broke off relations with the editor of *L'Action*, Henry Bérenger, and the last article she published in it appeared in late 1908.[8]

Family Fortunes and Misfortunes

As Roussel and the movements in which she participated attained greater success, the economic situation of her immediate family grew worse. Her small income from speaking, publications, and diction lessons certainly could not make up for Henri's sluggish earnings. Though his sculptures received positive reviews at exhibitions, his effort to sell them to Paris municipalities or to individuals proved mostly fruitless. In his frustration, he compared himself to a more famous contemporary whose sculpture he considered "very bad." "Rodin exhibited a fellow with no arms or legs, and he had the nerve to call this 'The Man Who Walks' [*L'Homme qui marche*]." (The sculpture does, in fact, have legs, but no arms or head.) That other art critics considered Rodin's piece to have "elementary strength" irritated him. "It's elementarily strong to walk without a head; even St. Denis at least had one, which he carried in his hands [after his martyrdom at Montmartre, as the legend has it], but this one?" He mocked Rodin's *The Thinker* as "a sort of large fellow, who is sitting there in the garden and has the air of making fruitless efforts—I call this 'Constipation by M. . . . .'"[9] Belle Époque tastes were evolving toward modernism, but Godet's sculptures remained traditional in their style and themes, celebrating the female body and, ironically, the joys of motherhood (see figs. 5 and 6).

One sculpting project that kept Henri busy during these years was a bronze statue of Clémence Royer (1830–1902). A Freemason, freethinker, and self-taught scholar of economics, politics, philosophy, biology, and anthropology, Royer was best known for her translation into French of Darwin's *Origin of Species,* accompanied by a provocative social Darwinian introductory essay that went beyond Darwin's own work and misinterpreted him into the bargain.[10] Émile Darnaud ranked Royer among the three or four intellectuals he most admired. Royer was a heroine among freethinkers because of her anticlerical, libertarian ideas, and among many feminists because she advocated equality between the sexes. Despite her "genius" and her prolific publications, the Parisian intellectual establishment had never accepted her, and their rejection provided even more reason to memorialize her in a monument. The project became a mission for both Nelly and Henri, as well as for Georges Clémenceau, Aristide Briand, René Viviani, Émile Levasseur, Anatole France, and other celebrated intellectuals and politicians whose support they solicited, as well as a large array of feminists, such as Hubertine Auclert, Amélie Hammer, J. Hellé, Parrhisia, Marbel, and Nelly's sister. This project remained a major concern for several years; Nelly organized a committee of supporters that met regularly. In addition to subscriptions, Henri managed to obtain 2,000 francs from the government for it.[11]

In 1907, Godet came to the realization that he had to abandon any hope that sculpting would support his family. Although a deeply committed socialist, he uncharacteristically turned his efforts toward becoming a capitalist. With the counsel and financial help of Montupet and Andrée's husband, Paul Nel, Henri undertook the project of forming a joint-stock company for the sale and transportation of marble from the quarry in Carrara, Italy, to various clients in France and Belgium. Nelly and Henri had gone to Carrara during their honeymoon, and it retained significant sentimental value for them, which eased this profound transition. His sculpting had put him into contact with the Giromella family, who distributed marble from the Carrara quarry. Their business was bankrupt, and with Montupet's help, Henri, who was fluent in Italian, was able to step in and take it over. He kept the family as employees while he ran the business from Paris. His time became increasingly consumed with soliciting shareholders and clients for this company.

Initially, Henri suffered great difficulties in working with the Giromellas and attracting shareholders. In the winter and spring of 1908, he complained bitterly of working day and night "like a Negro." He had to make frequent trips to Carrara, where he would stay for several weeks, and traveled to see clients and seek shareholders throughout France and in Belgium. Henri complained of a perpetual and "insurmountable grumpiness" over his difficulties. His new obligations meant that he could not be as good a "barnum" while Nelly was on tour, for now it was he who lacked time to write to her, let alone to respond to her usual requests. Moreover, it was now his turn to ask her to make contributions to his career. He requested that she meet some of his clients while she toured in Belgium. Henri's success, like Nelly's, hinged on family support; Montupet not only secured shareholders through his own business contacts, he loaned Henri 10,000 francs, presumably to allow the family to live until the business generated income. Henri was most grateful, and for the first time ever wrote about Montupet in glowing terms.[12]

As Henri struggled with his new enterprise, Nelly traveled as much as ever. She was absent from Paris for fifty-one of the first ninety days of 1908. In February, she embarked on a tour that in many ways marked the pinnacle of her success. Although she was well-practiced in traveling and lecturing, this trip posed the greatest challenge, for she ventured for the first time alone into countries whose language she did not speak. She began her tour in Lille, went on to lecture in Brussels and several other Belgian cities and towns, and then traveled to Budapest. After lecturing there, she visited Nuremberg and Vienna; and on her return trip, she stopped in Trieste, Venice, Milan, Genoa, and finally Carrara, where she met Henri. Although she traveled alone, Roussel's only complaints were the usual ones about the weather and fatigue. From Lille and Belgium, she reported "great success" in her lectures and in the sale of *Quelques discours*. On her way to Budapest, she delighted in conversing with two German men in her compartment, one of whom spoke adequate French. Roussel loved to dazzle unsuspecting strangers. After disarming them with her bourgeois dignity, charm, and feminine beauty, she gracefully set about astounding them with her knowledge, relentless logic, and personal charisma. She knew that private conversations on trains—or anywhere—would resonate, for they would be repeated when her acquaintances recounted their stories of meeting this unusual stranger.[13]

Roussel also continued to relish her public victories. One of her greatest came in Budapest, from where she wrote:

> I am pampered, feted, admired, visited, invited, taken out, interviewed, and I do not have a single minute to myself. My lectures are events. The first provoked long articles in *all* the newspapers. And the second just obtained a more considerable success. . . . I received congratulations from the consul-general of France, "happy with the success of their compatriot." The most eminent journalists, whom one never sees at feminist lectures, were present today, to the great joy of the ladies. . . .

In Hungary they swallowed her whole, your phenomenon. Moreover they adore the
French language, "the most beautiful," say the cultivated who know a lot of it. . . .
How your phenomenon wants to tell you this, and so many other things in person,
dear Barnum.

She provided her grandfather with a similar description, proclaiming "Glory is
beautiful!"[14] After meeting Henri in Carrara, traveling with him to Monaco and
resting there for several days in the "Villa Nel," she spoke in Nice at an event
organized by Dr. Danjou, where she earned "warm and numerous congratulations." As before, her audience in Nice included members of the wealthy elite,
in whose acquaintance she delighted—especially that of a marquise. Her grandfather again attended, and he told her that each time he heard her speak, she
had made immense progress. "Where will this end?" Nelly queried Henri with
evident self-satisfaction.[15]

Roussel's question has a sad irony to it, for she did not know that with this
tour she had, in fact, reached the peak of her career. For the moment, however,
her daily activities continued at a frenetic pace. She met frequently with leaders
of the neo-Malthusian movement and with politicians such as the radical senator Alfred Naquet, author of the 1884 divorce law; wrote articles for *L'Action*; gave
diction lessons; and, inasmuch as she and Henri would be spending time in Carrara, started teaching herself Italian. With Henri, she attended a session of the
Chamber of Deputies. She also regularly went to meetings of the UFF, convened
the patronage committee for the Clémence Royer monument, and helped organize a feminist congress to be held in June.

Nelly did not attend the feminist congress, because, for once, her private life
took precedence. She tended to the ailing members of her family, all of whom fell
sick with the flu at the same time. On June 20, when Henri was still recuperating, they embarked on a trip she had begun planning a year earlier—while on her
relentlessly long and demanding 1907 tour—to celebrate their tenth wedding anniversary. They traveled through Geneva to the Alpine resort of Combloux, where
they vacationed together for the unprecedented length of two months. There they
spent afternoons sipping tea on the terrace, reading, and writing letters. Nelly
continued her study of Italian and took long walks alone or with others in the
pine forests; Mireille and the Montupets joined them for a week in August. At the
end of their vacation, Henri returned to Paris alone, and Nelly thereafter explored
the glaciers on her own, although saddened by her husband's departure.[16]

Nelly then implemented the next segment of her long-term plan: to pay for
the Alpine holiday they had just taken by lecturing. On September 4, she went to

Switzerland, where, over two weeks, she presented "Libre maternité" once and "L'Eternelle sacrifiée" five times. Meanwhile, upon his return to Paris, Henri set about looking for an apartment to rent. Montupet's generous loan the previous spring now permitted Nelly and Henri to move out of André and Paul Nel's apartment. Henri did his best to meet his wife's request for a "convenient bathroom and a dining room that can be turned into a salon-office"—-a workroom of her own (fig. 14).[17]

Henri looked at apartments in their own neighborhood, not only to be near his workshop, but to remain close to the Montupets, Andrée and Paul, and, of course, Mireille. He finally found an apartment at 107 bis boulevard Soult, one block east of their current residence on rue Michel Bizot. The apartment had two bedrooms, which they would apparently occupy separately, and a dining room that would suit Nelly's work needs. Henri was quite pleased that it was on the third floor, "not on the fourth floor, like the poor," and that a cellar came with it, as well as a *chambre de bonne* (maid's room) on the seventh floor, so that the domestic they planned to hire would not have to live on their premises. Moreover, it was the least expensive of the apartments he had looked at, costing 800 francs per year. Meanwhile, Henri also undertook the task of hiring a maid at the rate of 45 francs per month, which he thought too expensive; but Andrée assured him it would be impossible to find one for less. He then arranged to have gas outlets and carpets installed to Nelly's specifications.[18]

By the time she returned to Paris on September 20, Nelly had spent more than five of nine months away; they had seen Mireille briefly in Combloux, but neither she nor Henri had seen their son all summer. When Henri returned to Paris at the end of August, Nelly asked, "How do you find Paris and Nono?" to which he responded, "Nono is really nice, he speaks all the time about his mama, and says to me, 'Faut zy dire que je l'emboie' [in baby talk: 'Tell her that I hug her']." In subsequent days he uttered many more such expressions of affection through his father. Embarking on his fifth year, however, Nono continued to be ill-mannered and difficult with his parents, servants, and strangers alike. Thus while fretting over which apartment to choose, Henri wrote to Nelly,

> Another question, no less burning and just as perplexing—Paul and Andrée have proposed to me that we leave Nono [with them]—my father's heart is without doubt stone, because it is not torn at the pronouncement of this proposition. Of course, we would pay them for boarding this tenant, and this would be on condition that they declare themselves absolutely satisfied with the situation . . . the question is to know whether your heart as a mother is as untearable as my heart as a father. I, who

have already reflected on it, think we are going to have a lot of difficulty rehabituating ourselves to Nono's roguish pranks, judging by the first days of my return. He is very nice—when he climbs on top of me it's usually to hug me—but that isn't always enjoyable, one has to be in the mood for it. It's not that he doesn't express himself in a very distinguished fashion—I heard him this morning say to Marie [the domestic]: "Ta gueule—-ta bouche bebé" [Shut your face—your mouth, baby].[19]

Upon receiving the letter, Nelly responded briefly in the fourth paragraph, "We have time to talk about this more. My heart as a mother does not seem to me to present any serious wound, . . . [her ellipsis] but there are other questions involved." She wrote this letter on her son's fourth birthday, but she made no mention of it.[20] For the next few years, Marcel continued to live with his aunt and uncle.

Once Nelly and Henri settled in the new apartment, their domestic life stabilized. She continued to see her children regularly for meals and Sunday outings, and Marcel usually spent one night a week with them. Montupet's loan also allowed Nelly to continue the Parisian bourgeois lifestyle to which she was accustomed, with laundresses, seamstresses, and hairdressers coming to her home to provide their services; she shopped at department stores regularly and spent hours getting fitted for tailor-made dresses. They attended the theater regularly (though almost always free of charge, having been given tickets by friends), went to the cinema, and always ate at restaurants on the maid's day off. Meanwhile, Godet's nascent business continued to preoccupy him and cause severe stress. Consumers were installing central heating instead of buying marble for fireplaces, he complained. He felt intensely uncomfortable as the head of the joint-stock company; potential shareholders were so "materialistic" that they wanted to be assured of dividends: "they never planted the flag on the summit of the ideal . . . they are louts."[21]

Roussel continued the political activities mentioned above, but she sharply reduced her speaking engagements, doing only one three-week tour in Belgium and three minor engagements in Paris during the first half of 1909.[22] As capable as ever of drawing large crowds, she put her usual energy into her performances and continued to sell copies of *Quelques discours*. The press lauded her performances, with the usual comments on her impeccable diction, irrefutable logic, beauty, and qualities as a wife and "perfect mother." Her reputation also continued to provoke her enemies. At the Third Catholic Congress of the Gospel in June 1909, M. Taudière, citing statistics that were certainly exaggerated, blamed her for the fact that the French produced only 12 babies annually for every 1,000 marriages, while the Germans produced 141.[23]

But by that winter, neo-Malthusians had begun to feel the distinct effects of the changed political climate. In February 1909, Eugène Humbert and Liard-Courtois were prosecuted in Rouen. Roussel was on tour in Belgium at that time, and while there she visited her childhood friend Jeanne Tilquin, who lived close to the border in Revin (Ardennes). The campaign against neo-Malthusian propaganda had become so intense in that region, Jeanne warned Henri, that "Nelly could have enemies if she gives a neo-Malthusian lecture. It appears that in Belgium [the persecutions] are even worse."[24]

Malthus Before the Judges

The police and courts brought charges of "affronts to moral decency" against neo-Malthusian propaganda almost from the start of the movement. The original law of July 29, 1881, on the freedom of the press made citizens accountable for "abuse" of freedom of speech as legally defined. The law of March 16, 1898, extended the definition of obscenity from the printed word to objects and also made it illegal to violate a private domicile with leaflets or other forms of propaganda. This enabled anyone—such as the infamous "père-la-pudeur," Senator René Bérenger (not to be confused with Henry Bérenger of *L'Action*)—to file a civil law suit if any neo-Malthusian propaganda came his way. The law of April 7, 1908, subsequently authorized preemptive searches for and seizure of obscene materials.[25] These laws sponsored by legislators such as Bérenger and Gauthier de Clagny coincided with the more aggressive and graphic campaigns of Humbert and others. Indeed, immediately upon the appearance of Humbert's *Génération consciente* in November 1908, Gauthier de Clagny denounced the paper as "detestable and anti-French" in a long debate about depopulation in the Chamber of Deputies. He urgently called for its repression, and his proposition received enthusiastic endorsement from the Right.

When Humbert split from Robin in 1908, he brought two changes to the movement that at once gave its detractors more grounds for prosecution and more reason to fear it: his approach became more sexually explicit, and he launched a more serious campaign to spread methods of contraception among workers— the most fertile element of the French population, and the class upon which national defense depended for soldiers. Humbert enjoyed immediate success in his reinvigorated efforts to distribute neo-Malthusian propaganda. He and Paul

Robin's son-in-law, Gabriel Giroud, published and distributed posters, stickers, and brochures. Unlike the earlier Dutch *Means to Avoid Large Families*, which had merely illustrated birth control devices, the new brochures graphically explained their use, and particularly the placement of rubber pessaries and sponges in the female body. Among these brochures were 20,000 copies of Fernand Kolney's *La Grève des ventres* and Dr. Fernand Elosu's *L'Amour infécond* (Infertile Love). Most successful was the publication by Gabriel Giroud (writing under the pen name of Georges Hardy) of *Moyens d'éviter la grossesse* (Means to Avoid Pregnancy) in 1909. This 96-page booklet also contained graphic instructions and devoted an entire chapter to the rubber pessary and its application. Thousands of people purchased this clearly written manual, and it was reprinted several times prior to 1914.[26] Humbert sent these publications gratuitously to all the deputies and senators, as well as to writers, journalists, directors of reviews, and members of well-known organizations. He opened a "sexology" library, which, in addition to these brochures, included fiction and nonfiction writings on population growth and sexual problems. But Humbert primarily occupied himself with the sale of contraceptive devices, profits from which helped pay for printing and distributing the propaganda.

The seventh issue of *Génération consciente* announced the group's commitment to reaching the most "miserable" workers in the poorer and most overpopulated sections of Paris and the suburbs. In this era of continued labor unrest, and increased international tensions, which raised concerns about the strength of the French military, the neo-Malthusian movement focused all the more stridently on working-class progeny as victimized "fodder" for factories and cannon. In the face of a nationalist revival and the birth of a new radical right wing, the neo-Malthusians preached antimilitarism. At the first meeting sponsored by *Génération consciente*, in 1908, undercover police agents mingled with an audience of 500 in the filled-to-capacity hall of the Hôtel des Sociétés savantes, listening carefully for language that would subject the speaker to prosecution for violating the laws against indecency. The police admitted, however, that nothing of the sort had been uttered. "They even openly opposed abortion, and Gabrielle Petit herself abstained from pronouncing the words 'pessaries,' 'contraceptives,' and others." The agents recorded the purpose of the meeting with words that echoed Roussel's own campaign (even though she was not there): "to indicate to women of the people that they must remain free in their bodies and only procreate when they want to . . . [the rate of] mortality is frightening among children of the people in their first year of life . . . the opposite is true among [bourgeois] capitalist women who only reproduce for economic reasons[;] but on the other hand, every night the fetuses they reject are carried away by the thousands in Paris gutters."[27]

As president of the League Against Licentiousness in the Streets, Senator Bérenger had succeeded in obtaining many condemnations of artists and literary figures—among whom he was known as "Father Chastity" and the "Madman of Pasquier Street"—on the basis of the law against "affronts to public decency." Calling the neo-Malthusians' frank treatment of sex and their illustrated instructions on the use of birth control devices "pornography," Bérenger now filed a formal complaint against them. This led to a search of Humbert's offices where Elosu's *Amour infécond* was found, which was treated as sufficient evidence for prosecution, because Humbert had been responsible for printing it.[28]

In February 1909, Humbert and Liard-Courtois crossed the legal line in Rouen. According to police, they had advertised a neo-Malthusian meeting by distributing leaflets to private residences and cafés. But they also did more: they glued neo-Malthusian stickers to mailboxes throughout the city, one of which belonged to a Protestant pastor and lawyer named Gast. Gast, in turn, filed a complaint to his local section of the League Against Licentiousness in the Streets.[29] In the meantime, such tactics proved their worth: 500 people went to the meeting. The undercover police who also attended recounted that Liard-Courtois had spoken first, explaining why workers should use contraceptives, and emphasized the sexual exploitation of women. Then Humbert took to the stage and announced that "anyone fearing realistic demonstrations" should leave. No one did. He then presented a picture, in color, of the cross-section of a woman's pelvis, "with details of genital organs"; at this point, he declared that the lecture was private and again urged those who might be shocked to leave. Again no one left, so Humbert proceeded with visual aids in his graphic instruction on the use of contraceptives. The police observed that he "placed his fingers in the apparatuses" to demonstrate their use. At that moment, the lawyer Gast and M. Widener, an engineer, appeared, along with the local police. Humbert continued his demonstration of sponges, douches, and other apparatuses. He further offended the intruders when he said that for twenty centuries, Christianity had created a "monstrous prejudice" and shame against "the most adorable parts of the woman," and that he wanted to see women "redeemed."[30]

By declaring the meeting "private," Humbert frustrated the efforts of Gast and the police, circumventing the letter of the law, while violating its spirit. The current law nonetheless gave Gast what he needed: Humbert and Liard-Courtois had placed "indecent" leaflets in the mailboxes and under the doors of private residences—an act that the revised law of 1908, directed explicitly against neo-Malthusians, had prohibited. In May 1909, Humbert and Liard-Courtois were tried and convicted in Rouen. In July, they appealed their conviction in court. The logic of the court decisions is telling because it recalls court decisions in the Cassagnac affair based on the presumption that women did not have the right to sexual pleasure without suffering. The judges in the Rouen trial found a leaflet entitled *Aux Femmes* (To Women), which was widely distributed in the hall during Humbert's lecture, to be immoral, because it contained the statement: "You are absolutely mistress of your fate; you should not be ignorant of the fact that science puts at your disposal the means to avoid pregnancy at will, without depriving yourself of love, and thus to avoid the unnecessary dangers of abortion." The judges decided that such propaganda had the purpose of "exciting the unhealthy curiosity and awaking the senses by encouraging the public to undertake immoral practices." They found other culpable acts in Humbert's demonstrations: he had "no fear" before an audience of "at least 500 people, among whom were minors of both sexes, of explaining, with suggestive gestures, the functioning of condoms, injections, sponges, and other devices in which he traffics to favor contraceptive fraud." His demonstration of how to introduce contraceptive devices into a woman's pelvis "could only arouse sensual desire and lewdness."[31]

The judges decided this time that such actions fell under the letter of the law. Humbert and Liard-Courtois were also found guilty for distributing propaganda to private homes: Gast, "as the master of his house, and father of a family, incontestably had the right to demand reparation for damages to the inviolability of the home." Finally, Humbert was found guilty for having printed the leaflets. The decision of May 12, 1909, by the magistrate's court of Rouen was upheld. Their decision regarding Liard-Courtois is noteworthy, for his role in promoting birth control was the same as Roussel's: explaining why, rather than how, to use it. The court admitted that under the law, they could not convict Liard-Courtois for what he had said in the meeting, but the leaflets he had distributed—"Ayons peu d'enfants" (Let's Have Few Children), the same title as one of Roussel's lectures—made him more than a simple accomplice of Humbert's. The court decided that the "why" aspect of having fewer children could not be separated from Humbert's role of explaining "how." It therefore believed it had enough evidence to condemn Liard-Courtois to a month in prison and a 300 franc fine. Humbert was sentenced to two months in prison and a 500 franc fine.[32] If Liard-Courtois could be convicted, so could Roussel.

Unnamed Ailments

As the proceedings against Humbert and Liard-Courtois began in February 1909, Roussel showed signs of weakening health. For years, she had occasionally complained of digestive problems; after she first met Dr. Danjou in 1904 and ate a vegetarian meal in his home, she converted to vegetarianism and kept to her diet through these years, apparently for reasons of her personal health rather than of ideology. But she also followed the advice of her mother, who believed fervently that illnesses could be cured or prevented with purging and sent Nelly to a professional healer, Mme Azéma. In 1908 and 1909, Nelly saw this healer as frequently as two or three times a week for consultations and treatments. Azéma guided her in self-purging, and massaged her, both manually and with electrotherapy. Though Nelly was adamant about sticking to her vegetarian diet, even while traveling, Henri urged her to "gobble down" raw eggs and to drink fresh milk while in the countryside. She also frequently underwent "milk cures," consuming nothing but milk, sometimes for several days at a time.[33]

In the summer of 1909, Louise Nel rented a residence for the family in Montigny-sur-Loing (Seine-et-Marne), near Fontainebleau—close enough to Paris for Henri to be able to commute there on weekends. Nelly, suffering from bouts of insomnia, considered her time away a "rest cure," where she would do no work, and where she would be able to escape to the forest for solitude. When she first arrived, Andrée, Nono, and their cousin Suzanne had already installed themselves. Paula Ripert, a professional Parisian vocalist, as well as her husband and children, joined them. Nelly complained bitterly about her inability to sleep, being surrounded by too many people and too much noise. Even the walks in her beloved forest tortured her, for she could not bear being with other people. She only wanted to be alone with Henri. She particularly lamented her sister's presence, for Andrée "made more noise than everyone else put together" and "screamed at the top of her lungs about how much she loves the silence of the forest." She wondered if she had the morale to return to Paris to attend a meeting that Jane Misme, editor of *La Française,* had called for contributors to her journal. But she lacked any motivation, saying that if she went, she would just be performing her "cancan."[34]

Henri did not join her in Montigny for several weeks, because business demanded his presence in Carrara. From there, he wrote to her with deep nostalgia about their trip in Italy the previous year, suggesting she that join him. He referred ironically to a conversation he had with three priests about the curative powers of Lourdes and quipped that Italy would be their "Notre Dame de

Lourdes," where they would both regenerate themselves. But Nelly sought out the curative powers of the forest instead. She said it helped her attach less importance to her "petty" preoccupations and reconnected her with her spiritual side and her enduring love for Henri: "You [and] the forest are evidently the most wonderful of all that the good Lord produced. . . . Soon, I hope, [I'll have] the joy of seeing one in the other." Unfortunately, Andrée kept prolonging her stay in Montigny, and by the end of June, Nelly said she needed several days to recover from the first ten days of her "rest cure."[35]

While in Montigny, Nelly wrote the dedication to a collection of articles she had previously published in newspapers, entitled *Quelque lances rompues pour nos libertés* (A Few Lances Broken for Our Liberties). Although the title used the violent and implicitly masculine metaphor of battle, Roussel again framed her feminist politics in the softness of motherhood, childhood, and femininity, as she had done in her earlier collection *Quelques discours*. The frontispiece of *Quelque lances* was a photograph of Godet's dual bust of Nelly and Mireille (fig. 9), a portrayal of motherhood more radiant than the photograph of Roussel and Mireille in Godet's workshop used as the frontispiece of *Quelques discours* (fig. 11). Once again, too, Henri gently took issue with the dedication, this time to Mireille. "You write," he noted, of the "liberties that she will enjoy. Don't you think it would be prudent to add . . . perhaps or I hope [?]" The final version read, "To my daughter, To my dear little Mireille, so that later she will remember that her mother was among those who battled to conquer the liberties that she perhaps will enjoy." Darnaud wrote the preface to this volume, describing himself as "one of her best friends," lauding her virtues as a spouse and young mother, and identifying her as one of the "above-average individuals, precursors troubling the general somnolence and pushing the world ahead" of whom Charles Letourneau had written (epigraph, Introduction, p. 1 above).[36]

One might wonder that Nelly did not include Marcel in her dedication, given that her greater goal was a new social harmony based on "equivalence" and better relations between men and women. "Nono" was, after all, living with her that summer. At first, Nelly got along well with her son, describing him as a "little fawn trotting over the rocks." But she soon found him to be "like the weather, changing and uncertain." He woke her up too early in the morning and lacked respect for her. In July, she sent him to Paris to stay with a friend for a week or so, but when he returned in August, she thought his being there would "kill" her. Nono was far more a distraction than an inspiration for his mother.

Marcel may have been a difficult child, but Nelly's depressed state of mind lowered her tolerance for what may have been the normal behavior of a four-year-old seeking his mother's attention. Four days after one of Henri's visits, Nelly wrote that she had hardly slept at all since he had left. She begged him to "bring me above all sleep, if you know where it hides itself." She wrote that she experienced nothing but "dreadful nights of exasperation, and lamentable days of despondency—that is the summary of my existence—the existence of a martyr, I assure you. Ah! It's all very nice, this 'rest cure'! Even though only delightful things surround me—the sky is splendid, the air exquisite, the garden so fragrant—I see nothing: my head spins; I hear nothing, my ears ring; I feel nothing but the stiffness of my limbs; and I only desire one thing: to sleep, to sleep, to sleep."[37]

Nelly's torment made a strong impression on Mireille during her brief visit. Almost ten years old in the summer of 1909, she already started to become a spokesperson for her mother's pain. When writing to her grandmother, she said "Marcel is still very bad [*méchant*], Tatadée [Andrée] is right to be very severe with him, but she is unable to make this wild devil obey. He doesn't spend a day without making a scene, most often about making him go to the bathroom." And in another letter, Mireille wrote, "I am getting along very well [physically] . . . this is fortunate, because Mama is so sick that she can hardly take care of me; she has not been able to sleep for a week now, and Marie [the domestic] hasn't slept either. The housekeeper can no longer come, but Mama says it doesn't matter, because things would not be much better if she could come . . . Marcel is still tiresome even when he is good." Nelly was still ill toward the end of her sojourn in September. Henri urged her not to worry about her health and said they would consult a doctor upon her return. "Surely you will be cured," he assured her, "and quickly."[38] Roussel returned to Paris in October, after having spent four months in Montigny. Weekly visits with Azéma and a Dr. Bonnier through the end of the year, and a much lower level of activity recorded in her dairy, indicate that her ill health persisted.

The abundant documentation offers no concrete clues about what provoked the insomnia that caused her such sustained agony in the summer of 1909. Two obvious changes in her life may have depressed her: her first experience of having the primary responsibility for parenting her son, and the new political climate that more aggressively criminalized and prosecuted neo-Malthusian works.

Roussel nonetheless continued her political activity. In November 1909, Humbert once again landed in court because of "affronts to decency" in specific articles he had published in *Génération consciente*. Roussel presented herself as a witness for the defense at his hearing, where she spoke about the benefits that lower fertility would have among the poor. The trial took place behind closed doors for fear of its effects on public morality, but newspapers reported its out-come, and named Roussel as one of the witnesses for Humbert. Upon learning the news, Darnaud kindly wrote that she "must have impressed the court." But he reiterated his conviction, just like that of the judges in Rouen, that teaching "young girls the art . . . [his ellipsis] of loving without fearing pregnancy" would result in profligacy. Moreover, word had reached him of her weakening health through their mutual friend Dr. Danjou, and he cautioned her to avoid this sort of activity. Then in his meandering epistolary style, he made a tactless remark: having witnessed the births of his three sons, during which his wife had not ut-tered the least cry, he did not see how childbirth itself could be a deterrent to hav-ing children. Like Nelly, he had had three and lost one—and "like her," he could criticize those capable of having three children but who "limited themselves to one or even none." This last comment enraged her.[39]

Because of her declining health, Roussel undertook no public activity in the subsequent months, but her ambition remained unabated. Still ill, she was then drawn into public life once again. In February 1910, the Group française des études féministes (French Feminist Studies Group) organized a meeting to dis-cuss *recherche de la paternité*. Roussel was not on the program, but she spontane-ously spoke about the need to provide government support for single mothers so that they could be independent of their seducers. Minister of Labor René Viviani presided, flanked by several deputies and senators, among them the infamous "père-la-pudeur," Senator René Bérenger. Roussel was curious to know what im-pression she made on the latter.[40]

That same month, Roussel received more unexpected publicity. With great fanfare (and accompanied by her pet lion), Marguerite Durand announced that she would present herself as a candidate for the Chamber of Deputies and ex-pressed the hope that Roussel and Hubertine Auclert would do the same. *Le Matin*—the third largest circulating newspaper in Paris—covered the story, but when more than thirteen other newspapers, including *The World* of New York picked up the news, they misreported that Durand had announced the actual candidacies of Roussel and Auclert. The news continued to spread even after *Le Matin*'s clarification two days later.[41] Roussel explained that she had neither the time to run for public office nor any interest in doing so, and that she thought female candidacies would serve no purpose—but she savored the publicity. Her reentry into public life was salve to her self-esteem, which had been waning since the previous summer because of her health. The following month, she spoke at a huge meeting organized by several feminist groups at the Hôtel des Sociétés savantes. The room was overflowing with a "very mixed audience," turbulent and vibrant. "I knew I was quite a celebrity," she wrote to Henri, "with its advantages and its inconveniences: the thrill of [audience] curiosity [as she rose to speak], then the impressive silence that fell with the announcement of my name, even though I spoke after others who are so well known; wild applause, and murmurs of protest, because there were many enemies in this frenzied crowd. . . . I had the impression, and others told me the same, that I was *the* sensation, as was expected." Like an actor awaiting the next day's review of a play, she noted impatiently that the papers had not yet covered the event. An impressive array of them soon did, however. Although Roussel did not hold as central a place in the press coverage as she must have hoped (several articles gave pride of place to the eloquent lawyer Maria Verone), *Les Nouvelles* reported that her "magisterial speech was the success of the evening," and noted that the hall had been so full that three hundred people were unable to get in.[42]

Later that month, March 31, Roussel spoke at yet another meeting to protest the persecution of neo-Malthusians and to make an appeal in their defense. Two thousand people crowded into a room at the Hôtel des Sociétés savantes. Sébastian Faure spoke first, arguing in moderate language that one should exercise caution in the serious act of bringing a human being into the world. Roussel then further explained neo-Malthusian doctrine in language far less measured than that of her anarchist colleague, in a speech that was frequently interrupted by applause. She railed against "the race of Bérengistes" and the hypocritical tactics they used to convict her colleagues of pornography. The meeting grew controversial when a priest, Abbé Violet, presented an opposing view, which met with indignant protests. Faure attacked the institution of marriage, which provoked "a large number of women and a few men" to stand up and heckle him. Faure then withdrew, and the meeting was "suspended in the midst of brouhaha and lively protests from a large part of the audience."[43]

The journalistic attention this meeting attracted was more important than the event itself. *L'Autorité*—reflecting the persistent and widespread anti-Semitism of the Right and its tendency to associate any perceived evil with Jews and republicanism—declared Malthusianism to be "a republican and Jewish doctrine, with the distinction that Jews, being prolific, are assured of power to nurture their offspring . . . and republicans, by their organization of the regime that exploits the wealthy, have every interest in diminishing if not eliminating those who rank among the miserable." The article concluded that France's depopulation, "so agonizing, so troubling for patriots and sociologists, impotently watching the extinction, the disappearance, the decrepitude of the French race" was "the attentive work of Jews and of the republican regime." Meanwhile, the speeches presented at this meeting were published in a 32-page brochure, *Défendons-nous*, which later came under further attack.[44]

Three years earlier, Darnaud had written to Henri about his fears that Nelly—quite healthy at the time—was overworking herself: "You have told me that Madame Henri Godet never feels better than when she is launched, as Nelly Roussel, on a vertiginous lecture tour. So be it! But this overexcitement seems dangerous to me." Nelly Roussel's identity depended on her public audience. After months of depressive reclusion from public life, her sudden activity in late 1909 and early 1910 inspired her to attempt a lecture tour. In May, against Henri's wishes, Nelly embarked on a tour to Bordeaux. They were both so concerned about her fatigue that she scheduled only four lectures in twenty days. Her travel descriptions were a far cry from what they had been previously; instead of delighting in the landscape or in conversations with fellow travelers, she complained of the "dirty countryside" and the "filthy train." But worse, she experienced stomach pains so severe that she could barely sit up and had to clutch her stomach "with all her strength" to counter the vibration of the train. Fortunately, she stayed with her friends Dr. Fernand Elosu—author of *L'Amour infécond*—and his wife Thérèse, who took care of her. Henri was so worried, however, that he asked Dr. Elosu to write him a letter conveying in detail his medical opinion about Nelly's condition so that he could take it to a doctor in Paris. He instructed Nelly not to write to him at length, so as not to exhaust herself.[45]

Henri took Elosu's letter to Dr. Bertz Maurel, whom Nelly had begun consulting just the previous month. Meeting him for the first time, Henri found Maurel to be "very nice," a doctor who loved his *métier* "with a passion." He spent more than an hour questioning Henri; he wanted to be sure that his own observations were in accord with what Elosu and Nelly described, and that he was not going astray in diagnosing her pathology. "It's extraordinary how he already understands everything you must feel," Henri wrote to Nelly when he left the doctor's office full of hope and excitement. "I am convinced that he will cure you . . . if you follow his prescriptions." The prescription was a rest cure in the country. Maurel recommended that as soon as Nelly returned, they rent a place in Garche (Hauts-de-Seine), where he spent his own summers; there he could observe her regularly. "The doctor conveyed so much confidence," Henri said, "that I am now sure that with a little discipline and a few sacrifices, and the help of your mother, we'll be able to afford [it]."[46]

In his correspondence to Nelly, Henri did not name the pathology Maurel diagnosed. Whatever she understood of her ailment, she behaved with both denial and optimism. Feeling better after the initial ordeal in the first few days of her trip, then gaining more confidence with her public speaking, she ignored her husband's remonstrances and carelessly allowed herself to become drenched in a rainstorm. Henri was furious at this news and insisted that she take better care of herself. He repeated Maurel's prescription that she make every effort to be idle, get moral and physical rest, perfect nutrition, and fresh air night and day, and avoid dust, including the rice powder she used as makeup, "a campaign [against which]," he added, would be "more beneficial than [that against] the corset," which Nelly also persisted in wearing. He went on to say, "In sum, you have nothing, but you have everything to fear, depressed as you are." She then painfully declined requests from her tour organizers to commit herself to another trip the subsequent year. By the end of her tour, she acknowledged her fatigue and lamented how sad it was, "after having made the tours I did during many years, to be reduced . . . to taking precautions for four miserable lectures! What a setback!"[47]

Unfortunately, the Roussel-Godet correspondence provides few clues about Maurel's diagnosis. The prescription for rest, and Henri's comment that Nelly "had nothing" wrong with her, but had "everything to fear" because she was depressed, indicates the belief that her illness was psychosomatic: her mental depression caused fatigue, anxiety, and intestinal cramping. These symptoms, Maurel's prescriptions—even his stated desire not to go astray—and subsequent events are ample evidence that he diagnosed her as suffering from neurasthenia.[48] One of the most common diagnoses of her time, neurasthenia was defined as a nervous disorder whose symptoms included headache, dyspepsia, insomnia, painful menstrual periods, and "cerebral depression, sometimes accompanied by peculiar mental symptoms." By 1904, neurasthenia "was on everybody's lips." It was "the fashionable new disease," whose diagnosis expanded "to accommodate every physical symptom imaginable and a number of mental ones as well."[49]

In 1899, Gilbert Ballet, professor at the Paris Faculty of Medicine and president of the Society of Neurology, published *Neurasthenia,* his lengthy explanation of the disease first diagnosed by the American George Beard in 1869. This volume saw three editions and translations into other languages, including English. Ballet "corrected" some of what Beard said, particularly as regards the main cause of the disease. Rather than the vague "conditions of modern life" that Beard had proposed, Ballet narrowed the cause to "over brain-pressure" (as translated in the English version), in turn caused by "excess of intellectual work."[50] Such work primarily burdened men, and indeed neurasthenia was originally associated more with the work pressures to which men were subjected. But Ballet devoted two sections of his book to women's experience with the disease, which, he said, had "been best observed and best described by Weir Mitchell," whose "rules of a rational treatment" had shown "incontestable efficacy." Women's neurasthenia, Ballet said, sometimes followed "painful disorders of the utero-ovarian apparatus," but more often was the "result of physical, intellectual, or moral over-pressure." The circumstances that created the "over-pressure" were the care women gave to men and children.[51]

All Nelly's symptoms fitted the diagnosis of female neurasthenia, though in her case, the source of the "over-pressure" was, of course, her work, particularly given the increasingly hostile political climate in which she was trying—with real risk—to conduct her neo-Malthusian campaign. Ballet systematically set forth and strongly recommended Weir Mitchell's rest cure for women neurasthenics. Fortunately, Dr. Maurel did not insist on all its most stringent elements—complete isolation, confinement to bed, total immobility—but he and subsequent doctors and health professionals did insist on rest, offered endless advice about diet, and administered electrotherapy—all common treatments for the disease.[52]

Upon her return to Paris from her tour of the southwest, Roussel immediately followed Dr. Maurel's recommendations. On June 26, she began a three-and-a-half-month rest cure in Vaucresson, near Garches, a short distance west of Paris, where she shared a boardinghouse with the landlady and several other women. Henri came every week and spent two or three days with her. Nelly passed her time socializing with the other residents and receiving visitors from Paris—her mother, her sister, occasionally the children, and a few close friends. Otherwise, she rested and took walks. Dr. Maurel came to see her every Sunday. In her third month there, she wrote Henri that she had just "spent my fourth good night! Four good nights in a row! This makes one believe in miracles!" She added, however, "there always has to be something that torments me, for I had intestinal pains all day yesterday, and they have not completely gone." A few days later, Mireille visited, and she then wrote to her father expressing guilt that she had contracted a cold and passed it on to her mother. Nelly added that she had caught the cold "just at the moment she was beginning to feel better" and had then relapsed into sickness.[53]

Roussel returned to Paris on October 3, 1910. That fall she made no public appearances, but she did attend a few meetings of the UFF, and on November 26, she read a new playlet *Pourquoi elles vont à l'église* (Why Women Go to Church) publicly for the first time. On the surface, this piece represented the essence of Roussel's arguments in her lecture on women and freethinking, and it drew concretely on her observations in the provinces of the relationships freethinkers—including Darnaud—had with their wives. This play also represented the deadly boredom of a Madame Bovary, a state of frustration Nelly herself felt with her re-trenchment from public life. The scene takes place in the home of M. Bourdieu, "a modest employee, a civil servant, or a well-off worker," located in the administrative center of a canton—in other words, a midsized town populated with the sort of people to whom Roussel brought her lectures. M. Bourdieu serves as the vice-president of the local association of freethinkers. The play opens with Mme Bourdieu, a young, plainly but "correctly" dressed woman, setting the dining room table for Sunday lunch, anxiously looking at her watch. Her husband, out at the café having an apéritif with his freethinking friends, is late, and she fears the roast she is cooking will be overdone. Suddenly, her "gay, exuberant, stylishly dressed," neighbor, Mme Rosier (Rosebush) drops by on her return from Sunday mass. Mme Rosier describes the religious spectacle of lights, music, flowers, excellent brioche, and most exciting, a female singer from Paris (a version of Roussel herself). She urges her neighbor to come with her to vespers, where the singer will be performing again. Mme Bourdieu protests that it would be hypocritical for her to attend, since she professes no religion. Mme Rosier replies that one does not go to church for religion; rather, one goes to "be able to get dressed up, to see people, to hear music, to be entertained." After all, there is little to do for amusement in their town. She pities Mme Bourdieu for spending her Sundays alone and bored and promises to stop by again on her way out that afternoon.

Monsieur Bourdieu finally returns. He complains bitterly that the roast beef is leathery. When his wife attributes this to his tardiness, Bourdieu responds, "It seems to me you can easily arrange not to overcook a roast, especially when that's all you have to do." He proceeds to eat in silence while reading the newspaper. When she asks him for news from his morning, he replies "Nothing, or at least, nothing that interests you. We only spoke about serious things"—politics, propaganda—"not women's business . . . one returns home to eat his soup tranquilly, without worrying about anything else. That's how I understand family life."

M. Bourdieu then says he will spend the rest of the afternoon in the café, as usual. His wife mentions that she would like to go out too, but cannot go alone, and tells him about Mme Rosier's invitation to attend vespers. Bordieu assumes she is joking. She protests that she is bored; he replies that surely she can find plenty of household chores to do. Furthermore, he forbids her to go to church, because it would compromise his position as vice president of the freethinkers. After he leaves, Mme Bourdieu picks up the newspaper he has been reading and discovers that it features a story about her husband speaking at a banquet on the virtues of freethinking principles: "the respect of human individuality, freely in bloom. It is necessary to *interest all those who surround us* in our efforts, in our ideal, and render them sympathetic to it *by a personal conduct beyond all reproach.*" Seeing through his hypocrisy, Mme Bourdieu changes her clothes and goes off to vespers with her neighbor.[54]

The rebelling wife and tyrant husband had become "well-established theatrical types" by 1910.[55] But Roussel's portrayal came from her authentic experiences in the provinces, where the separation between gendered spheres was far more entrenched than in Paris. It also went to the heart of her dispute with the assumption of freethinkers that women were irredeemably dominated by priests and were "by nature" attracted to religion, as well as with the hypocrisy she perceived in the gap between ideals and their implementation. When Darnaud—whose wife regularly attended mass—read the play, he told her it was a "little masterpiece," a "fine pearl," and her other friends paid similar compliments. "What a genius you have for a wife!" Darnaud told Henri.[56]

"A Jaurès in Skirts": Revival and *Rénovation*

Roussel's rest cure had positive results, because from December 1910 through May of 1911 she made eleven public presentations, a marked increase over the previous year. Press coverage of these lectures, moreover, indicates that her ability to dazzle audiences remained as strong as ever. In early March, for example, she gave a lecture in Gray (Haute-Saône) on "Women and Freethinking." The posters advertising her appearance had an "excellent effect," drawing 700 people—including 150 women—from as far away as forty kilometers. Roussel spoke to them for an hour and twenty minutes, and toward the end, she gave a "poetic, ardent peroration" bringing "the audience to the edges of their seats, hands in the air, ready to break into applause, piously waiting for the end of the sentence that was unfolding." Many in the audience, one witness attested, would have asked her to continue longer. Though she did not perform *Pourquoi elles vont à l'église*, she sold seventy copies after her lecture.[57]

Roussel, it would appear, had regained her previous health and energy. Now thirty-three years old, she enjoyed her reputation more than ever, and had little reason to believe that her career would not continue its successful path, albeit at a much slower pace than previously. On April 1, she undertook a two-month tour, more highly packed than those of the previous two years, on her now familiar route to Switzerland, then the south, with her usual long stop in Monaco. Not only did she recapture her past glory, but this time, the act of speaking made her "fatigue vanish," unlike her previous tour, which had caused so much fatigue.

And despite the incompetence she encountered among some of the provincial organizers, she claimed she would never become "disgusted" with tours, because she had "a love for propaganda and travel that had a phenomenal hold on her heart." She continued to draw sustenance from her ability to dazzle audiences, noting that her "new dress produced its little effect." A worker in Millau (Aveyron), an industrial town in a "lost and inaccessible region" specializing in the production of gloves, commented "She's a Jaurès in skirts," comparing her with the famous leader of the Socialist Party. Nelly compared her successes with those of Sébastian Faure, who easily attracted audiences of 4,000. She also drew satisfaction from the continued sales of *Par la révolte, Quelques discours, Quelques lances rompues,* and *Pourquoi elles vont à l'église;* she read her new play with great success after her lectures on this tour.[58]

While in Monaco, Roussel received a speaking invitation from the newly constituted Fédération des groups ouvriers néo-malthusiens (Federation of Neo-Malthusian Worker Groups), or GONM—whose very existence confirmed the success, especially in the eyes of the police, of the neo-Malthusians' efforts to reach the working classes. One of the founders of this federation, Luis Verliac, was a member of the mechanics' union and a former member of the League of Human Regeneration. When the latter organization folded, he assumed Robin's mission—independently of Eugène Humbert—of taking birth control methods to workers; he established a cooperative to reduce their cost, and along with others, organized a series of public lectures. The GONM had its start in March 1911, and consisted of small groups of workers, primarily in Paris and in the regions around Brest (Finistère) and Auxerre (Yonne). As its name suggests, it had a syndicalist base. It included some key people, such as Dr. Sicard de Plauzolles of the League of the Rights of Man, and Georges Yvetôt, head of the General Confederation of Labor (CGT), the federation of French syndicates. The GONM advertised itself and its ideology—which included anti-militarism and anti-alcoholism as well as neo-Malthusianism—through its monthly newspaper, *Rénovation.*

With the exception of Francis Ronsin, historians have paid no attention to the GONM, because its membership was small and dispersed. The police and anti-Malthusian groups paid a good deal of attention to it, however, because they considered it a serious threat to social order. The group in Brest originated among militant workers in the naval arsenal, and the police regarded it as a dangerous, subversive influence on a conservative, traditional, Breton population, with healthy fertility. In Auxerre, the group posed an opposite danger. The population of the Yonne already had an exceptionally low birthrate, and the neo-Malthusian message there sanctioned and strengthened the practices of an already converted audience. In both cases, although many in the labor movement vehemently opposed birth control, government officials soon viewed the network of labor syndicates as a conduit for the further propagation of ideas and practices that would, in turn, cause the French race to degenerate further.[59]

In response to this threat in Auxerre, Luis Toesca, a philosophy teacher at a private school in Joigny (Yonne), member of the League of the Rights of Man, and former member of the Socialist Party, planned to present a "public and contradictory" lecture against neo-Malthusianism; women especially were encouraged to attend. "Public and contradictory" meant that others opposed to his views would be sponsored and put on the agenda. The GONM immediately invited the "best orator who could treat the subject in a fashion that would not offend the delicacy of the women present."[60]

Roussel had never before put herself in the position of debating a featured speaker whose position diametrically opposed to her own, and whose audience would also presumably oppose her. Upon arriving in Auxerre, she wrote Henri, himself embattled with business affairs in Carrara, "Here I am, my noble warrior. . . . This evening is going to be a battlefield for me." But in fact, there was no battle. Toesca came across as a fool throughout, further weakening the pronatalist cause in this region. The GONM had suggested getting a larger room, knowing that Roussel—though invited at the last minute—would draw a large crowd. But Toesca refused, precisely because he wished to deter that larger audience, so 500 people jammed into a room that could accommodate only 200.[61]

The audience consisted of workers of both sexes, "ladies in superb finery, with flowered hats as large as the wheels of a cabriolet, employees and civil servants, young girls, soldiers, and children. And this crowd filled the benches, pressed together, stepped on each other's feet, . . . raised themselves onto the walls so they could see and be seen." And at the last minute, according to police, "a crowd of workers, led by members of the neo-Malthusian group and leaders of the Auxerre Bourse du travail [Labor Exchange], invaded the room." Shouting and protests ensued between those who thought the event should be moved to a different venue and those who wanted to stay where they were. Roussel intervened, commanding silence. Only then was Toesca allowed to speak. Even *L'Indépendent auxerrois,* one newspaper favorable to him, had little good to say about his talk and acknowledged that his words had been lost on the audience. Reading passages from the historian Fustel de Coulanges, poets, and the Bible, Toesca spoke for an hour about "every subject but neo-Malthusianism" to an audience that listened in polite silence with "mocking smiles, malicious looks."[62] Only five or six people clapped at the end. Roussel, by contrast, spoke with her usual success.

The undercover agents conceded that "at no moment" did her speech "offend her audience, which, on the contrary, applauded her frequently."[63]

The press and the police alike noted the irony that this event, intended as anti-Malthusian, ended up greatly benefiting the local neo-Malthusian movement. The police regarded this success with particular seriousness and blamed the pro-natalist organizers for allowing the event to be "invaded," for "the working-class element" had come specifically to hear Nelly Roussel, "a habitual orator at social-ist meetings." What really threatened them was the systematic diffusion of neo-Malthusian propaganda through an already-organized working class. Although the GONM had only come into existence that spring, the prefect of the Yonne subsequently blamed its activities for the very low birthrate in that department, and for a decline of 12,000 in the population, shown in the 1906 census. Statistics of-fered proof that neo-Malthusian theories were spreading "in the most numerous class, the working class," a phrase government officials repeated often.[64]

The GONM differed from other working-class organizations because, through birth control and anti-alcoholism, it sought to empower workers as individuals, and not just as a class; indeed, the individualism in its message made many so-cialist groups turn against it. Its anti-militarism, however, fueled resistance to the bourgeois desire for "cannon fodder." The phrase "the most numerous class, the working class" in the police reports thus acknowledged how much rested on the need to retain a sizeable working-class population for military purposes. So the prefect of the Yonne concluded some months later, "this campaign in the future, and by the contagion of example [among workers], may have serious effects on depopulation. I add, finally, that the theorists of this neo-Malthusian movement are recruited almost entirely from the antimilitarist groups." That same month, another report summarizing the history of the movement and the sentences im-posed on Humbert, noted that, in general, prosecutors "deplored the insufficient repressive legislation . . . as propaganda extends in the centers of the working class and is little by little considered as a corollary to the [revolutionary] syndical-ist propaganda; some magistrates think neo-Malthusian associations should be dissolved."[65]

Relapse and Resurgent Anti-Malthusianism

Although Roussel derived tremendous ego gratification from her 1911 tour and her victory with the GONM in Auxerre, traveling did not offer her the plea-sure it once had. She was fearful that her lectures would not go well and felt depressed when she thought they had not gone as well as they should have. As in the past, her schedule kept changing, to Henri's frustration, More than ever, he was concerned about her health. She did too much and did not know when to stop, he said, when she was on her way to Millau, "and now you're going to go and lecture in a horrible place, where there are horrible trains and probably horrible people." Nelly apparently had little problem with her physical health during these weeks of travel, unless she was trying to hide her symptoms. She told Henri that she was more afraid of falling sick than of any specific illness. More than in the past, though, she missed Paris, she said repeatedly. And she especially missed Henri more than she ever had. She wrote in terms of endearment ever more romantic, sending him "voluptuous kisses," and he returned the affection, writing of how he "looked at the moon, thinking you were looking at it too, and that our two regards meeting in infinity would create a new star, which would upset astronomers."[66]

The summer of 1911, as the second Moroccan crisis developed, marked another turning point in family relations and in Roussel's career. In early July, Paul and Andrée, still fighting incessantly, finally separated (though for less than a year), and Marcel came to live with Henri and Nelly. That same month, Henri fell seriously ill. His doctor came to their home to treat him with suction cups, a common application meant to draw blood from an organ afflicted with congestion or inflammation. He was bedridden, and Nelly became his caretaker, devoting all her time to him. In early August, they both moved into a sanatorium far from Paris, in Montigny-en-Gohelle (Pas-de-Calais), where they stayed until the end of September. Mireille and Marcel stayed in Beurey (Meuse) with Andrée, where the Montupets owned a summer home. Apparently unaware of the gravity of her father's condition, Mireille worried more about her mother becoming fatigued in caring for him.[67] Henri remained bedridden during most of his stay at the sanatorium, but he finally recovered at the end of September. After a two-week business trip to Belgium, they returned to Paris in mid October, having seen neither friends nor family for two months. Ill health continued to plague the family; shortly after their return, Marcel, now in boarding school, fell ill with a cold and entered the Lamotte-Beuvron sanatorium, where he underwent surgery to have his adenoids removed; he remained there for more than three months. Roussel recorded having visited him only once, the day after his surgery.[68]

Roussel's own health problems persisted, especially her fatigue and digestive difficulties. She continued to see Dr. Maurel several times a month for "stimulation shots," and she purged herself regularly with sodium phosphate. Mme Azéma treated her for neck and back pain. The absence of activity also indirectly signaled the state of her health. Throughout 1912, Roussel gave a few lectures in the Paris region, attended meetings of the UFF, and socialized with family and friends; but the sharp reduction of activities in her diary and the increased number of days for which she recorded only "rest and correspondence" indicate her withdrawal from public life. She also noted a new activity: crocheting. She became more involved with her children as well; she saw to Mireille's singing, piano, and acting lessons and spent more time with Marcel when he was home from boarding school.

Roussel's retrenchment from public life coincided with the growth of an increasingly aggressive nationalism that further inspired the enemies of neo-Malthusianism. The increased pressure they exerted on the government to outlaw the movement's propaganda infuriated her. One of the most influential efforts came from Paul Bureau's report to the Second Congress of the French Federation of Anti-Pornographic Societies in 1912, "La Propagande néo-malthusienne et sa répression." Bureau was a devout Catholic, professor of law at the Institut catholique and the École des hautes études, a leading "repopulationist," and member of Senator Bérenger's League Against Licentiousness in the Streets. He began his report by proclaiming that "no social ill is or ever has been as serious as the perversion of sexual relations." Neo-Malthusianism, he declared, had become "not only a doctrine . . . [but] a practical reality as well for unhappy individuals abandoned to their egoism and frenzied desire for pleasure." Its doctrine justified "control over physiological activity" that gave each individual complete ownership of his or her own body. The same logic, Bureau argued, could be used to justify suicide, abortion, and infanticide. Moreover, because the "anticonceptional recipes are not always infallible," their use in fact contributed to abortion and infanticide. Contraceptive devices would also destroy marriage, the foundation of society. "Thanks to science," Bureau claimed, "seduction and adultery have at last won their place in the sun."[69]

Bureau set the tone of his report by returning to the Cempuis scandal. He noted that Paul Robin, the founder of neo-Malthusianism, had not only provided a sex education at Cempuis for both boys and girls when they reached puberty but had suggested that little girls be "be initiated by older men, 'more gentle and more expert,' in order to avoid the brutishness of young men and prepare women for their proper role." There is nothing to suggest that Robin's ideas went beyond the theoretical realm in this regard—there is no evidence he was a pedophile—but anti-Malthusian propaganda kept alive the association of Robin's presumed sins with birth control advocacy. Bureau then traced the history of the movement, whose initial success, he claimed, was the result of foreign support. But he attributed its victory in winning over public opinion to the "supple and ingenious power" of the modern mass media.[70]

Neo-Malthusians could easily reach their chosen audience—workers, women, and the young of both sexes—with inexpensive pamphlets containing practical information. More effective in their brevity than a long book, these publications insulted and vilified marriage, family, individual property and work, country and army, and religion and traditional morals. Bureau also pointed to the use of *papillions*—the gummed stickers that Roussel had placed on statues in Le Puy and that Humbert and Liard-Courtois had been prosecuted for distributing in Rouen. Neo-Malthusians, he claimed, used these stickers "by the hundreds and thousands"; they were effective as propaganda, because they bore "short formulas that instantly catch and retain the attention."[71]

Bureau expressed particular concern that this propaganda was reaching workers. A police search at the Brest (Yonne) labor exchange had led to the discovery of various contraceptive devices, and an arsenal worker had openly admitted during a public meeting that they were for sale on the premises. "What grief . . . to see [manual workers] put their energy into the service of luxury and of licentiousness, [energy] that in previous times upheld the noblest causes: to realize their ideals of justice and of fraternity [over which] their ancestors spilled blood," Bureau lamented. "Who would have thought that the capitalism they detested would . . . easily conquer a proletariat disorganized by debauchery and weakened by the crudest pleasures?"[72]

Bureau also bitterly lamented the legal limits to stopping the spread of this propaganda. He recalled that in 1907, Minister of Justice Darlan had promised vigilance and "energetic action" to end neo-Malthusian activities, but without result. In 1910, Minister of Justice Girard submitted a bill to strengthen the laws of 1882, 1898, and 1908 against affronts to good morals; the bill was still under examination in 1912. Bureau insisted that if such propaganda were allowed to continue with impunity, "it will become obvious that France definitively renounces all hope of sustaining its place among the great nations." Both the doctrine and the practice of neo-Malthusianism were "crimes against the fatherland."[73]

The same year of his report, Bureau appealed directly to workers when he presented a talk at the popular university of the Faubourg Saint-Antoine; Roussel, Madeleine Pelletier, and Humbert (who had just been sentenced to six months in prison) attended. The title of Bureau's talk was "A Scourge for France and for Humanity: Neo-Malthusianism." He presented statistics proving that Germany would soon have an army twice the size of the French. Again, however, he stressed most strongly the moral question, as well as the relationship between sacrifice and female sexuality: "To suppress the fear of motherhood is to destroy the home, the family, the country. . . . The individual is not made for pleasure, but for devotion, sacrifice, and heroism. The bourgeoisie is largely neo-Malthusian [it practices birth control], and this is deplorable, but the people close to nature [workers] will not allow themselves to be counseled by the criminal doctrines of neo-Malthusianism and will continue to give children to France and to humanity." It is both curious and telling that Bureau and other pronatalists openly recognized that the bourgeoisie practiced birth control but seemed to accept it as an inevitable fact. The audience received Bureau's lecture politely, but when Humbert directly asked Bureau whether he thought Malthusians should be prosecuted, the law professor equivocated. The audience stood up and shouted that he had to respond "yes or no." Bureau effectively threw down the gauntlet in his answer, advocating restrictions on freedom of speech: "All acts are not permitted, all opinions should not be either."[74]

It would take another eight years for the National Assembly to outlaw neo-Malthusian propaganda, but Bureau's report and subsequent ones like it helped influence the decision, particularly with the argument that contraceptive methods—in their fallibility—actually promoted abortion.[75] But apart from his and other natalists' ultimately successful influence on the National Assembly, their efforts also reveal the perceived success of the neo-Malthusian movement. A twofold concern stands out in this rhetoric: the perception that this doctrine had reached the working classes, and a fear that female sexuality, untempered by motherhood, would destroy the national moral fabric. Indeed, this latter concern seemed to carry at least as much weight as the fear of depopulation.

The same year that Paul Bureau and others escalated the anti-Malthusian campaign, a sad event occurred that had symbolic value for neo-Malthusianism, as well as for Roussel personally: on August 31, 1912, the anniversary of his being fired at Cempuis, Paul Robin killed himself with multiple doses of chlorhydrate of morphine dissolved in alcohol. Two years earlier, Robin had written, "I feel my role is finished . . . I must die, put myself to sleep, without nightmares, without dreams, from which there will no longer be an awakening."[76] Already feeling terrible physical pain then, his state of health had further deteriorated, with loss of eyesight, memory, and motor faculties, all of which contributed to a severe depression. While his health and his philosophical beliefs drove him to suicide—even with this act, he did not abandon his highest principles: he donated his body to science, and even tried to record for posterity the effect of the poison on his body as he died. Robin had carefully prepared his family for it, but they were nonetheless deeply moved by his death. Roussel wrote an obituary, in which she lauded Robin as her "New Christ."[77]

Only a few months later, Roussel's health took another turn for the worse. In

February, she escaped the Paris winter and accompanied Henri on a business trip to Lyon and then went to Monaco. While Henri made excursions to see clients and to attend to affairs in Carrara, Nelly consulted her old friend Dr. Danjou about her health, and spent most of her time resting. Meanwhile, Marguerite Durand wrote to her about the performance of Maurice Donnay's *Les Éclaireuses* (loosely translated, "Women Trailblazers"), a play whose main character was one of the first Frenchwomen to receive a *baccalauréat*. Married to a tyrant, the heroine divorced him and took up a life of independence and friendships with other independent, professional women. To celebrate the fiftieth performance of the widely acclaimed play, Durand organized a panel of "real" *éclaireuses*, with herself, Roussel, Maria Vérone and Suzanne Grinberg (both lawyers), and Mme Cayrol (a doctor). Each participant was to speak for ten to fifteen minutes. Durand wanted Roussel to take as her subject "woman in the battle against the human misfortunes for which feminism can have a powerful influence, such as the battle against the misery of alcoholism and war." Durand was "enchanted" that Roussel was resting, but nonetheless urged her to "enter into the battle" at the Théatre Marigny, where the play had opened with brilliant success, with President Raymond Poincaré in attendance. Durand assured her that there would be a "rich and elegant" audience, one that held "fashionable teas."[78]

Roussel finally accepted with deep reluctance. One account of the event noted of Roussel's presentation, "To speak after Maria Vérone was not an easy task. Applause punctuated almost every sentence of Nelly Roussel's . . . she spoke magnificently. When she spoke of the horrors of war, and women's role in leading the reign of peace, she was greeted with wild applause." Another account, this one authored by a woman and supremely sarcastic, said of Roussel, "It was certainly with premeditation that this *éclaireuse* put a large black lace scarf on her shoulders to ensure that her indispensable gestures would take off in flight. And in this pathetic fashion, she supplicated men to give women power." Most newspaper accounts were positive. Roussel's own description revealed, not only the difficulty this performance posed for her, but the measure to which performance influenced her mental and physical state: she had been "dazed, stupefied, overwhelmed by fatigue," she wrote to Godet. "I went there as I would go to the scaffold; as always, as soon as I felt myself on stage . . . I recovered all my lucidity and all my composure."[79]

This event had significance well beyond Nelly Roussel's subjective experience. The play featured female characters who were not only independent in their professions but sexually independent as well—women who exemplified natalists' worst fears. After her divorce, the heroine's female doctor—herself unmarried

and with a lover—advises her patient that she has physical needs requiring gratification; the heroine then takes a lover. The popularity of this play, with its explicit
female sexual liberation, simply confirmed Bureau's assessment that neo-Malthusianism had "conquered public opinion." But also noteworthy is the fact that
Durand asked Roussel to deliver a pacifist message rather than the one about
"conscious motherhood," for which she was best known. The increasingly bellicose national and international climate may have justified Durand's choice. The
audience of givers of "fashionable teas," moreover, might not have so easily applauded Roussel's rhetoric about control over reproduction, even though it was a
theme more relevant to the play than pacifism. The *Doll's House* theme of rebel
wife had become widely acceptable in France, however, and received official support from members of the government during a period considered the height
of French feminism.[80] But the tide was rising against neo-Malthusianism, and
French feminism would meet similar challenges.

The energy Roussel derived from the stage did not last. From the beginning
of April—traditionally a month of lecture tours for her—her health took a turn
for the worse, and she did little more than rest, often in bed. On May 21, 1913,
she entered Humilimont, a sanatorium in Switzerland, for a cure she and Godet
could ill afford. Initially, Nelly felt deep repulsion for her surroundings, in part
because the sanatorium was run by nuns. From the outset, Henri wrote loving,
encouraging letters that included much about Mireille (Marcel was in boarding
school), detailed descriptions of his meals (no doubt to encourage her appetite),
and stories about her sister Andrée's air-headed antics—she was now reconciled
with her husband Paul and the mother of a year-old son, Jean. His letters also
suggest the gravity of her state. "In effect," he said, "you must have been a gro-
tesque figure upon arriving, and the doctor did well not to delay it." He and other
family members insisted that she move to a nicer, more expensive room.[81]

Nelly remained in the sanatorium until October 20, a total of five months.
Henri visited her occasionally, sometimes staying for an entire week. In between
visits, he experienced deep loneliness and wrote romantic letters in which he told
her, in unusually explicit terms, how much he wanted to make love to her.[82] She,
meanwhile, underwent a regime of diet, showers, bathing, milk cures, and walks,
and formed enduring friendships with the other patients. Her stay in the sanatorium, in addition to Henri's sluggish business, took a harsh financial toll on
them. By the end of the year, they were nearly broke. Moreover, within a month
of her return to Paris, Henri had to go to Carrara, where he remained until mid-
January, thus renewing their long separation. Roussel's symptoms persisted—
she complained of headaches, digestive problems, arthritis, and "sclerosis"—

apparently from poor circulation—and she continued to purge herself with various substances. In January, she wrote of how much she wanted to be "cured" prior to Henri's return, and said: "Now that I am better, I no longer have any scruples in telling you that I was atrociously sick, more sick than ever. I didn't dare write to you, not wanting to worry you, [not wanting you to] see in my letters my infinite discouragement and my frightening despair." Her despair came after she had written of her wishes for "a year of sun, from every point of view" on New Year's Day, 1914.[83]

Misdiagnoses and Missed Diagnoses

Roussel suffered from abdominal and digestive disorders, as well as insomnia, acute anxiety, depression, and menstrual pain during the last twelve years of her life. The symptoms fluctuated, however, and were not always acute—she had good days and bad, and her mental and physical states were closely intertwined. Apart from insomnia, the symptom she most frequently mentioned was intestinal pain, which showed its first acute signs in 1910—a symptom in keeping with the popular diagnosis of neurasthenia, as were several of her other symptoms. Some of the remedies Roussel pursued did seem to help at times, but the persistence, and indeed aggravation of her symptoms caused her and those around her further distress. The cure most frequently prescribed for her—rest—suggests Roussel's doctors believed that mental and physical fatigue (neurasthenia) caused other symptoms. But what if they had the etiology of her disease reversed? What if Roussel's intestinal pain was the sign of a real physical disorder that not only remained undiagnosed but itself caused her other symptoms—indigestion, insomnia, depression—for the last twelve years of her life?

A few months prior to her death in 1922, Roussel was diagnosed with pulmonary tuberculosis. Her doctor told her that the disease had come from her stomach disorders. Although tuberculosis primarily attacks the lungs, the medical and scientific world had known since the early nineteenth century that tuberculosis could originate in and attack any number of organs. The problem with extrapulmonary tuberculosis—then and now—is that it is exceedingly difficult to diagnose. Since the origin of Roussel's tuberculosis was in her digestive system, it is logical to deduce that the recurrent digestive disorders from which she suffered beginning around 1910, later followed by other symptoms, might have been caused by abdominal tuberculosis. The term applies to several different possible sites of infection in the abdomen, and it is impossible to know precisely which of her organs might have been attacked. But many of the symptoms she described match those in current clinical textbooks.[84]

Abdominal tuberculosis is a comparatively rare form of the disease. From 1975 to 1990, for example, it constituted only 3.6 percent of the total number of extrapulmonary tuberculosis cases in the United States. Even today, it is difficult to ascertain its patterns and symptoms. Its primary source is bovine, coming from the bacteria in unpasteurized milk. Thus it was more prevalent in the past, but because it was impossible to detect, its symptoms were attributed to other disorders. Ironically, Roussel may have been infected by one of the "milk cures" in which she so often indulged at dairy farms, where she drank unpasteurized milk, straight from the cow. Today, abdominal tuberculosis is treated with chemotherapy. Even if it had been more readily detectable in the early twentieth century, there would have been no cure for it.

In her pursuit of a cure for an illness she and everyone else misunderstood, as in her relentless pursuit to relieve female pain more generally, Roussel never lost faith in science. *La Faute d'Eve* (Eve's Fault), another short play she wrote in 1913, which was performed only for private audiences, embodies that faith—and her knowledge that progress could not come without struggle.[85] The "Eve" in this play is very different from the one in *Par la révolte*. Rather than being a victim of institutional oppression, this heroine is already liberated, and she is eager to enter into battle from the outset. The play begins with Eve complaining to Adam of her boredom in their perfect Paradise. She has carefully examined each flower to try to perceive its soul and the source of its perfume. She has explored all of Paradise in the same manner, and now that she is finished, nothing more can hold her interest—nothing new will reveal itself to her. Only one thing tempts Eve, and that is the beautiful, mysterious, and forbidden flower of science.

Against Adam's protests and to his deep anguish, Eve picks the forbidden flower and smells it; the world about her transforms completely. Suddenly, it is complex and fascinating. "We thought we could see, but we were blind! We thought we knew the limits of the world, but the world is infinite," Eve shouts. Initially terrified, then curious, Adam also smells the flower—but as he does, with a clap of thunder, an Angel appears to tell them that because they have disobeyed the Lord, they will now suffer fear, hunger, and cold; they will live among unchained instincts, blind forces, and countless perils. Adam falls to his knees in supplication, bursting into tears of regret and anger at Eve, the temptress. Resolute and proud, Eve says, "No, Adam, I saved us. Stand up. . . . What is called punishment, I call deliverance." Taking his hand and leading him, she continues,

"Let us enter fearlessly and without regret into the immense, unknown world." She beckons him to follow her to the battles that murder, the anguish that tortures, the love that consoles, toward pain and toward hope. "Come! We have not yet lived; we are going to live." Upright, proud, holding hands, eyes looking into the distance, they pass in front of the immobile and implacable angel.

When Roussel wrote this play, she did not know that she had yet to face the greatest personal and political battles of her life, and that France was about to enter a war—a new "unknown world"—that would destroy her faith in science and progress.

CHAPTER SIX

The Great War

Pacifism, Censorship, and the Disease of a "Weary, Wounded Heart"

I believed in Progress, Justice, and Good.
This belief was my joy and my support,
My profound reason for living
But faced with the dreadful madness of the World
I fear I no longer believe in anything.

Nelly Roussel, "Invincible Croyance"

One of the enduring questions in feminist historiography is whether the Great War, in its destruction of traditional modes of thinking and in the creation of new occupational opportunities, advanced women's status. Even if we set aside the matter of her health, the war did not offer Roussel emancipation, at least not in the ways most important to her. It completely silenced the already persecuted neo-Malthusian movement. Eugène Humbert fled to Spain just before its outbreak to avoid the draft, and the last issue of *Génération consciente* appeared in August 1914. Humbert's wife, Jeanne, remained in Paris, where, she said, the atmosphere was full of hatred: "No one spoke anymore, they only whispered. Everyone distrusted one another . . . our friends were taken over by panic."[1] War seemed to vindicate the populationists, who had long argued that the defense of the nation depended on its fertility. Jules Breton, a member of the Chamber of Deputies, proclaimed that Germany would never have declared war if France's birthrate had been as high as its own.[2]

Feminists were less receptive than ever to the issue of birth control; even prior to 1914, the patriotic impulse had caused them to focus more directly on motherhood as a justification for women's full citizenship. The importance of motherhood only intensified when the war broke out, rendering the climate openly hostile to Roussel's "freedom of motherhood" campaign. On the other hand, most feminists expressed optimism that the war would benefit women in the recognition and respect they would receive for shouldering the home front burdens. However, as social commentary indicated, female war activities could easily be read through the lens of the "eternal feminine." Women's performance of masculine jobs became emblematic of their eternal, self-sacrificing nature, peace would quickly restore prewar gender roles. By 1918, Roussel herself appeared to have yielded to this gender imperative. Having faced the outbreak of war with considerable political bravery, she ended it all but cloistered from the outside world.

The war and related events at once drew Roussel's family closer together emotionally, while geographically dispersing its members, resulting in a richer and more abundant correspondence. The Roussel-Godet wartime family correspondence also reflects a keen self-consciousness about the act of letter writing. Authors apologized for letters that were too long and rambling or too short and abrupt, or simply "improper." Correspondence became a source of contention in Marcel's relationship with his parents, sister, and grandparents, all of whom scolded him for not writing "proper" letters and not writing frequently enough; indeed, Godet especially considered daily composition of letters an essential part of Marcel's education. Even Roussel's letters changed. Hers had always conformed to rules of grammar and etiquette, and in the hundreds she wrote prior to the war, she crossed out only one line. Those she wrote during the war frequently had crossed-out sentences, sometimes to the point of making them impossible to read. Her "messiness" resulted from her fatigue, weakness, and fuzzy-headedness, she explained; but correcting mistakes in her word choice was for her an important means of maintaining dignity.[3]

Indeed, Roussel's health turned letter writing and reading into a collective endeavor. Often too weak to write on her own behalf, Nelly appointed Mireille or Marcel to write to Henri, her mother, or other family members and friends, and then often added a note of her own. Mireille also added notes to letters her mother wrote. No boundaries of privacy existed between Roussel and Godet, for in her absence from Paris, he routinely opened her mail—excusing himself for his "indiscretion"—out of curiosity about the welfare of her friends.[4] This body of correspondence yields a microcosm of the French war experience, as well as being a window into the complexity of their contentious family relations.

The Outbreak of War

Nelly, Henri, and their domestic Mathilde spent the summer of 1914 in a rental home in Dainville (Seine-et-Marne), approximately twenty-seven miles east of Paris. There they passed five tranquil weeks, though Nelly continued to suffer ill health to the point that she could not receive visitors other than family. Mireille joined them in the last week of July. They received the news of mobilization the day it was announced, August 1, 1914. Though Henri, at age fifty-one, was in no danger of being called up, the announcement nonetheless took an immediate toll on Nelly, causing insomnia and plunging her into a state of fatigue so debilitating that she could do nothing but rest for two days. Three days later, she mustered the energy to write her sister Andrée:

> I do not know what sentiment dominates in me, anger or boundless contempt for a humanity capable of such a monstrous madness! Ah! The pretty phrases of public meetings!! We have received an abominably sad letter from poor Juliette [her sister-in-law, whose husband Fritz Robin had been called up]. I think also of Mme Fonsèque [a member of the UFF and mother of her close friend Germaine Lambert], whose two sons are leaving! And then of Tilquin [her friend's brother], and Philippe [Nel, her cousin], and so many others!! This prevents me from thinking too much about ourselves, who risk no immediate danger, but for whom the future is no longer anything but a somber question mark. I am very happy to have Mireille with me, and I would really like to have Marcel. As for the other Marcel [Noble—a close family friend], it is useless to tell you how Mathilde [their domestic] cried over him; but she has regained her calm and her insouciance.[5]

Godet retrieved Marcel from Paris on August 11, and the family remained in Dainville for the rest of the month. The material impact of the war hit them immediately: oil, sugar, and salt supplies became depleted within three days. They began dining at the early hour of 6:30 in order to save on lamp oil. The locals asked them to prepare to help with the harvest, because the farmers had been called up, and they saw military trucks charging through their village, going east to meet the invading Germans.[6]

In these shocking early days of the war, Émile Darnaud, now eighty-eight years old, conveyed his optimistic impressions from the Ariège, in the southern tip of France, remote from the palpable impacts of German invasion. Because circumstances so prodigiously favored their nation, he wondered whether it was France that wanted this formidable European war. Darnaud noted that the Allies outnumbered the Germans, who would have to fight a two-front war, and he thought the French mobilization went "marvelously well—calmly, methodically, and with proud satisfaction." Despite the rise in prewar nationalism, few French people shared either Darnaud's optimism or his patriotic enthusiasm at the outbreak of war; indeed, surprise, worry, sadness, and resignation characterized general public opinion. The Germans first set foot on French soil on August 3. By the end of the month, they had occupied Lille and other northern towns and had invaded as far as the Somme river. Information about this latest advance did not reach most people until August 29: it was the first news indicating that France had been invaded. It was met with shock and disbelief. We can only wonder whether Émile Darnaud's sanguine vision dissolved as the horrors of the war unfolded. This was his last letter to Roussel; he died that September.[7]

Meanwhile, Roussel and Godet abruptly decided to give up their summer rental a month early. They returned with their family to Paris on September 1, arriving one day after the first German shells fell on the city, killing an elderly woman (a fact concealed from the public). Airplanes also dropped messages stating: "The German army is at the gates of Paris. All you can do is surrender." The day after their return, the French government decided to move to Bordeaux, a measure that hardly inspired confidence.[8]

The French had not anticipated the Schlieffen Plan that sent German troops into France through Belgium, and the first several weeks of the war went very badly for them. They culminated in the Battle of the Marne (September 6–10), which took place not far from the summer home Roussel and her family had fled the previous week. Though this key battle seared itself in French memory because it succeeded in driving the Germans back, by November the fighting had stalemated. The troops became entrenched, with the Germans occupying most of northeastern France. The first two months of the war turned out to be its most deadly period: the French lost 329,000 soldiers.[9]

President Raymond Poincaré's immediate call for a *Union sacrée* (Sacred Union) had its intended effect, particularly as the Germans drew closer to Paris. Its purpose was to integrate into the Third Republic all the political groups, institutions, or communities that had opposed the government and warred among themselves—the Army, the Church, socialists, syndicalists, and even anarchists, as well as the extreme right wing. The collective sense of innocent victimhood at the hands of unjust German aggression made this appeal compelling. Propaganda portraying Germans as murderers, rapists, torturers of civilians, and especially of children fed the impression that they were cruel beasts. Moreover, press censorship prevented the spread of antiwar sentiment, as well as any accurate knowledge of early military defeats and the numbers of dead. Laws extant even prior to the outbreak of the war allowed the military authorities the right to ban newspapers "likely . . . to have a bad influence on the morale of the army or of the population," as well as "anything that might be taken for peace propaganda." But the law of August 5, 1914, gave local police the power to silence virtually anyone.[10]

The *Union sacrée* and the censorship muted or realigned the vast majority of feminists and pacifists. Most feminists became caught up in the spirit of national defense and believed that advocating women's rights would be selfish and anti-patriotic; many thought, moreover, that women's contributions to the war effort would ultimately advance their cause of full citizenship. As Margaret Darrow has noted, women's patriotic role invoked their "natural" disposition for self-sacrifice. Wartime female patriotism meant sacrifice—suffering the loss of fathers, husbands, sons, brothers, lovers, and members of one's extended family. In the interests of national defense, women were told to "hide their tears and stifle their sobs" in order not to undermine soldiers' courage. Beyond stoic silence, they could exhibit their patriotism through an array of services, ranging from working for the Red Cross to knitting and crocheting clothing for the military and sustaining soldiers' morale with regular correspondence. Indeed, in the spring of 1915, the press promoted *marraines de guerre* (godmothers of war), a campaign that encouraged women to "adopt" soldiers as pen pals. Mireille Godet adopted one such soldier. The entire family took such an interest in him that the Montupets began sending him money.[11]

Nelly and Mireille willingly dedicated themselves to wartime projects. Once back in Paris, they donated old clothes, purchased wool, and began knitting. Caroline Kauffmannn, through the Grand Orient, organized an *ouvroir* (sewing room) of "republican feminists," and she and other members of the UFF attended training exercises for Red Cross rescue dogs. But Kauffmann was not content to abandon prewar feminist goals. In December, she wrote to Roussel remarking on how enfeebled the feminist movement had become, adding:

We would like . . to see you regain your health so that you can work on the sacred cause of feminism whose soul you incarnate with enthusiastic force, admirable eloquence that awakens those who are unconscious, and makes them share, almost without their knowing it, the inspiration that you [ignite], yes! You awaken obscure thoughts that suddenly become clarified. . . . Earlier feminists often had a forbidding appearance. [Your poetry and grace] . . . ennoble feminism as the cause of justice and truth; you add to it beauty, and by this means it will be better understood and more accepted. That is why [both] old and young feminists place all their hope in

you and ask you to take precious care of yourself, because your strength and health
are so useful to the world.

Attendance at meetings had dwindled to a handful of people. Were Roussel able
to attend, she would attract women "like a magnet," "dissipate the torpor," and
inspire new motivation.[12]

Battling the War and Censorship

Although Roussel succumbed neither to the appeal of the "Sacred Union" nor
to the image of Germans as any less human than the French, the war led her to
reorder her priorities, as it did other feminists. Within two weeks after its outbreak, she sent antiwar articles to the mass circulation *Petit Parisien* and to Marguerite Durand's newly revived *La Fronde*. Neither of these submissions, however, was published. The police had already begun to crack down on *La Fronde*.
Marguerite Durand had stated in her newspaper that German soldiers had no
"monopoly on cruelty," and early in September, she wrote an editorial calling for
peace. The police even forbade Durand's ironic observation that the first victim
of shells launched on Paris had been a woman. Indeed, they found even the title
of her newspaper (which translates as "The Insurrection") seditious, and Durand
stopped its publication that same month.[13]

In subsequent months, Roussel combined her feminism with war-related issues: women's work, pacifism, and internationalism. Mobilization meant that
many women immediately lost their husbands' incomes. Eventually, the government did provide allowances to the wives of men who had been called up, and
other women's situations eased as they began to perform men's jobs. But prior
to those developments, Roussel opportunistically used the crisis of women's economic situation to stress the inequities they faced more generally: "The question
of female economic independence," she wrote in a letter to *L'Humanité*, "is going
to pose itself with more urgency and acuity than ever before. Let us consider for
the moment only the practical side of the problem, without resorting to feminist
arguments based on the dignity and liberty of the female being, which would
only result in indifference. This atrocious war has mowed the husbands of young
women down by the thousands, obliging them to survive on their own. They
must be . . . assisted in sustaining the bitter battle that awaits them."[14]

In January 1915, an editorial assistant for the left-leaning feminist newspaper
L'Équité urged Roussel to contribute an article about women who had taken on
responsibilities "for which they had been previously thought incapable." They

loved the article she submitted, but it was "ruined" by censorship, according to the angry editors.[15] The article that finally saw the light of day in April said that while it was suitable to talk only about "the nightmare [of war] that haunts us, and the pains that restrain us," the "loyal silence" of feminists should not be interpreted as abdication. Roussel compared the war to a storm that surprises the traveler and forces him to stop, but does not distract him from the path to his destination: the goal of pacifist, socialist, rationalist, Malthusian, and feminist ideals. Did the war mean that women would have to wait to implement these ideals? "Oh, to wait!" she answered, "A simple word that can designate the supreme degree of suffering and of courage. But women are not just waiting. They know when it is necessary to act." Roussel said she was not referring here to "brilliant heroines" who commanded the admiration of crowds or to female ambulance drivers who fell on the "field of honor" (a phrase she always put in quotes) under a hail of bullets; rather, she was referring to the countless women workers who everywhere in public and private enterprises, without any previous training, had replaced the men who had been mobilized; and to the peasant women who had had to undertake harvests without either the men or the farm animals commandeered by the war. For all these women, "we must not ask for laurels," she said, but "instead [we must] demand citizenship."[16]

Other observers interpreted women's new work roles quite differently. Her journalist friend and colleague Urbain Gohier, who was neo-Malthusian and antimilitarist, also believed women should not receive laurels for their wartime contributions, but for reasons opposite of Roussel's. He wrote in *Le Journal*—one of the four largest Parisian dailies, with a circulation of close to one million—that such self-sacrifice was not only inherent in the female "race," it was woman's duty:

The Great War is causing civilization to assume the characteristics of primitive societies. The man takes up his role as warrior, hunter, nomad; and the woman once again finds herself sovereign of the home. . . . Rural and urban workers have adapted themselves to all sorts of new jobs; from the fabrication of shells to the tramway and Metro services, there is only one idea: duty. The man is gone? Well, the home must survive, the little ones must be fed, family life must continue. This is the duty toward the country, toward the husband who is at war, in short, *duty*.

And this race has always done its duty; it does so by instinct, without thinking about it, with no need of glorification; something that is closest to her being would be torn away from her if she were diverted from it. Devotion, sacrifice, courage in the face of peril or pain, an effort above and beyond reasonable limits is natural to our women.[17]

This article was one among many that treated the issue of women's work in this manner. Rather than viewing female performance of traditionally male tasks as a sign of strength and ability, most commentators instead naturalized it as new variant of "eternally female" self-sacrifice. It was against this very notion that Roussel had directed her entire career. As she clipped and saved these articles, she had good reason to doubt that women would win citizenship as a reward for their wartime contributions.[18]

Early in the war, Roussel became just as committed to pacifism as she was to feminism. She published her thoughts in the Geneva-based *La Libre Pensée internationale,* in December 1914, saying that she was unequivocally *not* launching herself into "the hymn of universal love":

> I do not dream of a world of inert peace, of beatific bliss, which is neither possible nor desirable. I know the necessity and also the beauty of the eternal instinct of battle, to which every living species owes its survival and progress. Violence itself, to my eyes, is not always inexcusable. But international war seems to be an absurd deviation from this primordial instinct, the work of a false civilization. Certainly, it is necessary to fight! But to fight consciously and freely for an idea, even for a wild dream; to fight against natural disasters, against social tyrannies . . . against an enemy that has been recognized as such, not one that is hated [just] because of tradition, prejudice, or obedience.

Roussel argued that the "enemy" could never be an entire people, because a "people" includes diverse elements, individuals who are soul mates with those in other nations. Hatred between peoples is neither natural nor instinctive, but instead systematically manufactured by those invested in armed conflict. She applied Le Bon's theory of crowd psychology—to which Darnaud had so often referred in his correspondence—to explain the modern means of coercion, an explanation that anticipates Gramsci's theory of hegemony and postmodern thinking two generations later: "Neither friendship nor antipathy come from profound instincts; they are political affairs. It is so easy for those who hold the press and education in their power to create an atmosphere favorable to their designs, to give birth . . . to contrived sentiment, collective and momentary passion that carries crowds away." The distinction between "defensive" and "offensive" war is inane, she argued, because the people on both sides believed that "the enemy" had started the war. Despite what the French had already suffered, she suggested, they should regard the first victims of war—the German people—who had been "led astray by perfidious educators [and] abominably sacrificed to the ferocious appetites of a madman [Kaiser Wilhelm II]"—with pity and indulgence.[19]

Roussel contributed another article to *La Libre Pensée internationale* early in 1915, which caused the French government to ban its circulation from France; but it received considerable notice in Switzerland and was sent to Germany as well. Her article lamented the official publicity about the atrocities of murder, rape, pillage, and destruction that Germans had wrought on Belgian and French soil. She feared such reports would incite French soldiers to horrific reprisals and would inspire more enmity. "Overshadowing the consciences of even the best," she said, "the war transforms into ferocious beasts the bad or doubtful elements of which modern armies cannot purge themselves . . . what [German] soldiers are doing in France and Belgium is no different from what invaders have always done in the countries they have invaded. The current war is distinguished only by the reach of the line of fire, the number of combatants, and the improved engines of destruction."[20]

Roussel's pacifism might have seemed antipatriotic to some. She cleverly deployed patriotic sentiment as a guise for her pacifism, internationalism, and feminism. She gave a talk entitled "Pour le salut de nos blessés" (To Save Our Wounded) in Paris on March 15, 1915. She delivered it at the prestigious Hotel Continental, under the presidency of Dr. Troussaint, doctor-in-chief of the army, to an audience that included Henri, her mother, Montupet, Marcel, her sister Andrée, her aunt, her friends the Wolfs, and other members of the Montupet family. Ostensibly, Roussel spoke on behalf of the Women's Committee of the Society for Rescue Dogs (sponsored by the Red Cross), to raise funds for the purchase and training of dogs to rescue injured soldiers on the battlefield. But she used this opportunity to criticize the war, referring to the "dreadful upheaval" that was "digging an abyss between the past and the future." Prior to the war, men and women had been "animated by the single passion of universal progress and of hope; but henceforth, the noble battles of ideas . . . will be victim to the bellicose aspirations of the civilized world." Now "philosophers and artists have made way for soldiers [and] the pen and the spoken word [must] temporarily abdicate in favor of the sword." Roussel then said that she was raising her "weak voice in the middle of the tempest's roar" so that she could speak about the only thing now in the thoughts of her audience: national defense and the salvation of the Fatherland.[21]

Roussel's task on behalf of the Women's Committee of the Society for Rescue Dogs was to explain that how these canines—whose senses made them more efficient than human rescuers—were trained to find soldiers on the battlefield. Roussel seized on the opportunity to portray the battlefield through the sensibilities of the stretcher-bearer—what he saw, heard, touched, smelled, and felt. Her description divested the battlefield of any honor or glory. To the stretcher-bearer, she said, the war is

> stripped of all its glitter, appears naked, shameful. For him, when the tumult of
> combat fades, when the exaltation and exhilaration that encourage and sustain fall
> away, when the mirage of glory fades . . . the "field of honor" is nothing more than
> a mass grave. No voice other than that of the pain that exhales in an immense, infi-
> nite moan; no movement other than the heavy black flight of ravens, drawn by the
> tragic odor of death. Who could be astonished that, in the lugubrious night, among
> the piles of ragged cadavers, the upheaval of an earth disemboweled by cataclysm,
> a man, reduced to his human means, cannot always—however highly strung all his
> faculties—discover the poor quivering, mutilated body, from which a breath of life
> escapes, too weak to become a signal, an appeal or a moan . . . so many martyrs have
> died alone, unknown and despairing.[22]

She also made more subtle points in her genuine effort to raise funds for the purpose of saving lives. For example, Roussel admitted that as a lover and owner of cats, she had previously disliked dogs. She had not only thought them "noisy, clumsy, brutal, malodorous creatures" but had seen their "passive obedience" and "ability to forget injuries," traits other people admired, as evidence of "a ser-vile spirit, without grandeur" (similar, perhaps, to that of the "eternally sacrificed woman"). Her observation of rescue dogs in training had changed her estimation of this species completely, however. In fact, the experience had brought "tears of tenderness and appreciation" to her eyes.

Throughout this lecture, Roussel manipulated the metaphor, if not the reality, of being silenced by war, patriotism, and censorship. Her own patriotism, she claimed, muffled her voice, for even though the Germans had many more dogs than the French, she "would never dare, for the honor of my country, make an avowal of such inferiority," if it were not necessary to do so. Finally, she paid hom-age to her sponsors by publicly expressing her fear of angering them by suggesting French inferiority in this respect. By acknowledging the mechanisms of silence, she evaded both official and unofficial censorship and gave voice to the illicit.

Roussel also used the speech as an opportunity to deliver a feminist message. The commitment to national defense gave her the excuse to highlight women's special contribution. After praising women's charitable work with the rescue dogs, she went on to say that woman would "repair the wrongs that men commit. Where he injures, where he kills, where he destroys, where he causes suffering and tears, she comes to heal, to relieve, to console, to cure. She is too familiar with pain not to feel pity." Woman, she said, was the "irreconcilable, eternal enemy" of war. Elsewhere, Roussel argued that only women could redress the horrors of war, for "it is we, creators, who know the price of life, who must come to abolish the works of war."[23]

Indeed, women across the world had already begun to undertake that effort. To establish principles to guide a peace settlement, Dr. Aletta Jacobs of the Netherlands (who as an advocate of contraception had a good deal in common with Roussel) and Jane Addams of the United States convened an International Women's Congress, which opened on April 28, 1915, at The Hague. French feminists refused to send a delegation, however, and even Hélène Brion, who would later be prosecuted for her pacifism, expressed reservations about this effort, because she thought that the Congress would call for immediate peace at any price, something the French could not support. Only 52 of the 1,100 women who attended the conference came from belligerent nations.[24]

Disappointed at the absence of Frenchwomen from this Congress, Roussel published a third article in *La Libre Pensée internationale*. She attacked the journalist Gustave Téry for congratulating Frenchwomen on their decision not to converse with "Austro-Boche shrews" (the French had derogatorily called the Germans "Boches"—wooden heads—even prior to the war). The "shrew" epithet resulted from the putative discovery of letters on prisoners and dead soldiers "in which German women encouraged their husbands and sons to exterminate our husbands and sons." Roussel wondered how, on the basis of a few "inferior individuals," Téry could conclude that German and Austrian wives and mothers were any different from their French counterparts. She recalled by name the women she had met in Hungary and Germany: "Oh! To see them again, to embrace them, to cry with them over the pains that torture us in the same way, to tell each other that in spite of . . . the men in arms who cut each other's throats, our hearts and minds have remained fraternal, sharing always the Ideal. . . . Perhaps this would give me consolation . . . for the few 'shrews' among us."[25]

In arguing that women—even across enemy nations—would collectively oppose war because they placed a higher value on life, Roussel appears to have been attributing an inborn pacifist quality to them. But she was not; rather, she was claiming that experience made women and men different: women gave life, men killed. Her argument nonetheless brought her into an apparent logical paradox. It was women's experience with pain, she said in her lecture "Pour le salut de nos blessés," that rendered them more capable of empathy. Ironically, this was the same argument Augusta Moll-Weiss had made in opposition to Roussel's campaign against female suffering. If women were emancipated from the maternal pain caused by nature, law, and society—as Roussel so wanted—they would no longer be "too familiar with pain not to feel pity." But Roussel saw a paradox or contradiction in Moll-Weiss's logic: if women had a share in public power, she argued, a new morality would emerge: war and war-related scourges that demanded female empathy would cease to exist, and female pain would no longer be necessary as a foundation for morality.

Enduring the War: Neurasthenia, Financial Stress, and Family Battles

Roussel presented "Pour le salut de nos blessés" three more times in March 1916. It was published in *La Française d'aujourd'hui* the same month. She planned to deliver it in the provinces, but never did—almost certainly because of her ill health. Indeed, this was her last public appearance for three years, until March 1918 when she testified at the trial of Hélène Brion, who was accused of distributing pacifist brochures.[26] The energy with which Roussel carried on her numerous activities in the first eighteen months of the war belied her ongoing physical ailments. Added to her worsening digestive disorders were increasingly debilitating menstrual periods and states of extreme anxiety. Her menstrual period became a routine subject in correspondence to Henri, Mireille, and her mother; she personified it as "Colcotar," a most "unwelcome visitor" who "terribly excited" her nerves. Her weight became another closely monitored symptom. By June 1915, she weighed only 99 pounds, wearing shoes and several layers of clothes.[27]

Roussel's abdominal pain set off a vicious cycle of anxiety, insomnia, and mental instability. She and others concluded that her symptoms resulted from overwork and a crisis of "nerves," even though writing and speaking had always been inherently salutary for her. She continued to pursue various remedies for her gastrointestinal disorder; she routinely purged herself with "phoscao," put herself on a milk diet for several days each month, sought and took rest cures, and took laxatives. In the last two years of the war she received abdominal massages, either manual or with the application of electric current, at one point on a daily basis. All these cures, with the exception of laxatives, constituted the clinically recommended treatment for digestive disorders that were wrongly attributed to neurasthenia.

In their concern for Roussel's health, family members sometimes worked at cross-purposes and caused further distress. The war directly contributed to family conflict in two ways: it fueled tensions over already existing political differences among them because Antonin Montupet favored the war and felt optimistic throughout, while Nelly and Henri persisted in their cynicism, pessimism, and internationalism. The war ruined Henri's Cararra marble business. By the spring of 1915, he and Nelly again found themselves almost broke, placing them at Montupet's mercy. Henri worked temporarily in his step-father-in-law's Paris office, alongside Paul Nel, Andrée's husband, for whom he and Nelly had long harbored contempt. Godet's sense of humiliation deepened with Montupet's repeated lectures to him about how to salvage the Carrara joint-stock company.[28]

Nelly and Henri's relationship with Antonin Montupet had always been tenuous and complex, not least because Nelly remained intimately close to her mother. Louise Nel and Montupet were, moreover, raising Mireille, and doing so with love and generosity. They had been generous to Henri and Nelly as well. Louise Nel frequently handed cash to her daughter, and through the war years, Montupet often sent them money orders, which cumulatively amounted to at least 3,000 francs. But tensions persisted, and each conflict revived past injuries. On one occasion, Montupet threw Godet out of his office for no apparent reason, and on another, Godet barged into the Montupet home without ringing the door bell and went straight to the master bedroom to see Louise Nel, an act that infuriated Montupet. In so tightly knit a family, lines defining appropriate intimacy with regard to space were often blurred. Anger at Montupet surfaced frequently in the correspondence between Nelly and Henri, and at one point, the latter started referring to Louis Nel's husband as "sontupet"—meaning something like "her angry old fart," perhaps. Nelly rarely referred to him as "Pépé," as their children, and even Henri (in third person) routinely did. In her diary, she always calls him "Mr. Montupet" or, even more frigidly, "my mother's husband." But the family correspondence also reveals that Montupet had the best of intentions, even if he was avuncular, condescending, and conservative. His generosity and genuine concern for Nelly, Henri, and their children made it impossible for them to extricate themselves from their reluctant intimacy.[29]

In the late spring of 1915, a family crisis erupted over Roussel's health. She wanted to go to a sanatorium, but investigations into such an arrangement led nowhere, no doubt because she and Godet could not afford it. When she accepted an invitation from her childhood friend Jeanne Tilquin to join her in the coastal resort town of Trouville (Calvados), relations with Montupet exploded. The resulting correspondence offers a rare glimpse into family dynamics and the nature of Roussel's multifaceted illness. When Godet initially informed Montupet of his wife's trip, he was "subjected to a lecture on expenses." But the stepfather's objections had deeper roots. For reasons not made explicit, he had had a serious dispute with Jeanne's father and said he could not bear to have Nelly "sit at the table of a bandit who wanted to ruin [my] family."[30]

This family affair became what Godet described as "good theater with too many acts." He concluded that his father-in-law had seized upon the first possible pretext for a conflict whose ulterior motive was to "get rid of us, since he finds us troublesome and expensive. After your return [from Trouville], if he wants to launch into the fifth act, my intention is to tell him straight out what I think, to put him at his ease and force him to speak frankly." Godet said he was going to investigate the possibility of employment in America through the Society of Artists. He would liquidate his workshop, and Nelly and the two children would move to the United States. And then using the wartime lexicon, Henri added: "If he sees us so entrenched, the enemy will retreat . . . and we must never be afraid." Roussel responded from the coastal villa that if Montupet persisted in his threat to ban her from his home, "tell him that I don't care, and that I am not at all fond of entering a house where I am obliged to encounter people who disgust me, beginning with my amiable brother-in-law [Paul Nel]. . . . I think it best that I not return until after the terrible ogre's departure to Fourchambault [of which he was mayor], and that way I'll see him again after the glories of his high municipal authority have made him forget all this." Even Louise Nel expressed deep concerned about her daughter's "lack of discipline." Henri's desire to escape to the United States—and to bring Mireille, to whom the Montupets were as deeply attached as her own parents—indicates how seriously relations had deteriorated. Henri continued to encourage Nelly not to fear her stepfather, a "wolf who snarls, but from a distance."[31]

After Trouville, Nelly went to stay with Henri's niece, Angèle Déraux, in Vaires (Seine-et-Marne), and then to a hotel near Dainville. New tensions arose as Montupet, Louise Nel, and, unwittingly, even Mireille pressured Nelly to stay with them at their home in Beurey (Meuse), which produced a rarely expressed sense of guilt about maternal and filial obligations—she especially worried about disappointing Mireille. It also produced a new "symptom" strongly associated with neurasthenia—indecisiveness—quite uncharacteristic of Roussel's former self. "Ah, my wonderful state of tranquility didn't last long, my sweet satisfaction of knowing what I want and must do!" She described herself in a state of despair at "*having to choose*, to fall again into the incertitude that has tormented me for three weeks." Still smarting from his stepdaughter's "disobedience," Montupet urged Henri to send her to Beurey for the sake of her health and blamed him for the family crisis. He claimed that Henri, if he had wanted to, could have prevented Nelly from staying with the Tilquins.[32]

Henri angrily drafted a response to his father-in-law in which he expressed his deep frustration over Nelly's condition: "Could I have opposed this trip? Yes, it's true, but the question for me was to know if this was wise, given the situation: Nelly having her [train] permit in her hands, and the idea in her head that this trip would improve the state of her health? That put me in the position of either upsetting her or annoying you—you to whom I owe so much and whom I like very much, despite [the fact] that it doesn't disturb you in the least to hurt me without any reason when something passes through your head."[33] On the subject of Nelly joining the family in Beurey, Henri stressed her need for the solitude: "I do not know if it will please her to go to Beurey, which is so far away, and where she will have stormy arguments with Marcel, because she does not know how to moderate her anger with humor, as it is necessary to do with children"; and then with reference to a fundamental aspect of her personality and the "overwork" that was causing her illness, he stressed: "she does everything with the same conviction—that is what is killing her—lectures, or discussions, or simple conversations, she uses all her strength in them—that is why the regime that suits her the best for the moment is solitude."[34]

The dispute also aggravated tensions between Henri and Nelly. As he argued against her journey to Beurey, she began to rationalize why she should go: she wanted to visit both Mireille and war ruins Mireille ardently wanted her to see. At the same time, she feared that the train would exhaust her and aggravate her gastrointestinal problems. But she further reasoned that a change of scene had always been good for her, and that it would compensate for the fatigue. She asked Henri's advice. He responded furiously: "I was . . . imagining that it was the solitude that suited you, and not Pépé's passionate conversation. The question is to know whether you are counting on taking care of yourself or treating your physical depression with contempt. . . . Decidedly, it is your lot to be pulled between contradictory projects."[35]

Nelly's indecision and sense of powerlessness deepened her psychological crisis; she wrote four or five letters to Henri over four days, but she was unable to send them. He in turn fell into depression because he had not heard from her. His fears about her health deepened, especially when he received letters from the rest of the family indicating that they anticipated her arrival in Beurey. When he finally heard from her, the physical appearance of her letters drove him to further despair. Although she had written in the same manner for more than ten years—neatly adding notes in the margins, sideways and upside down (in order to save paper), now her marginalia were scribbles that represented to Henri the disarray of her very being. But the content upset him more, especially when she wrote, "I just came through a ghastly crisis, a true torment of indecision, which aggravated my poor sick nerves." These words only fueled Henri's anger and frustration, already at a boiling point because of his overriding concern for her mental and physical health. Just thinking about the possible trip to Beurey, he claimed, had put her in a terrible mental state, and he blamed her for creating her own crisis. Still smarting from Montupet's suggestion that he had no control over his wife, Henri confessed that he had "surrendered as always to the desire not to oppose" her for fear of making her even iller; but in this case, Henri concluded, his own surrender only contributed to her crisis of indecision, and he felt "deeply discouraged."[36]

Roussel did not go to Beurey. Instead, she spent August and September of 1915 in a pension in Villiers (Seine-et-Marne, near Dainville). Upon her arrival there, she was in such pain that she could not even "read a newspaper and understand the meaning of the words" or write legibly. The proprietor, appreciative of her "celebrity," kindly told her it did not matter when she paid her rent. Her condition improved, but she was far from alone; she made friends with the other residents, performing *La Faute d'Eve* and reading her lecture on rescue dogs for them. Uncharacteristically, she engaged in séances with local friends from the previous summer, Mmes Bienaimé and Béal, whose husbands had been called up. Mme Béal, a "remarkable medium," made the spirit of Émile Darnaud, deceased a year earlier, appear in a hat. As Nelly recounted, "this spirit told us (using knocks) astonishing things, astonishing in that they were really from him, and could hardly be inspired by Mme Béal." Henri was not at all happy to learn that his mentally fragile wife was dabbling in spiritualism, fearing it would frighten her, put her into a trance, or otherwise psychologically damage her.[37]

Though Nelly's stay in Villiers proved salutary, her gastrointestinal problems persisted. Henri proposed she stop all laxatives and purgatives, and she tried this, resulting in "an intense gastrointestinal crisis."[38] By the end of August, he was convinced she needed medical intervention, and he visited a sanatorium, where a Dr. Hercourt and his assistant reiterated the now familiar refrain, as he told Nelly, that they had "cared for and cured sick people of just your type." Hercourt, who had examined Nelly on an earlier occasion, promised Henri that he would make "special arrangements" so that the sanatorium would be more affordable for them. It would be expensive nonetheless, Henri confessed, "but in the final analysis that doesn't matter as long as we get results." Henri insisted that Nelly could be cured if she set her mind to it and if she were far enough from Paris that she saw only family. But for reasons not revealed in the correspondence, she did not go into this sanatorium, and Henri concluded that Nelly lacked the conviction to seek the only thing he believed could cure her: complete rest and solitude, and isolation from everything that got on her nerves.[39]

The stress that Henri endured over his wife's health was intensified by the failure of the Carrara joint-stock company, his dependency on Montupet, and his need to find some other source of income. He was also forced to relinquish the sculpting workshop on rue du Rendez-Vous that he had occupied for twenty-five years; it was being converted to a factory for war production. He had to find places to store his large and unwieldy works of art, including the statue of Clémence Royer. After years of effort at raising money for the project, he had not succeeded in finding a public site for it. Henri felt a deep sentimental attachment to this space, and he compared his forced move to a bombardment.[40]

In the early summer of 1915, at a time when his antipatriotic feelings were most intense, Godet attempted to go into business selling postcards—photographs of bas-reliefs he created that represented patriotic allegories of war. He quickly failed because, as wholesalers told him, his cards were "works of art," and only "really stupid cards" sold.[41] He then pursued every possible industrial contact. Many among them, both family and friends, were profiting from war-related industries, especially Montupet, Paul Nel, and Fritz Robin. Indeed, the latter two, originally called up for duty, were returned home within a matter of months so that they could attend to their respective industries.[42] Their longtime friends the Wolfs also profited; Mr. Wolf was in the business of financing industrialists and was directly involved with a three-million-franc order for shells. Henri's desperation even drove him to consider asking Wolf for money. In the end, no doubt through Montupet's or Wolf's contacts, Henri settled on the production and sale of machine oil as a possible business, but again met with marketing difficulties. He hoped to get Wolf to introduce him to the socialist leader Albert Thomas, who had just entered Viviani's cabinet as undersecretary of state for artillery and munitions, so that he might obtain a government contract. But by the beginning of August, the situation looked grim. "I do not find the means of earning a penny, despite my work and my perseverance," Henri wrote frustratedly, fretting about what "Pépé" thought of this, just when Nelly had written that, to her surprise, she had little money left—not even enough to pay for her first week's stay at the pension. Their letters crossed in the mail. When Nelly received Henri's, she responded: "Since I hope that mother is going to think of sending me something, you don't have to think about selling your soul this time. It is true that we can sell the jewels first, which would be a lot easier—because your soul is too valuable to find someone who could put a price on it in the general mess of these times."[43]

Godet's luck then began to change. By chance, he ran into Billiard, an old acquaintance he assumed had been mobilized. Like the others, Billiard had more value on the home front in war-related production. Billiard put Godet in touch with an English oil company and a steel manufacturer, whose representative he became. While he did not make the millions he thought he would, his financial situation improved quickly. In 1916, he went into partnership with a man named Del Pozo, formed H. Godet & Company, General Factory Suppliers, and became an aggressive entrepreneur. Even while urging Nelly not to travel to the Montupets' home in Fourchambault in the summer of 1916, he instructed her to distribute his prospectus and price lists to the industrial establishments there. Times had changed for the antimodern Henri Godet, who had dismissed automobiles for always breaking down and believed that airplanes would never get off the ground. From the Taverne de Paris on the Place de la République, he wrote to Nelly about how bizarre it felt to be composing a letter in the midst of the noise of automobiles and the "soft perfume of gasoline." After a business trip in which he met with aviators, whose conversation "was not banal," Godet noted "it goes without saying, how lucky one is to be in living in a period where extraordinary things are happening." Despite his native cynicism, Henri Godet was finally "modern" in his sensibilities. By October 1916, he reported that his business was going "distinctly well." All the same, he continued to identify himself as a "sculptor."[44]

Mireille, Marcel, and Mathilde

No one in France escaped the ravages of the Great War, but people's experiences of it varied according to age, gender, and social status. This was as true in the microcosm of Nelly Roussel's family as elsewhere. About to turn fifteen when the war broke out, Mireille had already blossomed into a competent, serious young woman who shared many of her parents' tastes and passions. As with other young people, the war forced an early adulthood on her when the lives of close friends were struck with tragedy. Initially, she shared Montupet's optimism, and contrary to her parents' position, she openly expressed "anti-Boche" sentiments. She also expressed a keen fascination with troop mobilization and the presence of Germans on French soil. In the summer of 1915, about to leave for the Montupet home in Beurey, not far from the front, she felt excitement at the prospect of hearing cannon fire. Once there, she observed evidence of what she referred to as "kulture Boche" with contempt. Soldiers' outhouses became *salles à manger de Guillaume* (William's dining rooms), and henceforth *guillaume* became the family's word for toilet. "Admire the pretty color of the Eure [river]," she wrote; "it must be made with the blood of Germans."[45]

But Mireille then saw ruins from the Battle of the Marne, which transformed her: "I am beginning to see a little of what the war is; it's horribly sad, all these demolished villages . . . all that remains are chimneys or walls pierced with bullets. Everywhere one encounters soldiers' graves, French and German." A few days later, she sent another postcard of the village they had seen: "My dear Mama, this is what we saw yesterday; it is the most moving of what I have seen up to this point. . . . Not one house is standing, the region is desolate. Soldiers' graves are everywhere, both French and German, in the gardens, on the roads, one meets up with nothing but that. I have never seen anything so sad!" In principle, such postcards should have been censored, because they conveyed a stark reality to everyone who saw them that the censored newspapers and word of mouth could not communicate. Such images sank into Mireille's consciousness more profoundly as the sons, nephews, boyfriends, brothers, and husbands of close friends lost lives and limbs. Their close family friend Marcel Noble became a German prisoner of war and had his leg amputated.[46]

Throughout the war, Mireille not only found consolation in her studies but became nearly obsessed with them. Her academic awards and her letters demonstrate a lively innate intelligence. Throwing herself into the study of Latin, Italian, English, physics, chemistry, history, geography, and French literature, she worked to the point of exhaustion. Her efforts had such a deleterious impact on her health that at one point, she was forced to drop out of school. But she doggedly pursued her objectives in the face of increasing hardship and disruption. In 1916, at age 17, she decided to take courses to prepare herself for the baccalaureate examination, so that she could obtain a degree in philosophy and teach the subject. Such options had been unavailable to her mother's generation. Ironically, Louise Nel helped cultivate in her granddaughter a drive for the education that she had denied her daughter.[47]

Given his purported feminism and aesthetic sensibilities, it is also ironic that Mireille's father was far less keen than other family members on her idea of pursuing higher education. By the summer of 1916, his business was so successful that Henri imagined the opportunities it would offer Mireille: the "infinite diversity" of occupations, self-instruction, and possibilities of travel. She could use her English, and she would have the spare time to play the piano. He envisioned Mireille at some point replacing him in the business, "with her brother, or her husband, or even by herself . . . *independence is the most essential thing in life,*" he stressed. "The position of professor," he told Nelly, "even when admirably paid, *is a chain.* It's necessary to be on time, *to recite platitudes in order to advance,* one can get fired, etc." He, however, would offer Mireille "liberty, [but] not equality." She could learn to be a shorthand typist, for he would prefer a "patronne" (owner) to perform this indispensable labor rather than an employee. Emphasizing the seriousness of his proposal, he urged Mireille and Nelly, who were together in Barbizon at the time, to decide quickly. Instead, Mireille worked so hard studying for the baccalaureate that she again became ill and once again had to suspend her studies.[48]

Mireille's correspondence shows considerable maturity and an intimate, tender relationship with both her parents. Seeing her mother's declining health, she became worried and protective. During the family crisis over the possibility of Nelly going to Beurey in 1915, she first pleaded with her mother to come. Then, realizing her mother's psychological crisis, Mireille tried to assuage Nelly's guilt, saying, "you must not regret that you did not come to see me," and ended the letter with a tone of forced cheerfulness. Indeed, at times it seemed as though the mother-daughter role were reversed, as when Mireille wrote on the occasion of her eighteenth birthday: "I am happy to get your news, but above all, do not tire yourself out more by writing to me; that would make me feel bad. Take advantage this month of the solitude and come back to Paris with more energy."[49]

Mireille also provided emotional support for her father in the relocation of his workshop, and she aided both her parents by participating in the ongoing effort to discipline and cultivate Marcel. She tutored Marcel in English and chastised him when he did not correspond frequently enough, and when the letters he did write lacked proper etiquette. Mireille rarely wrote about her brother without biting sarcasm. Her attitude seems not to have derived from simple sibling rivalry, since she was five years older and they had not lived together under the same roof. Rather, it was a piece of the family dynamic, which included the perception that Marcel, unwanted from his conception, continued to cause disruption by his very existence, especially for Nelly.[50]

Marcel faced his own set of challenges during the war. It broke out shortly before his tenth birthday. Rather than returning to boarding school in the fall of 1914, he moved back to his parents' apartment and attended school in Paris. Henri, who was alone with him during Nelly's rest cures, generally had a much better relationship with Marcel than did his mother, Mireille, or their domestic, Mathilde. But Henri needed to discipline him, which he did maladroitly. He complained, for example, that Marcel was not diligent enough about his homework. One night "the animal" (meaning silly devil), as they regularly called him, returned home nearly two hours late, which infuriated Henri. In retaliation for his son's insensitivity to the worry and annoyance he had caused, Henri chose to do something that would "deliberately annoy" Marcel. "I fell on his green beans and pitilessly destroyed them," provoking "tears and grinding of teeth," he wrote Nelly. Marcel had carefully cultivated his potted *haricots verts,* and Mireille and

Henri had previously threatened to throw them out the window as punishment for his recurring misdeeds. Despite Henri's penchant to retaliate rather than to discipline, he, more than Nelly, understood that much of Marcel's behavior had to do with simply being a child.[51]

Marcel got on his mother's nerves more as her progressively worse illness further reduced her toleration for noise of any sort. In the summer of 1915, when Henri was making plans to visit Nelly at her summer pension, he asked whether he should bring Marcel. She responded that it would be better to leave him in Paris with Andrée, so that he would not miss school. But Henri cut to the truth of the matter: "It's not an issue of school; he doesn't attach importance to it; but the kid's presence would perhaps be a little too much for you [and would be] the opposite of solitude." And on the same subject a few days later, he wrote, "you seem to dread the presence of your son so much that I no longer know what to do." A year later, when Nelly was visiting her mother with the children at the mineral springs in Bourbon L'Archambault, she wrote, "however likeable my entourage is, I suffer from being *constantly* surrounded, above all, when the entourage includes Marcel, the terrible 'tormentor.'" A week later, from Montupet's house in Fourchambault, she wrote of Marcel's "laziness and *abominable character* that drives us all to despair. He can't say here that 'it's Mathilde's fault.'" The problem with Marcel was not just in Nelly's mind. When Henri read this last sentence to Mathilde, she emitted "shouts of triumph" that Marcel could no longer blame her for his bad behavior. Marcel was difficult for everyone.[52]

Mathilde Eyssartier was otherwise the glue that held the family together. Like all bourgeois families of the time, Roussel and Godet continued to depend on the help of a domestic servant—and more so as Nelly's health declined. They were fortunate after years of unreliable servants to hire Mathilde, who first came into their service in February 1912.[53] The war transformed relations between employers and domestic servants, not just because of supply and demand economics—domestic servants became increasingly rare during the war, while the need for them did not—but because the crises it produced in everyday life loosened some of the psychological, emotional, and class barriers between them. Such was certainly the case with the young Mathilde, aged twenty when the war began.

Mathilde attended Roussel's lectures, went on long walks with her in Vincennes and the forests of Fontainebleau and Barbizon, and corresponded with the family when she was away. The penmanship, grammar, and spelling errors in her letters reflect her lower-class background and a deferent attitude, but the letters also reveal a warm affection and genuine concern for her employers. They do not, however, indicate the power she wielded. Mathilde had control over when and for how long she would take time off to visit her own family in the provinces or to see one of her succession of *poilu* (soldier) lovers. Henri and Nelly had to "borrow" the servants of others when Mathilde decided to leave for several weeks at a time. Many of their own decisions had to take her wishes into consideration. Her willingness to accompany them determined whether Nelly or the family would go into a pension or rent a house or apartment while away from Paris. During one relocation crisis in 1918, Mireille wrote to her father, "Mathilde assumed direction of the [multifamily boarding] house and everyone must obey her here, including us." In the summer of 1917, when Mathilde was temporarily working elsewhere, Godet lamented, "It's the eternal question of maids at this moment; it's that way everywhere. We shall talk about it in Barbizon—and Mathilde will tell us what she wants to do." Mathilde was particularly fond of Nelly's company, which she found stimulating, and she especially enjoyed being with her in the forest.[54]

Roussel's Refuge: "Her" Forest

EXHILARATION

Hour of exaltation too brief,
Respite from my exquisite suffering,
Sublime happiness of a moment,
Reality more beautiful than a dream
I come, in the summer that draws to a close
To gaze upon your dazzling sight.
I come, vibrating like a lyre,
To proclaim my joy and my delirium,
Plunge myself, exhilarated, into your splendor,
Which in turn enchants me and tears me apart,
Autumn, heroic smile
of dying Nature.

Nelly Roussel,
Barbizon, October 15, 1917[55]

Nelly Roussel had always loved forests. She had spent hour upon hour walking and hiking through whichever one she came upon in her peripatetic existence. The forests of Barbizon and Fontainebleau (Seine-et-Marne) assumed such special meaning to her that she claimed them as her own ("ma forêt"). She measured every other natural setting by the standard of "her forest," and nothing was ever as good (fig. 15). Her devotion to the forest became more acute during the war, because it alone offered her respite and solace during these dark days of failing health and the suspension, if not complete failure, of all the principles to which she had dedicated her career. Thwarted from public speaking and political writing, forced into prolonged rest cures, Roussel found her voice in poetry; "Exhilaration" was one of seventeen poems she later published in a small volume entitled *Ma forêt*. Of these published poems, the first was written in 1909; but she wrote most of them in 1916 and 1917 while in Barbizon.

"Exhilaration," whose translation above loses the fine symmetry of her rhyme and form, exemplifies the mixture of dark emotion and sublime spirituality the forest evoked in her. "Hymne" is more explicitly spiritual: "O living temple! Cathedral of / Gold and emerald at every turn! / . . . I am your priest, your vestal virgin, / Whose love never sleeps / . . . " (Barbizon, October 29, 1916). The spiritual self Roussel expressed in her poetry is reminiscent of her youthful religious devotion, and of her first publication, a poem about the cathedral of Notre Dame. Although she had not completely abandoned her belief in science and progress, the horrors of war, added to the repeated failures of conventional and alternative medicine to diagnose or cure her worsening stomach ailment, magnified her need for a new kind of cathedral. The forest offered a tableau of beauty that constantly changed with the seasons and with the light of each day. It afforded her solitude and freedom from the noises that so enervated her, as well as the space for physical exercise and rest; and it gave her an outlet for literary self-expression as her former ones dried up. The forest, she claimed, made her feel sixteen years old.[56]

Marcel and Mireille both spent more time with their mother during the two summers in Barbizon (1916 and 1917). During that time she had unusually few complaints about her son; in fact, she wrote about him with warmth, and she genuinely amused herself with him. Godet and both children also visited her on weekends when her stay there extended into the autumn months—the season that held most meaning for her. Nelly loved sharing her forest with others. After one visit, Mathilde returned to Paris with "shouts of enthusiasm" about "Madam's forest," and recounted, to Godet's consternation, that she could not keep pace with "Madam," who, she said, almost turned a somersault scrambling through a ravine. Nelly subjected each of the many friends and family who visited Barbizon and Fontainebleau to her walking itineraries. She incorporated her family into the forest by naming her special places for them: "Mireille's and Marcel's Oasis," "Belvedere Henri Godet," "Tatadée Route." Because she considered the forest "sacred," she passed judgment on others based on the degree of respect—or lack thereof—they accorded to it. "Mr. Montupet" did poorly on this count, because he thought all trees were the same.[57]

If the forest offered Roussel solace, it could not stop her recurrent gastrointestinal crisis and other sources of physical distress. Her need for silence and solitude, moreover, sometimes made visitors unwelcome. As in the past, Nelly complained of her sister Andrée's loud, excessive chatter in the forest and expressed relief when she departed: "in the sudden silence, one hears all the songs of the meadows and woods better." In September 1917, Nelly's mood swings and Andrée's screeching voice caused a serious, long-term breach between them. Nelly felt "shattered," but she had no regrets. The two sisters had no direct contact for more than a year.[58]

If the forest could not cure Nelly, it alone was able to provide a measure of spiritual and emotional comfort, not only as a space, but as an outlet for her need to write and to perform. "Exhilaration," Henri thought, was among the best poems Nelly had written about the forest.[59] The autumn months that inspired it had special meaning for her because of the changing vibrant colors; but as her bittersweet poem indicates, nature inevitably "died with a smile." The autumn reminded her of her own mortality; death must at times have seemed imminent. But her literary production also revitalized her social contacts. She sent her poems to friends and family and read them aloud at a Barbizon dinner party in honor of an artilleryman home on leave. The hosts and guests seemed very pleased.[60]

Roussel extended her 1917 stay in the forest as long as she possibly could—until the end of October—when even the thought of leaving made her sob, caused insomnia, and gave her "black ideas." When she finally returned to Paris with her persistent digestive disorders, her routine centered on treatments by a therapist called Magnin, who massaged her stomach with electric currents to ease her digestion, the standard treatment for neurasthenia. She saw him nearly every day. When she was too fatigued to go out, he came to her home. If her weight is any accurate measure of the success of these treatments, they may have helped, for she gained five pounds from the beginning of November through the end of December.[61]

Paris Bombardment, 1918

On January 30, from 11:30 p.m. to 1:30 a.m., four squadrons of seven Gotha bombers each attacked Paris, each dropping more than 250 bombs. Some of them fell directly on the Godets' neighborhood: rue du Rendez-vous (where

Henri's former workshop was located), place de la Nation, avenue St. Mandé (where the Montupets and Mireille lived), and the cour de Vincennes. Altogether the Germans dropped fourteen tons of bombs, which killed 49 people and injured 206. Parisians suffered panic during several siren alerts through February, and they endured another bombardment on March 8. This time the bombs hit Nelly and Henri's street, boulevard Soult; 13 people died and 50 were injured. More bombs fell three days later. Then, on March 23, "Big Bertha," a cannon capable of hitting its target from 74 miles away, lobbed shells into Paris throughout the entire day. Parisians abandoned their city en masse. On April 1, Nelly, Henri, Mireille, and Marcel took a night train to Grenoble, where they arrived at noon the next day, three hours behind schedule.[62]

Roussel and Godet chose Grenoble because Mireille had a friend there who could help them find lodging. More important, they needed to go to a city where Henri could conduct his business and the children could resume their schooling. Mireille, who had once again decided to take the baccalaureate exam, felt particularly concerned about continuing course work to prepare for it, and Grenoble offered that possibility. The move was hard on everyone: the exodus from Paris produced chaos on the train system and led to price gouging in the cities to which Parisians fled. Hotels, boardinghouses, and apartments quickly filled up, and the few rooms available rented for outrageous prices. The trip itself was traumatic for Nelly. Already plagued by nervous anxiety and insomnia, the two months of bombardments and bomb alerts further destabilized her. Upon their arrival in Grenoble, she collapsed with fatigue. They managed to reserve a hotel only for the first night, and had no idea where they would stay thereafter. Henri complained to Montupet about the shortage in housing and high prices, and he was grateful to receive 670 francs from the latter.[63]

The following day, everyone but Nelly scrambled about looking for a permanent place to stay. It was Marcel—now thirteen years old—who found a convenient "villa" in La Balme, two and a half kilometers outside Grenoble, accessible by a tramway that ran every thirty minutes. The proprietors rented out three rooms, of which the Godet family occupied two. They were pleased that the house had electricity, and they appreciated the beauty of its location at the foot of the Alps. From one side of their rooms, they had a lovely view of the mountains. The other side, unfortunately, offered the unpleasant and ominous sight of munitions factories. At first, Nelly was able to endure the ugly sight of these factories by telling herself that they served the cause of national defense; but she later complained bitterly about the noise they emitted, and the railroad line running just below them that kept her awake at night. As Mireille described it to her grandmother, the cannon fire from nearby forts, and the "factory sirens that groan lugubriously several times a day, and even at night" made her think they were under attack, as in Paris.[64]

The family mobilized itself around Nelly's care, obtaining a chaise longue so that she could spend her days resting tranquilly in the sun. They immediately established a normal routine: Marcel started school in Grenoble, tutors were found to guide Mireille through her "bachot" studies, and Henri conducted business in Grenoble. The bombardment had shaken him too, for it brought back memories of 1914, when it had seemed that the Germans were on the verge of laying siege to Paris. Thoroughly cynical now, he saw no end to the war, and he feared for his own business if he lost its Paris headquarters. He came to view the move to Grenoble as a semi-permanent one. The attacks on Paris continued sporadically, and he worried that the Germans would soon invade the city. If they did, the same thing would happen there as in other places the Germans had invaded: refugees had to flee suddenly, leaving all their possession behind to be looted or destroyed. He thus decided to return to Paris as soon as it would be practical in order to shift the headquarters of his business outside of Paris and retrieve the family furniture and valuables. As he summed up their situation to the Montupets, "we have no choice but to be buffeted about by events."[65]

Because of Nelly's health, Henri had to remain in La Balme until they could find lodging for Mathilde and arrange for her to join them. It took two weeks for Nelly to emerge from her self-described "scatterbrained, stunned, numbed" state, during which she continued to feel head and stomach pain. Her "extreme weakness and nervousness" persisted beyond the first two weeks: every concern became an object of obsessive worry, and she feared her own mental depression as much as she did her physical state. Just as she thought she was recovering from the fatigue of relocation, Mireille came down with German measles. The proprietor was "crazy with fear about contagion," and Henri had to persuade him to let them stay. The maid refused to enter their rooms, placing on them the burdens of housekeeping, which Henri assumed. Nelly wrote to her mother about the sad month that had passed since their arrival in Grenoble—a month of "rain, cold, ennui, illness," and the "diurnal and nocturnal battles" with her stomach.[66]

Nelly began to feel better once she hired a masseuse, Mme Berthier, to treat her four times a week; she became strong enough to take 90-minute walks. They finally found a room for Mathilde in La Balme, and she joined them, which allowed Henri to depart for Paris on June 22, for what they—especially Nelly—assumed would be a brief trip. His departure sent her into a renewed state of profound depression and anxiety. She worried about what might happen to him in Paris, and she lamented, moreover, the worry she caused him. The day after he left, she wrote to him of the sadness and guilt she felt over her mental state: "When you are here, I worry you with my neurasthenia; when you are gone, I want you to think of me without bitterness, seeing me as I once was, and not as I am now . . . without forgetting that there are ways in which I have not changed, and shall never change."[67]

In the meantime, the ever-determined Mireille had decided, despite crucial time lost to German measles, to take the baccalaureate anyway, and she continued her tutoring in physics, chemistry, and English. She then took the exams—with great diffidence—at the end of June. Her other preoccupation was her mother's health.

Around 3:00 p.m. on June 29, Nelly was preparing to dress and go to Grenoble; she was still in her nightgown and slippers. Mireille was writing a letter to Louise Nel. She said that her mother was plagued by "Colcothar [her period], who is a person more and more disagreeable; [Mama] is not well these days, all the more so now that she is worrying about Papa being in Paris . . ."

Mireille's letter abruptly broke off in mid-sentence because the house started shaking violently; armoires with mirrors fell shattering to the floor as windows exploded, covering Mireille and Nelly with shards of glass. They tumbled down the stairs, out the door, and scrambled up the mountain into a meadow where, from under the shelter of trees, they witnessed the source of this calamity: the munitions depot across from their house had exploded. A second detonation followed fifty minutes later, and a series of others lasted until 6:30 p.m. Mathilde found them, and as night fell, they joined other neighbors and slept in a field. Mireille later wrote, "Apart from the worry over Marcel, who was at the *lycée* [in Grenoble], this marvelous summer night, soft and starry, illuminated by the fire was an extraordinary spectacle." The explosions shattered windows even in Grenoble, where people at first thought there had been an earthquake. All transportation between La Balme and Grenoble stopped, and Marcel was not even permitted to try to go home on foot. He spent two nights in a hotel owned by friends of theirs, wondering why no one in the family had come to get him. "It appears I was the bravest," he later told his father.[68]

The day after the explosion, Mireille, Nelly, and Mathilde miraculously found a new pension farther up the mountain in La Monta, a 40-minute tram ride from Grenoble. While not as elegant as their La Balme "villa," the setting was more beautiful. The following week, Mathilde, Marcel, and Mireille salvaged all they could from the damaged house they had fled. They found that they had lost surprisingly few of their possessions. Also surprising, Nelly came through the disaster more successfully than anyone would have thought possible, given her mental and physical state. She wrote her mother about how "*lucky* we are to have come out of the rubble of the house without the slightest injury, not to have been rendered crazy or deaf by this frightening day of cataclysm, not to have caught a cold while sleeping outside, not to have lost anything, lucky not to have been more shaken up, and the extraordinary luck of having found a new pension right away."[69]

In the midst of this disruption, Mireille learned, to her surprise, that she had passed her written exams, and was expected to appear for an oral exam within a week of the explosion. Henri received the news of his daughter's success by way of telegram when he was in his Paris office and in a fragile mental state. Fearing the continued bombardments in Paris and regretting his trip there, he was further unnerved by the news of the explosion—about which he had received only the barest of details through the press. His reaction to Mireille's unexpected success is noteworthy: "I who have endured everything since I left you so well, including your catastrophic story, without showing any emotion—become dizzy and am obliged to hide myself in the closet and cry like a kid . . . you are going to catch it for having made your father cry." He described Mireille as his baby duck who kept swimming toward the "bachot" in the middle of explosions.[70]

When Henri wrote this letter, he had been in Paris for about a week, and it had become clear to him that his stay there would not be short. Beyond tending to his business, his other task was to sort through the possessions in their apartment on boulevard Soult, obtain a long list of objects Nelly and Mireille had requested, store valuables in the basement, and decide whether to send their furniture to Grenoble. Most important, Nelly wanted all their photographs and the correspondence from Émile Darnaud. Entering the boulevard Soult apartment threw Henri into a state of reverie. Of a cherished photo, he said, "Mireille is still on the piano with her little doll in hand," and then referring to the bust he had so lovingly sculpted fourteen years earlier, "the other Mireille . . . seems to look out benevolently; and you, Nelly, you have the air of being in the clouds," a noteworthy comment, given that he had originally wanted to sculpt his wife's eyes cast downward on Mireille. Two weeks later—July 14—Henri still could not decide what to take and what to leave, for he could not determine which objects were most valuable and where they would be safest; moreover "everyone" now thought a "Boche" advance on Paris improbable.[71]

As Henri's stay in Paris dragged on with no clear end in sight, Nelly grew impatient and even angry, because she could not understand why he was unable to accomplish the few tasks they both deemed urgent and return to La Monta. She continued her obsessive worry about further bombardments. News of the bombardments always reached her sooner than his letters, the latter being further delayed because Paris had once again become a military zone.[72] Meanwhile a new cause for family conflict emerged: the question of where they would spend the winter.

The conflict that ensued highlights details of their wartime material life, their chronic, free-floating anxieties, and the fragility of Nelly's mental health. Montupet, ever optimistic that the war would soon end, wanted them to return to Paris. Godet, having just packed and stored their valuables in the cellar and divested himself of the Paris branch of his business, had now committed to a permanent residence elsewhere. Del Pozo had made Henri his sales representative for engineering supplies in both the departments of the Isère (Grenoble) and the Rhône (Lyon). Nelly and Mireille strongly favored the former, Henri the latter, primarily for reasons of business. A fierce debate ensued. Nelly viewed Lyon as city of "seagulls and sausages," a virtual cesspool with a damp, chilly climate and noxious air that would render the whole family more susceptible to disease, especially Henri, who was prone to bronchial infections. Mathilde refused to winter in either Grenoble or Lyon, and announced she would return to Paris, further complicating their choices between a pension and an apartment. The former were rare, expensive, and had less privacy; and proprietors, Henri claimed, skimped on coal. But an apartment would require furniture and a domestic.[73]

Henri eventually won the argument, but the protracted debate in their correspondence further undermined Nelly's nerves. Once again Marcel became impossible for her to bear. The move to La Monta had put him in a "foul mood." He also bickered constantly with Mathilde, and Mireille complained that no one could control him. Nelly complained to Henri of their son's "disobedience, his imprudence, and his lies . . . you might reprimand him . . . but you will be no more effective than I." In August, when they were all entrenched in the Lyon versus Grenoble argument, Mireille further described the family dynamics to her father: "At no price do I want to stay between Mathilde and Marcel, a situation that is going to become completely insane, since I have no authority over either one or the other. Moreover, I don't know who does have authority, because Mama herself renounces it, and as soon as they see that she is not very, very sick, they go at each other. When one of them behaves well, the other picks a fight." Mme Berthier, the masseuse, finally stepped into the vacuum of authority and told Marcel not only that he was making his mother too ill for her treatments but that his behavior would cause him to fall ill with peritonitis, typhoid fever, and cerebral congestion. Apparently, her threats had a positive effect.[74]

Godet finally returned to his family on August 11, having been absent for fifty days. He stayed only a week and then went to Lyon to establish his new headquarters; from there, he commuted back to La Monta regularly. During this month and the next, Roussel seemed somewhat revived, but the whole family, once again "buffeted by events," successively fell ill with a "ferocious flu" that ruined their final weeks in the Alps. They moved to Lyon on September 23.[75]

Lyon: The Spanish Flu

Had Nelly known that the misnamed "Spanish flu" had begun to spread in Paris when Henri was there, she would have had yet another reason to panic— she had already expressed fears about his health because of the unusual July heat. But in fact, the whole family seemed oblivious to the flu epidemic even as each member, including the Montupets while visiting La Monta, fell sick with an apparently less deadly strain. About 20 percent of the Spanish flu victims had a mild form of the illness. The more serious cases took one of two forms. The first began with ordinary flu symptoms, but within four or five days, the virus attacked the lungs, leading to severe pneumonia, which resulted in either death or a prolonged convalescence. The second, more frightening form filled victims' lungs with fluid and killed them within hours or days. It produced brown and purple blotches over the face leading many to conclude that the disease was cholera.[76]

The Roussel-Godet-Montupet family's complacency at first glance seems strange, given the high toll the disease had already wrought. In Paris alone, nearly a hundred people died in July and August—which was only the beginning of an epidemic that would take 240,000 French lives, and from 20 to perhaps 100 million worldwide. But for reasons of morale, as the flu spread through France in June, the authorities decided to wait until military victory was imminent before revealing the seriousness of the epidemic and taking preventative measures. The "hundreds of thousands" of soldiers who died of the flu on or off the battlefield were said to have died on the "field of honor." On July 6, the Paris press finally reported the spread of the flu in Europe, saying that the disease overcame its victims suddenly, but "disappeared in about a week without serious incidents apart from exceptional cases." The continued bombardments and threats of attack preoccupied the press and the minds of the Parisians. Flu deaths—especially since many were misdiagnosed—were less sensational fare.[77]

The Roussel-Godet-Montupet correspondence makes reference to ill relatives and friends, some of whom died. But in fact, the family knew little about the actual threat that this pandemic posed. The silence of officials, and thus of the newspapers, explains why Henri hardly mentioned the flu while he was in Paris that summer, and why it caused no panic as the family tried to make plans for their winter residence. They moved to Lyon just before the highest number of deaths occurred, and before officials lifted censorship about flu statistics. In Lyon, they settled into a furnished apartment in the center of the city. Mathilde went ahead to help Henri set up the apartment and stayed with them for the next few weeks until they could find a new domestic. Both children registered in their respective lycées—only to discover that the flu epidemic had forced a postponement in the opening of the school year.

Only in October were measures taken in Paris and Lyon to disinfect public places and advise the public of measures to be taken: isolate the sick, wear masks, brush teeth and wash hands, and avoid both indoor and outdoor public meetings. Those who fell ill were instructed to stay in bed, take aspirin, quinine, and lemonade with rum. In Lyon, the municipality kept schools closed and canceled public events. Even with these measures and the high rate of death in Paris—700 people a day by mid October—Nelly and her family did not appear very concerned—perhaps thinking that the flu they had had while in La Monta had inoculated them. When they arrived in Lyon, Nelly believed the epidemic was already fading. Instead, the death rate there spiked dramatically during these months.[78]

Like self-fulfilling prophecies, many of Nelly's fears about Lyon were realized. The weather was predictably cold and damp; she immediately fell ill with a cold; their apartment was mouse-infested; and their *guillaume* backed up, with a dead mouse in the overflow. In a very unlikely coincidence, the terror of La Balme revisited them when an explosives factory in St. Fons, eight kilometers away, blew up, in a series of explosions that shook their apartment and lit up the night sky. And by the end of October, Roussel began to understand the true impact of the flu. She became very worried when Henri traveled to Paris in October and advised that he check himself regularly for a fever. Meanwhile, she was consuming large quantities of rum, a precaution doctors recommended. But it was in short supply and very expensive—16 to 25 francs a bottle.[79]

Despite the end of the war—completely uncelebrated or even remarked upon in Roussel's archive—the reopening of school, and the family's apparent escape from the flu, Roussel once again fell into deep depression toward the end of November, even though her physical symptoms had improved. She sent apologies to her mother for not having written, saying, "The truth is that my depression jumps out enthusiastically with every pretext offered to it in order to torment me more." Nelly understood the vicious cycle of her mental state: it cut her off from people and she became more depressed in her isolation. She thus made a conscious decision to venture out, and indeed, the city environment seemed to stimulate and cheer her. Taking up her public pen for the first time in nearly a year and a half, she wrote an article for Madeleine Vernet's new journal, *La Mère éducatrice*. Meanwhile, the whole family went to a Chopin festival, in which Isadora Duncan and an "extraordinary pianist" performed. So compelling were they that even "the coldness of the Lyonnais" could not inhibit enthusiastic applause. But the experience of being in the theater—as a member of the audience rather than as a performer—animated a different passion in Roussel. In her desire for purity as both an auditor and actress, she stood up and yelled at the audience to "shut up or leave," because they were making too much noise when the program began. She subsequently determined to resume contact with human society by seeking out and visiting a schoolteacher who had organized one of her lectures in 1912. In this same period, she also took great pleasure in studying philosophy with Mireille.[80]

Lyon offered Roussel another theater for the revival of her public self. She attended a performance for the "People's Theater" of *Taming of the Shrew* by a syndicalist troupe associated with the Bourse du travail (labor exchange). She had read and appreciated Shakespeare but had not been familiar with this play. The inherent misogyny in it drove her to give a spontaneous speech after the performance. In addition, she wrote a letter to the head of the troupe and took it to the newspaper *Le Proletaire*—where, by chance, she was thrilled to attend a (syndicalist) union meeting at the Bourse du travail. With these activities, Nelly wrote to her mother that she felt herself "morally resuscitated" by this rebirth in her political involvement. She then made contact with the Socialist Youth, and she gave a second speech at the Bourse du travail.[81]

But once again events beyond Nelly's control intervened and turned her revival into what she described as "a flash in the pan," and "the gray cinders that embroil the soul" returned. Just as she reentered public life in Lyon in the middle of December, Mireille's philosophy teacher came down with the flu. Initially, the silver lining to this unfortunate event loomed larger than the cloud: it prompted Mireille to suggest that the entire family return to Paris as soon as possible, since she would be unable to pursue her studies. Henri decided that he could conduct what business he had in Lyon from a distance. The family made its decision in half a day, and that night, they celebrated with their close friends the Wolfs, who were passing through Lyon. Nelly made train reservations for December 24 and tenderly wrote her mother to "put a shoe under the chimney for Christmas so that you will receive a doll," wanting to surprise her with their beloved granddaughter's timely arrival. In the meantime, Mireille wrote to her grandmother about how happy they all were to be leaving their "foggy city," and of her "mad passion to see the streets of Paris again" and to move back into her "pretty pink room." But, she added, "I dare not rejoice because there can always be a hitch." Indeed, in this same letter, she mentioned that Marcel had a sore throat and fever, "symptoms of the famous flu," and then complained, "he could have waited until we got to Paris."[82]

Initially, they thought that Nelly and Mireille could go to Paris as planned, leaving Henri and Clothilde, their new domestic servant, behind to care for Marcel. But four days later, Mireille too had a fever. On December 23, a doctor came to see the children, both of whom were coughing badly. "In a word," Henri reported to the Montupets, "it's the flu." No one was going to Paris. Henri believed they had both contracted it at the *lycée*, Marcel from his English teacher, who had supposedly recovered, and Mireille from her philosophy teacher, whose flu had provided the excuse to leave Lyon in the first place. The doctor ordered a number of remedies, including quinine suppositories, tisanes, milk with rum, aspirin, and other medicines, in addition to the application of mustard plasters and suction cups. Both children had high temperatures; Marcel's peaked at 104 degrees (40° C) by December 24. The doctor considered his case the most serious, because he detected the lung congestion characteristic of the more deadly strain. Mireille's flu fostered the less serious secondary infection of bronchitis.[83]

As a sign of the Montupets' parental claim over Mireille, Godet promised he would report to them daily on the flu's course. While he tried to assure them— "don't worry, I am doing everything necessary"—the panic and fatigue in his letters are palpable. He took both children's temperatures around the clock and reported them to Montupet. Because they did not want their domestic to contract this highly contagious flu, she remained shut off from the children; Henri and Nelly both tended to them, a difficult task. "You have an idea of our occupations from morning to evening, without counting the fact that Nelly still is not well and that she has just entered into her critical monthly period. Of course, I have abandoned all other occupations." By Christmas Day, Marcel was out of danger, but his muscles had atrophied, and he could barely walk. It was only on December 29 that he was strong enough to write his grandmother about his sadness over not spending New Year's Day with them for the first time ever. By January 11, Mireille had recovered enough to walk outside on her father's arm. The family finally returned to Paris in mid January.[84]

From 1914 through 1918, Nelly Roussel and her family not only endured the terrible impacts of war but suffered through her physical and mental illness. Starting in the winter of 1917–18, they experienced the bombing of their Paris neighborhood, a spontaneous exodus and economic dislocation, and a terrifying epidemic that threatened their children's lives. What did these events do to Nelly Roussel's political and feminist sensibilities and the concerns that had previously driven her career?

After 1916, apart from making reference to her personal encounters with soldiers on leave, Nelly said very little about the war in her voluminous private correspondence, even though Henri often wrote about it. By cutting her venues for public speaking, the war colluded with her disease—and its misdiagnosis—to silence her and turn her sensibilities inward. These events, along with the daily physical pain she suffered, offered sufficient cause for depression, which in turn aggravated her insomnia and intestinal dysfunction. Neurasthenia was a logical diagnosis at the time. Labeling her ailment no doubt gave her hope and made her feel less guilty about her behavior. But it was also a suggestive diagnosis that may have increased her propensity for depression. The cure for it—rest—also silenced her. As her activities in Lyon suggest, she needed a public life. She hoped that returning home to Paris, to her former life and feminist colleagues, would revive her.

One of the poems she wrote after her return, however, points to the despair she continued to feel after these terrible four years. Her belief in progress, justice, and good gave way to a quasi-religious belief in "Beauty," whose only home was the forest "cathedral." Her poem "Invincible Croyance" (Invincible Belief) resembles the Catholic prayers of her girlhood, except that Beauty had replaced Christ in redeeming her from doubt:

> . . . seeing that you come to my tormented heart
> To offer, O my forest, your enchanted sanctuary,
> I feel that, amidst such doubt,
> This weary, wounded heart, this poor, defeated heart,
> Will always believe in Beauty.
>
> *Nelly Roussel, Samoreau, October 1, 1919*[85]

CHAPTER SEVEN

Last Battles

Words of Combat, Hope, and Pain

> To be only feminist, without linking feminism to some grand ideal
> of social transformation and human regeneration, is obviously an
> error, prejudicial to feminism itself. . . . Not to be feminist is an-
> other error, no less serious.
>
> Nelly Roussel, "Glanes" [Gleanings],
> *Voix des femmes, January 5, 1922*

After the family's return to Paris, Henri settled back into his office near the place
de la République and his partnership with Del Pozo in the sale of engineering supplies. Mireille, who had turned nineteen by the war's end, moved back
in with the Montupets. Without explanation (at least in Roussel's archive), she
terminated her studies and abandoned her goal of teaching philosophy. Godet
resumed his efforts to recruit Mireille as his secretary. She learned to type and
worked for him, but she quickly developed a distaste for her job. Marcel, who was
fourteen when the war ended, lived with his parents in Paris and resumed his
schooling. He too learned to type and worked in his father's office. Mathilde did
not return to their service, though she remained a good friend of the family and
visited often. Clothilde ("Clo"), who had begun working for them in Lyon, stayed
on. Roussel and the children, and sometimes Henri, spent long weekends in
Fontainebleau and its vicinity, where Fritz and Juliette now lived (at Samoureau),
as did the professional singer Louise Sauval, Roussel's close friend from childhood. The Montupets returned to their Paris villa and acquired another home
near Fontainebleau, in Vaux-le-Pénil (Seine-et-Marne). The children went there
often; Roussel and Godet visited reluctantly, calling it "Vo le Pépé" and "Vo le
Penible" since tensions with Montupet continued. Nelly resumed her long vaca-

tions in the forest during the summer months, either staying with family and friends or renting a hotel room of her own.

If the war's end revived Roussel, she also emerged from it angrier and more radicalized than ever. She took part in none of the victory celebrations. In 1919, Bastille Day celebrations also commemorated the anniversary of the turning point that had brought Allied victory the previous summer. Recoiling from the sight and sound of the flares left over from the war that local officials used as fireworks, which reminded her of the Gotha bomber raids and Big Bertha shelling of Paris, Roussel took refuge in her beloved forest. Meanwhile, Henri mingled with the boisterous revelers in Paris, which also repulsed her. Still harboring notions of the crowd theorists that Darnaud had impressed upon her, she feared her husband would be contaminated with (patriotic) "microbes." "I would have suffered to see Paris ruined by this carnival décor, and even more, to witness the warrior enthusiasm, because this celebration was really *a celebration of militarism.* As long as the victors are thrown flowers and smiles, War will not die."[1]

Despite her anger, once back in Paris Nelly's mental depression seemed to evaporate, and mention of her digestive disorders appears somewhat less often in her diaries and correspondence over the next two years. No doubt, the end of the war itself emotionally revived her, and either her physical symptoms improved or she spent less time dwelling on them as she resumed public life. From January 1919 through 1922, she published at least sixty-six articles in newspapers and gave twenty-six public talks. In 1919, she published her collection of poetry inspired by the Fontainebleau forest, *Ma forêt,* and reissued *Quelques discours* (1907) under a new title, *Paroles de combat et d'espoir* (Words of Combat and Hope), expanded to 64 pages with additional lectures and articles.

The cover of this new edition (fig. 16) reflected Roussel's transformation. It features a rough sketch of Nelly by Juliette Robin: she has a beautiful face, a slight, somewhat petulant smile; she is draped in a simple and shapeless dress and has a modest—almost masculine—coiffure, with two strands of hair falling out of place. Her hands are outstretched in a beseeching mode, aquiver with an intensity of purpose. The preface also reflected her transformation: she repeated the dedication to her husband in the 1907 version, but added: "And to those who will perhaps continue [my apostolate], to my children, Mireille and Marcel." Finally, in his adolescence, Nelly was able to include her son. But the war and its aftermath had made Roussel realize that the goals for which she fought might not even be won in her children's generation, for a new conservative discourse had taken root and grown to dominance. The "eternal feminine" emerged from the war more deeply entrenched than ever in the public imagination, as did the aspect of sacrifice associated with it. In the eyes of some of her greatest admirers, Roussel even became the victim of her own sacrifice as she waged her last battles against female pain.

Postwar Culture

Nelly Roussel was hardly alone in the despair she felt as the war ended. Despite initial celebrations at the announcement of the Armistice, joy over the end of hostilities only momentarily mitigated the years of suffering all had experienced. This conflict had been a war of attrition for both sides, and only two months before its end, the outcome had been unclear. So too was what it all meant. If German aggression had justified French engagement at the outset, the huge losses made it impossible for any of the combatant nations to end the war with honor—and mounting death tolls themselves became the reason to fight on. French soldiers had mutinied in 1917, and in that year and in 1918, workers went on strike. Pacifists joined them in publicly demanding an official explanation of war aims. In the end, the expulsion of Germans and the return of Alsace and Lorraine failed to compensate for the staggering losses so many had suffered.[2] The French, like those in other belligerent nations, had to affix meaning to the unprecedented tragedies of war. One of those meanings was a deepened sense of population decline and national decay.

Although it had been on the side of victory, France, unlike its allies Britain and the United States, suffered the consequences of prolonged enemy occupation. It had also mobilized a higher proportion of its male population than any other country, and suffered the highest percentage of casualties among them—78.3— in contrast to the total average of 51.8 percent among both Allied and Central powers. The 1918 flu further raised mortality rates, particularly among young adults. The war and the flu ended marriages and prevented new ones. From 1914 to 1918, French couples produced 1.75 fewer children than in the four years preceding the war. The war also left an excess of women; those of childbearing age outnumbered men by more than one million, further reducing the potential to repopulate the nation. Even with the reacquisition of Alsace and Lorraine, which added almost two million people, the French population had shrunk to 38.1 million from nearly 40 million in 1911. This fact alone was a major source of worry and humiliation, one that gravely undermined any sense of victory.[3]

The occupation caused yet another source of suffering, less commonly discussed: hundreds of women in occupied France had been raped by German soldiers, which resulted not only in physical, psychological, and emotional damage but in pregnancies as well. What to do with the pregnancies and children born from them became yet another national preoccupation that raised issues about abortion and notions of the importance of biological nationality versus the possibilities of nurture and the natural instincts of mother love.[4]

To cope with these losses, the French had to understand them. Recent historians concerned with the formation of collective memory, most notably Daniel Sherman, have emphasized the central role that commemoration and mourning practices played in the creation of postwar culture. Many of them also sought to "correct" memories of wartime experience, particularly with regard to gender. Women's performance of men's jobs had disrupted traditional beliefs about feminine identity. The battlefield upset long-held assumptions about what it meant to be a warrior and a man. In the trenches, soldiers had difficulty fighting according to the traditional codes of masculinity that depended upon hand-to-hand combat, movement, and conquest. Instead, they found themselves immobile, the passive victims of artillery shells. This kind of war resulted in the distinctly unheroic symptoms of shell shock, lost limbs, and "broken faces."[5]

Commemorations thus sought to reconstruct male heroism. War monuments, poetry, fiction, posters, journalism, memoirs, celebrations of the Armistice, and other cultural products celebrated virility and reinvented a heroism that most soldiers had not experienced in the trenches. Best-selling postwar literature, such as Henri Barbusse's *Le Feu* and Roland Dorgelès's award-winning *Les Croix de bois*, depicted soldiers as virile and attributed virtue to violence. But another strong theme in these novels, as Mary Louise Roberts has shown, was the humiliation soldiers experienced because of women who had abandoned them through sexual betrayal. Female betrayal, she argues, became a focus for the more nebulous anger and humiliation at an inexplicable war experience.[6]

If trench literature portrayed woman as a symbol of home-front decadence, it also portrayed her as everything that represented the opposite of war: the "very principle of life itself," a symbol of peace, gentle beauty, motherhood.[7] Feminists across the political spectrum contributed to this image—as Roussel had during the war—by setting up a Manichean dichotomy between woman as the bearer of life and man as its destroyer. That effort, moreover, can be understood as a logical compensatory response to the emergent trope of the home-front woman as fun-loving, frivolous, and unfaithful; the motherhood image also appealed to a population that dreamed of demographic regeneration.

Postwar commemorations also effaced female heroism and independence; women were never remembered in their own right or held up as models for the tasks they had performed in the war effort. Monuments portrayed women as weak, grieving mothers "who gave birth to heroes and nourished sacrifice" and paid tribute to the men who "assumed the ultimate burden of citizenship." Such representations stressed the "unnatural aspect" of women's real wartime labors. Even the suffering of those who had been raped was eclipsed, according to Ruth Harris's poignant analysis, because "the actual victimization of women was transformed into a representation of a violated, but innocent, female nation resisting the assaults of a brutal male assailant." Margaret Darrow has shown that a "French women's war story misfired during the war itself." Memory about women's experience was not lost in the postwar era; it had never been created to begin with. "What women did in the war," Darrow argues, "or what was done to them by the war was explained—or explained away—as minor adaptations of a traditional feminine destiny. Thus, the feminine war story became simply the Eternal Feminine, and both the war and the [real] story [about women] dropped out."[8]

The postwar culture to which commemoration contributed so significantly thus reinforced the concept of womanhood Roussel had been battling against most of her life: she who is "eternally sacrificed" for the benefit of the society, state, and Church, but who receives neither tributes nor rights. While other countries granted women the vote in recognition of their wartime contributions, the French debated the issue but continued to withhold it. The war and postwar culture, moreover, infused pronatalism with an unprecedented virulence, which was buttressed by maternal imagery in commemorative monuments and literature. Natalism was more ubiquitous than ever.[9]

Thus as the French sought to honor their dead and their veterans, Roussel took the opposite path. Combating war, shaming warriors, and honoring women for their real actions and experiences rather than their commemorated ones became central themes in her revived campaign. These themes infused other issues that she again took up: neo-Malthusianism, pacifism, education, anticapitalism, the rights of mothers, and female pain. Her politics also shifted further to the left: she became a self-declared revolutionary and sympathized openly with Bolshevism. In every respect, Nelly Roussel battled the mainstream postwar culture and politics.

Postwar Feminism: *The Voice of Women*

Roussel resumed her contacts with feminists immediately upon her return to Paris. In February 1919, she attended a meeting of the Union fraternelle des femmes (UFF), the one feminist group in which she had consistently participated until her retreat from public life in 1916. There she gave a talk publicizing

"L'Enfance heureuse" (Happy Childhood), a children's education program that her close friend Germaine Lambert had recently launched. But the war had so radicalized Roussel that the UFF no longer met her needs; having committed herself to the group for nearly twenty years, she apparently abandoned it and began attending—and presiding over—the monthly meetings of a rival organization, L'Action des femmes (Women's Action).[10]

Although feminists had suspended their demand for rights during the war, most of their groups remained intact, and new ones emerged. L'Action des femmes originated in July 1915 with an unusual mixture of feminists who adhered to the matriarchal and bizarre, pseudoscientific theories of Céline Renooz (1840–1928). At its origin, the group had socialist leanings, but it was also patriotic and even pronatalist. Its program integrated demands for political and civil rights with equality in the workplace. What distinguished it most from other feminist groups in Paris was its decidedly antibourgeois stance and its base of support: the "popular classes"—proletarians and *travailleuses*—in addition to schoolteachers and artists. Céline Renooz even complained to the conservative feminist Amélie Hammer, long-serving president of the UFF, that the lower-class membership of L'Action des femmes would give feminism a bad name. The course of the war further radicalized its members. In 1917, it became pacifist, and one of its leaders, Anne Léal, identified militarism as "the most tragic stigmata" of what she called "masculinism": "War is the culmination of masculinism, because pan-masculinism engenders all the 'pans': pan-Germanism, pan-Slavism, pan-Americanism, etc., all the pandemoniums."[11]

Roussel also found "masculinism" problematic among men of the Left, as she had discovered among the freethinkers in her earlier career, and she adopted the term. The war and the Bolshevik Revolution changed the terms of what it meant to be revolutionary in France. Members of the Socialist Party were forced to decide whether to become communists, join the Third International and pass into the orbit of Moscow, or stay independent. In 1920, the majority of the party became communists. Since women did not vote, party membership counted less for them than ideological commitment. Nonetheless, the Bolshevik Revolution appealed to radical and socialist feminists in France because Bolshevists had granted women full civil and political equality. Their ideology attracted the interest of many feminists with whom Roussel had closely collaborated: Séverine, Marguerite Martin, Hélène Brion, and Caroline Kauffmann, among others. It also meant that bourgeois feminists—regardless of their ideological stance—once again came under attack. The personal and the private, more than ever, became political. Debates of previous years—such as the one Roussel had had with

Duchmann—reemerged with more vigor. The new radicalism split the feminist movement, leading some of its supporters to renounce feminism as detracting from the overall goals of a socialist or communist revolution.[12]

Bolshevism made Roussel more than ever committed to working-class women. She began collaborating with the journal *La Voix des femmes*, founded by Collette Reynaud and Louise Bodin in October 1917, and speaking at the meetings it sponsored, causing something of a breach with her former UFF colleagues. Like Roussel, Reynaud and Bodin had been radicalized by the war. From its origins, the journal defended peace as well as women's rights, and it was heavily censored for its pacifism. The charismatic Bodin—the "anticonformist" wife of a medical professor on the faculty at Rennes—collected a diverse group of women and men around the paper, some of whom were already very well known, among them Séverine, Marthe Bigot, Hélène Brion, Magdeleine Marx, Madeleine Pelletier, Marianne Rauze, Romain Rolland, Henri Barbusse, Léon Werth, Georges Pioch, Georges Yvetôt, and Victor Méric. The variety of personalities made it both impossible and undesirable for the journal to articulate a singular feminist viewpoint, but its general political orientation was distinctly radical: it defended equality between the sexes in every realm, published articles advocating sexual emancipation, and encouraged feminists to join political parties on the left.[13]

La Voix des femme's dramatic, allegorical masthead symbolized its goals: in the foreground stood a bare-chested, stoic worker-revolutionary, facing forward with his arms resting on a hammer and anvil. At his side stood a woman, also bare-chested, a sheaf of wheat stuck in her belt. Holding a sickle in one hand, her other hand is outstretched, pointing toward a crowd behind her, composed exclusively of women whose arms are raised in gestures of protest. Leaning closely to her comrade's ear, the woman says, "Listen to my voice, and we'll save the world!" Indeed, this allegory could not have contrasted more sharply with others that typically pervaded postwar visual imagery. Far from being a weeping widow, and without the slightest hint of the maternal, this woman is an action figure who shares work equally with her male companion. Moreover, hers is the authoritative voice. Another evocation of Marianne, she is a warrior. The newspaper her image represented gave women a voice through the printed word—words that substituted for swords, but that were often violent and even militaristic. Despite the plurality of voices contributing to this paper, its title suggested that women spoke with one voice. *La Voix des femmes* quickly approached a circulation of 5,000 as a bimonthly; it organized huge mass meetings and became the "loudest voice on the women's Left"—loud enough to become the subject of several police reports. In 1922, it became a daily paper, and it survived as such until 1939.[14]

This was the first newspaper since *La Fronde* with which Roussel could fully identify. In the spring of 1919, never having met Bodin, she wrote her a letter of support, and she subsequently sent her a copy of her 1907 collection of speeches, *Quelques discours*. Bodin immediately asked her to collaborate on *La Voix des femmes* if her health permitted. In Roussel, Bodin found a friend who shared a similar lifestyle, as well as her own disdain for bourgeois feminism. After receiving and reading *Quelques discours*, Bodin wrote, "We are, it seems, very close to one another, not only because of the dedication that you put in your brochure indicating that you are, like me, a happy and understood wife, but because of all the ideas you express [especially about women workers] . . . I await you at the *Voix des femmes* with an impatience all the more intense since your health, you tell me, is the reason for your silence."[15]

By October 1919, Roussel began contributing to *La Voix des femmes* regularly. Her first article, "Les Femmes et la guerre" (Women and War), responded to that of another contributor, Magdeleine Marx, who—partially echoing literary and commemorative representations in postwar culture—argued that women had not suffered during the war, had done nothing to stop the war, had remained indifferent to the martyrdom of men, and had only themselves to blame for their inferiority. In response, Roussel launched her "war against warriors." She enumerated all the ways in which women had suffered between 1914 and 1918—morally, physically, and materially—and noted their contributions as well. She made the rather unsettling but true point that the mothers and spouses of the ten million young men who had died would suffer longer than those over whom they shed tears. Moreover, because women had no rights, they had no responsibility for the war. Men were "infinitely more responsible for a catastrophe that we [women] have suffered almost as much as men, [but it was men] *who committed the crime of making war* . . . do they have a right to our compassion?" In fact, she noted, women should refrain from admiring "useless martyrdom and malevolent heroism." Women who opposed war should stop giving birth to cannon fodder, refuse to honor warriors, and disdain military parades: "if men have the stupidity to allow themselves to be taken to a massacre, we shall treat them, not as heroes, but as cowards and assassins . . . we must not just say 'down with war,' we must say 'down with warriors.'"[16]

Roussel took up similar arguments in subsequent articles, where she extended the blame to noncombatants. The "true assassins" were not just military chiefs, but "poets, historians, novelists, philosophers, who have sung and celebrated war." She attributed other social ills such as "physical deformities, tuberculosis, anemia, neurasthenia, and all that depresses and destroys the race" to men's subjection of women, because the "forces of love, pity, and peace" (womanhood) have been "enchained, gagged, and reduced to impotence." Roussel called on men of all classes, and of all parties, to "make your 'mea culpa.' You are not all equally guilty. But none of you is innocent."[17]

Indeed, not all men were guilty. In her antimilitary, pacifist politics, Roussel won an unlikely ally and friend in Colonel Jean Converset, who had served in the Infantry Division of the War Ministry and had been stationed in Rennes. He blamed the government, not the army, for the war. Converset was pacifist and author of an antiwar brochure, *Contre la guerre.* He was also a poet. He and his wife had attended Roussel's lectures at every chance they had while in Paris from 1902 to 1913, and though they did not meet her at the time, they had common friends in the Wolfs. "Then the war came," he wrote to her, "and we only heard the voice of cannon." He thought about Roussel often during the war, and when he observed the beaten-down "human prey" taken from the battlefield each day, he thought women should not bear children only to give them up to that fate, especially when they had no power in "things of war and of peace."

In 1919, Roussel sent Converset *Paroles de combat et d'espoir,* and he wrote to her of his profound admiration for her having had the courage to write pacifist articles during the war. "What a field that remains open to your activity after this terrible crisis, which left France almost at the bottom rank of nations regarding the terrain of feminism!" Even before he met her, she had inspired his poetry, and with this first letter, he sent a sonnet dedicated to her. "What is very sad is that there are not more women who think as you do, and that is one of the greatest disillusionments that have struck me with these terrible events of the war and the postwar [era]. But we must not be discouraged by that, I only regret that you may not speak as often and as purely, in the conditions in which I heard you before."[18] Converset himself began to contribute antiwar articles and poetry to *La Voix des femmes.*

Converset shared Roussel's fundamental assumption that if women were included in public life, it would be easier to prevent war and other social ills. But not many men, especially other veterans, agreed with him. The postwar cultural climate as a whole—particularly the memorialization of war heroes—did not offer a "field" for cultivating women's rights; nor did political life, once it resumed a year after the Armistice. The first elections to replace the wartime regime occurred in November 1919, and Frenchmen elected the most conservative Chamber since 1871, giving moderates and conservatives more than two-thirds of the seats. A large number went to war veterans. For the first time in the history of the Third Republic, a majority of the deputies were practicing Catholics.

Several factors explain this dramatic shift to the right. The separation of church and state in 1905, the nationalist revival prior to the war, the *Union sacrée* and the battle experience itself had enabled right-wing Catholics to accept the secular republic, and the clerical issue faded into political irrelevance. In addition, prolonged difficulties in the Versailles negotiations, labor unrest, the revolutionary appeal of Bolshevism, and the bitterness former combatants felt toward the deputies elected in 1914 contributed to the conservative coalition that formed the new "National Bloc." Catholicism immediately influenced the new government's actions: it reestablished diplomatic relations with the Vatican and it refrained from applying the 1905 law separating church and state in the recovered departments of Alsace and Lorraine. As would be seen in its future actions, it also accepted the Catholic theory of conception by enacting legislation that would severely restrict women's reproductive rights.[19]

The election results incensed Roussel. In an article published in both *La Voix des femmes* and *La Libre Pensée internationale,* she called the electorate a "herd" that had voted masters, exploiters, and killers into the government. She blamed her former allies and supporters—freethinkers—for handing power over to the Right, stating, "we know the refrain with which our good radicals invariably responded to our strongest feminist demands: 'Women's votes will bring back the priests.' And now, without women's votes, the priests are coming back." She said the Radical Party was dead, proclaimed herself a Bolshevist, and invited her compatriots to join her if they did not want to remain slaves.[20]

Neo-Malthusianism and the Law of July 1920

Neo-Malthusianism remained a cornerstone of Roussel's ideology and an explicit part of her propaganda. The human toll of the war and its long-term demographic impact on France hardly made conditions for a birth control campaign auspicious. In March 1917, Gabriel Giroud courageously and defiantly launched a new newspaper, the *Neo-Malthusien.* Roussel immediately wrote a letter of support proclaiming her "joy" at its appearance and promised she would dedicate herself to the dormant neo-Malthusian cause as soon as her health permitted. She believed more than ever that neo-Malthusianism was an issue that dominated all others.[21] In 1919, she published several articles in the *Neo-Malthusien* and *Voix des femmes* in which she turned the postwar pronatalist argument on its head. The war proved that "battles are won less with men than with cannons." Despite its larger population, Germany had lost the war. She also argued that Germany's larger size had actually contributed to its defeat after the naval blockade began to starve its civilian and military populations. The postwar period, she said, would be the worst time to bring infants into the world, for food was scarce, prices were high, and many people were suffering from disease and deformities caused by battle. The population was, quite simply, too worn out to take on the responsibility of putting children into the world. Women should demand that as a condition for bearing children, they would no longer be asked to "grease the battlefields" with them. They needed the assurance of peace and the opportunity to participate in public affairs. In the absence of such assurance, Roussel again called for a "strike of wombs."[22]

Roussel knew that her words would be unpopular in the postwar political climate, but she was determined to prove the Malthusian axiom that overpopulation—not underpopulation—caused war. In one article, she wrote,

I know I am saying "subversive" things and embarking on a "prohibited subject," which has for fifteen years earned me the insults of bourgeois *bien pensants,* salon feminists, and parade revolutionaries. It doesn't matter to me. Nothing will stop me from ceaselessly returning to this subject, from proclaiming this truth that is so misconstrued: that all the ills we suffer—the misery, the competition, the struggle for life, the physiological defects, the exhaustion and resignation of the masses, the subservience of women, debauchery, hatred, and war—have as a cause, if not the unique cause . . . immoderate and thoughtless procreation. No progress can be made without conscious motherhood. We must not expect anything from the lamentable heap of waste that is our current humanity. It is necessary to select, to regenerate. We must throw away the bad seeds and prepare the soil so that the good can germinate.[23]

Roussel had previously used the metaphor of germination, but within the postwar commemorative culture, the term assumed even greater meaning because of frequent references to soldiers' "seeds" and the sacrifice they had "sowed." Germination and fertilization also had a literal meaning in addressing the food shortages and returning men to the fields that women had plowed, sowed, and reaped during the war. Explicit here too is her thought that some seeds were "bad" and should be cast off, suggesting a eugenicist element to her thinking—one that she never developed systematically.[24]

Roussel also mocked official efforts to honor the mothers of large families when the public was asked to help support a week-long vacation for them, or when bronze, silver, and vermeil medals were respectively offered to mothers of five, eight, and ten children. Nothing could better underscore the "stupidity of our leaders who demand large families," she said, than their own request for public charity to support them. But she was gratified that mothers were finally being acknowledged. "Is this proof that our vehement protests have begun to be heard? . . . Let's hope that women, more sensible than men, do not allow themselves to be dazzled like [men] by the shine of a medal; that they will not show themselves ready to give life as unconsciously as men show themselves ready to take life [just] for the pleasure of hanging a little piece of ribbon on their chests."[25]

Roussel may have overreacted when she stated that the new Chamber would undo fifty years of republican reform, but her fears about clerical influence were well founded. Within months of assuming power, the Catholic legislature resumed work on a bill—in the making since 1909—that would outlaw birth control and all propaganda related to it. It did so largely in response to Roussel and ongoing neo-Malthusian propaganda. In December 1919, after the fateful November elections, Gabriel Giroud pasted thousands of posters throughout Paris that called on proletarians to have fewer children. Abbé Violet followed in his wake, tearing them up. *Le Figaro* denounced the poster, and the Catholic *La Croix* insisted that such freedom of expression could no longer be tolerated, and that its producers were "Boches."[26] *La Démocratie nouvelle* condemned the posters and wondered why the government manifested such "impotence, indifference, spinelessness" in the face of a campaign that was supported by German money. The "German genius, we saw so well during the war, excelled in its attempts at social dissolution and collapse."[27]

In the minds of many conservatives, the Germans continued to wage war on the French—not on the battlefield, but covertly—deploying Bolshevism and Malthusianism as their weapons of mass destruction. From 1896 on, the police in Paris and in the provinces had been compiling files on the activities of Paul Robin, Sébastian Faure, Eugène Humbert, Gabriel Giroud, Nelly Roussel, and others, with special attention to their influence on workers and on women.[28] But the German attack on France from 1914 to 1918, and the sudden appearance of Bolshevism, according to this theory, turned neo-Malthusians into pawns of a far greater and more dangerous conspiracy. One lengthy report in the police files, summarized the history of the neo-Malthusian movement and named Roussel among the leading participants. The report contended that the propaganda had caused incalculable ravages and that the government's failure to intervene was incomprehensible. It further collapsed this menace with a threat of global proportions: "Malthusianism and Bolshevism are the methods of a war without mercy that Germany has undertaken against the entire world, whose aggression in 1914 was only the [logical] result. Against the[se] secret weapons, all the nations of the world, except perhaps for the United States, found themselves defenseless and still do today."[29]

The most vulnerable elements of the population, according to this report, were the wives and daughters of workers, who for twenty years had been told not to have children. The author had personally investigated Malthusian demonstrations within the working-class milieu and witnessed how propagandists "sought to educate women during the absence of their husbands at the front." The report concluded that although the "Boches were chased from our frontiers, they continue subterranean attacks under the shelter of liberty of thought . . . the war is not over, it continues . . . more dangerously because it is elusive among us, as well as among our allies." The author urged the government to reinforce and clarify its authority. Only in this manner would the war really be won and thus "give to all our brave tombs on the Field of Honor the only compensation truly worthy of their heroic sacrifice." Invisible enemies posed more danger than those of the battlefield and required sanctions within the very population that was threatened.[30]

In May 1920, in an article entitled "Contre les ennemis de la race française" ("Against the Enemies of the French Race"), the extreme right-wing *Action française* singled out Roussel's propaganda as typical of the sort that should be outlawed. The author expressed outrage that a bill in the Chamber of Deputies prohibiting birth control propaganda had been languishing since the previous December. The disciples of Malthus were continuing their "murderous, detestable propaganda" with impunity, as proven by posters plastered on all the walls of Saint-Ouen (Seine-Saint-Denis) announcing Nelly Roussel's "criminal" lecture, "The Madness of Repopulators." Had the bill already become law, the article said, Roussel would have been imprisoned for up to three years and fined up to 3,000 francs.[31]

Shortly thereafter, Nelly Roussel delivered the lecture advertised in the posters. She spoke about Malthusian theory to a working-class audience of 1,000. Although weakened by her chronic disease, she had not lost her talent for public speaking: "in an auditory surge, she swept up her audience," telling women to unite and to show men that they were a force that could no longer be ignored. "A law is being prepared to suppress our propaganda," she said; "it will be unenforceable because the truth cannot be suppressed; one can hide it for a long time, but it always reappears."[32]

The following month, Senator Gustave de Lamarzelle launched a Senate debate about neo-Malthusianism. He attacked Gabriel Giroud for his journal and resurrected the ghost of Paul Robin to argue that neo-Malthusian propaganda amounted to pornography. Reading the debate in the *Journal officiel* and reactions to it in newspapers, Roussel was outraged by the silence on the Left. She lambasted hypocrites in the Senate—especially her former freethinking colleague and supporter Henry Bérenger:

> Everyone is keeping their mouths shut, even those who don't have the excuse of ignorance or stupidity, even those who knew Robin and who can appreciate him— those who fraternally shook his hand in the Masonic lodges—even Henry Bérenger, ex-director of *L'Action*, where during many years I led an ardent Malthusian campaign, which he does not [now] disavow. . . . Men such as he know well that neo-Malthusianism has absolutely nothing in common with pornography.[33]

Roussel also attacked the right-wing pronatalists. The most recent circular of the National Alliance for French Population Growth, addressed "to *industrialists, capitalists, and bosses,*" sought to motivate employers to encourage large families among workers, saying that a higher birthrate would make political strikes and labor stoppages less common. Roussel quoted it in *La Voix des femmes* so that others could see the open cynicism of the pronatalists. "Troublemakers" and their followers were always single or childless, it asserted. "Fathers of large families do not go on strike . . . and [they] change factories less frequently, because they are more fearful of not being able to find work. You should do everything possible to make your workers decide to have children."[34]

On July, 23 1920, with a vote of 500 to 53, the Chamber quickly passed a law prohibiting the sale of any birth control devices and the distribution of any form of propaganda or advertising that encouraged birth control or abortion. In order to help prevent the spread of venereal disease, which had become a major problem during the war, condoms were not outlawed. Anyone convicted of violating the law would be subject to a maximum of three years in prison and a fine of 5,000 francs, depending on the article(s) violated. Only two deputies expressed vocal opposition to the bill, one of whom used rhetoric similar to Roussel's. Most of those who voted against it were socialists.[35]

No major newspaper bothered to inform its readers about a law that "suddenly prohibited any possibility of sexual education" and made possible an unprecedented incursion into private life and individual rights, especially freedom of speech. The day after its passage, even *L'Humanité* devoted only twenty lines to it on its second page. The pronatalists had won a massive victory, and they continued to preach their message. Months later, a specialist in legal medicine again evoked Robin's alleged misdeeds in his course at the Faculty of Medicine, blaming neo-Malthusian propaganda for the drop in the birthrate. Purporting to cite Nelly Roussel, the professor referred to her as "Madame Lévy Rousset," not only mistaking her name, but making it Jewish and thereby reinforcing the association of birth control with menacing un-French, foreign elements.[36]

But what of French public opinion, especially given the near silence with which the passage of this law was met? Mary Louise Roberts notes that the parliamentary debates took on an apocalyptic tone because depopulation had become a focus for all the economic and military anxieties from which France suffered. France itself was seen as a dying body, so that "the right to seize the female body was . . . legitimated by the need to regenerate the social body."[37] (But did ordinary people think so metonymically?) An example from visual culture further suggests how the French had been made susceptible to an association between reproduction and national defense. Marie-Monique Huss's study of wartime postcards reveals, to a stunning degree, how French popular consciousness linked higher birthrates with military virility and home front patriotism. In stark contrast to the prewar neo-Malthusian campaign that sought to separate sex and reproduction, these cards—particularly images of the *poilu* home on leave—identified love (sex) with procreation, and procreation with military victory. One highly favored genre of cards portrayed baby *poilus* born (or growing out of cabbages) in 1915 and 1916 as future "classes" of conscripts in 1935 and 1936. Many of these postcards strongly associated virility/fertility with weapons. One prewar example portrayed seven babies suspended from a rifle with the caption, "It's just what we need for repopulation." The theme took on numerous other variations during the war, exploiting ample opportunity for double entendres, such as the postcard with the caption "Un bon coup de baïonnette" ("A good bayonet thrust"), which showed three happy babies hung comfortably in carriers dangling from a bayonet—the product of a soldier's patriotic "good thrust" while home on leave. Other such examples abound. In the context of this particular facet of popular culture during the war, we have better insight into the postwar comment from a mother of thirteen children—with another on the way—who, upon receiving the Cognac Foundation Prize, publicly proclaimed that she wanted another boy "for France," even though she already had nine.[38]

The mass production, consumption, and popularity of these postcards does not mean that the French population became converted to pronatalism. But it does suggest, as Huss argues, that the public values of patriotism became linked in the popular imagination with the private values of marriage and reproduction. The public became passively disposed to thinking that a higher birthrate would be a good thing for France, even if, as in fact happened, individuals continued the old habits of having few children. The gap between private behavior and public acceptance helps explain both the absence of protest when the Chamber finally passed the July 1920 law and the complete failure of the law to stimulate the birthrate.

It was the silence around the passage of this law—especially among politicians of the Left, syndicalists, feminists, and women—that embittered Roussel. She took to task the very men who most championed human rights, and the women who, like their male counterparts, deemed feminism secondary, if not irrelevant, to revolution. In particular, she targeted Ferdinand Buisson, president of the League of the Rights of Man—the league her husband had helped found in defense of Dreyfus, which, in principle, defended the individual rights of all citizens. Why, as a member of the Chamber of Deputies, had Buisson voted for this law of July 23, 1920? Roussel posed the question in print and wondered if there had been some mistake—Had the *Journal officiel* incorrectly registered his vote? She implored him to correct the error if so.[39]

The law for the most part silenced neo-Malthusianism. Although Giroud, Humbert, and others ceased publishing newspapers and tracts, in March 1921, police searched their respective premises on the pretext that they had sold to an undercover agent an old edition of Jean Marestan's *L'Education sexuelle* that had not been purged of instructions on the use of contraceptive devices. They did not find enough evidence to arrest them, but the police commissioner realized that Humbert was in an "irregular situation" with regard to the military—having dodged the draft in 1914—and he was taken to the Invalides to be indicted through the military justice system. At a preliminary hearing, the judge was about to drop the charges because of Humbert's age—he had been 44 in 1914 and probably would have been able to avoid the draft anyway. But the judge changed his mind when, upon receiving the police file, he saw that Humbert had been a neo-Malthusian militant and had continued to wage the birth control campaign from Barcelona during the war, while expressing antimilitary sentiments in his correspondence. At his trial in May 1921, Humbert was accused of "having, by his action, taken battalions from France." He was sentenced to five years in prison, the maximum allowed by the Military Code. In the following months, Jeanne Humbert and several other neo-Malthusians were tried before civil courts and received two-year prison terms and fined 3,000 francs.[40]

The July 1920 law was quickly dubbed a *loi d'exception*, or *loi scélérate* ("atrocious law"), a term first used with regard to the deliberately anti-anarchist laws of 1893–94 because they denied civil rights to a specific group of people.[41] Roussel renewed her attacks against Buisson when the League of the Rights of Man, the left-wing press, and the CGT declared yet another bill under consideration—one that would prohibit freedom of expression among antimilitarists—to be *super-scélérate*. She figured that militants on the Left remained indifferent to the law on birth control and abortion because these issues concerned primarily women, who did not figure in revolutionary programs, and noted bitterly that "measures against others are never as harmful as those against oneself."[42] Unable to attend a public meeting called by the *Voix des femmes*, Roussel wrote a letter that was read aloud at it. The audience broke into repeated applause throughout the reading. She compared the silence and calm after the passage of the July 1920 law with agitation over the antimilitarist legislation. It saddened and worried her that those who so championed justice, freedom, and rights did not demand these rights *"equally for all. . . .* Antimilitarist like them, and like them, threatened by the new law, I cannot thus associate myself *with the form* that our male comrades give to their protest. I rebel with all my strength against the adjective "super." Because in my eyes . . . *all* laws of exception, *all* laws that crush liberty are *scélérate to the same degree."*[43]

Pushed yet further to the left by these events, Roussel again proclaimed herself a "revolutionary" and rendered homage to the Soviet Union in the distinctly unrevolutionary journal *La Mère éducatrice*, where she admiringly described Moscow's coeducational system. She quickly learned, however, that Bolshevism—or at least its adherents—offered only more of the same dogmatism she had already encountered. When she saw how communists in France sought to indoctrinate young children, they reminded her of Christians trying to "save souls"; she yearned for the anticlerical, freethinking discourse of fifteen years earlier. All convictions, she argued, had to be the product of experience and reflection—not blind indoctrination—and children needed educations that would make them think for themselves—"to watch, listen, and reflect"—so that as adults they could choose their own paths. Roussel hated capitalism, and she applauded anything that opposed it. But she had little taste, she said, for "organizing brigades and party spirit."[44]

Nor were communists, male and female, any more sympathetic to feminism than prewar radicals and revolutionaries had been. Revered women revolutionaries, such as Clara Zetkin in Germany and Alexandra Kollontai in the Soviet Union, preached that women could never be emancipated in a bourgeois order, and many female militants in France agreed. "Most male militants," Roussel declared, "have not yet understood that the social question does not pose itself in the same manner for [women] as it does for them . . . it is infinitely more complex, since to the common adversary—the capitalistic and bourgeois order—are added injustices, vexations, prejudices from which we alone suffer." Such injustices would not disappear with capitalism, she argued, because they were produced by the male mentality common all classes and all political parties. "To be only feminist, without linking feminism to some grand ideal of social transformation and human regeneration, is obviously an error, prejudicial to feminism itself," she wrote. "Not to be feminist is another error, no less serious."[45]

Small Victories: Giving Voice to Others

To use the pervasive metaphor of her time, Roussel sowed the seeds of her doctrine on mostly infertile ground, especially after 1914. Even though she and her neo-Malthusian colleagues could not produce a mass movement, Roussel did have a transformative effect on individuals. One such person was Charlotte Davy, whose example illustrates the power Roussel could have in changing one life. We know about Davy because she wrote an autobiography, but surely there were others similarly transformed among the tens of thousands exposed to Roussel's doctrine who left no record.

Davy was born in 1883 to parents who could not nurture her, and for most of her childhood, she was raised by relatives. Her father was a low-level railroad employee and former Communard. Her mother was depressed and mentally unstable from the time that she gave birth to Davy, and she later became gravely ill with tuberculosis. According to her autobiography, Davy had an "exasperating" childhood that set her on a path of self-destruction. Her lugubrious young adulthood was filled with romantic disappointments, affairs with married men, incidents of sexual harassment, and sexual exploitation. Her various employers cheated her financially, and she suffered periods of dire poverty. Davy finally married a lover with whom she had previously had an adulterous affair. He soon went to war, and in view of her earlier misfortunes, she was lucky that he came home in one piece. She never had children and does not mention why—but the behavior of her own mother hardly offered her a positive model of motherhood.[46]

In the spring of 1920, Davy began reading *La Voix des femmes*. She decided to attend a meeting it organized, at which five speakers addressed an audience of 4,000. Roussel swept Davy off her feet. She later wrote, "I listened to [Roussel] stupefied; never had I heard such language: it seemed to me that it was my own personal suffering she was proclaiming to the entire audience, that it was my feelings she was translating; she was avenging me a little, and this was very sweet for me. In truth, from the height of her platform, she . . . changed me; her hands randomly threw the seed, and I felt that I was the fertile soil, that my heart was the furrow ready to receive the seed and [it] would germinate a little more goodness."[47]

Davy wrote an open letter to Roussel in July 1920 that was published in *La*

Voix des femmes. By this time she had read *Quelques lances rompues pour nos liber-tés,* which *La Voix des femmes* distributed to subscribers as a premium. She emphasized how deeply she had been touched by what Roussel said about female pain. Roussel responded immediately, and Davy became a collaborator on *La Voix des femmes.* Through Roussel and the newspaper, she found her voice.

Davy began writing her autobiography, and Roussel edited the manuscript from 1920 through 1922. In the process, they developed a rather extraordinary relationship. Davy revealed her innermost secrets, sexual and otherwise, which she feared would offend Roussel's sensibilities. Indeed, Nelly's capacity to take in Davy's life story testified to her true compassion. She understood Davy and lent her emotional support despite their different backgrounds and sexual mores—and indeed, if the content of this rather steamy biography may have exceeded Nelly's better judgment, the end result certainly benefited from her editing. Henri Barbousse, author of the best-selling *Le Feu,* wrote a glowing preface. Davy included a dedication to Roussel that credited her with changing her life. In a final paragraph to her last chapter, which was written after Roussel died, Davy thanked her again. She ended the book with the words (italics in the original): "*As long as I have the strength, guided by you, which will help enlighten me, I shall fight for a better world where goodness will triumph over hatred, and I shall be able to say, O Nelly, that it was you who made the sparks flash!*" She later told Godet what Nelly had meant to her: Davy had suffered as a "victim of prejudice, of injustice, of the rancor on the part of individuals." She would have remained—like so many others—resigned to her victimhood, "content to cry over a lost youth and a ruined life" if she had not one day heard Nelly Roussel. Roussel made her understand the need for feminism and gave her the power "to do something with the lessons of my hard experience." She published four books after her autobiography.[48]

Davy was unique in her opportunity to articulate the way Roussel had given her a voice, but she was not alone in having received close mentoring. Particularly in the postwar period, Nelly was angry that militants rarely asked women to speak publicly. Frustrated at the continued rarity of talented female public speakers, she established a "School of Propagandists" with Alice Jouenne and Marguerite Durand, under the auspices of *La Voix des femmes.* Its purpose was to "train a phalanx of active, audacious, well-informed militants, always prepared to set forth the ideals and program" of *La Voix des femmes:* feminism, socialism, pacifism, and internationalism. Beginning in early December 1920, they offered classes every Monday at 6:30 p.m. at a cost of six francs per month. Roussel taught the classes regularly, and two of the students also took private diction lessons from her.[49]

That same month Roussel also revived an event that had been dear to her past and was now more necessary than ever, given the renewed power of French Catholicism. She took up the earlier battles of freethinkers, "the fruits of which [had] been torn away" after the war, and once again organized the *Noël humaine,* or "Human Christmas," that had previously been organized under the auspices of *L'Action.* This time, she and Henriette Sauret organized the event with *La Voix des femmes.* It took place the morning after Christmas in the great hall of the Grand Orient and consisted of a three-part celebration of the "rebirth" in nature, humanity, and society; events included various poetry readings (Victor Hugo and Converset, among others), music (Liszt, Chopin, Beethoven, Gluck), dance performances, and a production of Nelly's own *Par la révolte,* in which she played the part of Eve.

Roussel gave an opening address in which she explained the meaning of this winter celebration. All religions, she said, had adapted, and thus demeaned, eternal symbols that predated them. She wished to return to their prereligious meaning. The *Noël humaine* celebrated the winter solstice, the birth of a "New Spirit"—nature—and childhood, the awakening of a sleeping consciousness and the dawn of better times. In her presentation, Roussel not only drew on her understanding of the sensuality behind Church ritual and crowd behavior, she uncannily understood how nationalist ritual could substitute for the religious. Her description portended the rise of fascist movements and totalitarian governments when she asked her audience to understand the crowds that

> kneel before the tabernacles, under the religious impulsion of the glamorous Gothic arches, in the soft dim light where the clergy illuminate their trembling stars, in the intoxicating fragrance of incense and flowers, in the lulling, pealing harmony of the organs, in all this sumptuous and mystical apparatus where pains are numbed and hopes exalted; let us understand as well that these crowds also rush frenetically to the fleeting passage of the powerful of the day; they applaud, with drunken cries, the flags flapping in the wind, fireworks, clashing sounds of men in arms, regulating their steps to the rhythm of high-sounding music, and all the jumble, and all the flashing of official, patriotic, and military ceremony–

From her own religious background, Roussel knew how the sight, sound, and smell of Church ritual made isolated individuals into a community of senses and spirit. And she understood how pomp and circumstance created patriotism. At the same time, she knew that "these crowds obey the basest need in them," one that is common to all of humanity: a need "to forget our daily miseries, monotonies, sorrows, to live for a moment a life that is larger, more intense, more complete"; most human and most noble is *"the need to have communion in a unique thought and in a similar ideal."* She said that it was the task of militants to show the crowds an ideal worthy of this communion, to offer them joyous subjects worthy of this great desire. Roussel concluded by returning to her own perpetual theme, the compelling imagery of childbirth, maternal pain, and redemption that she made into a metaphor of revolution itself: "We shall turn toward the East, from which the first light always comes . . . we shall see the fetus Liberty who tormented the sacred womb of the Revolution, its mother; we shall hear the great people in the process of giving birth, which under the frozen sky proclaims the formidable pains of its immense labor."[50]

Last Words of Hope and Pain

In the first half of 1921, Roussel spoke publicly seven times in Paris and its environs. She gave her last talk on June 12 at a large demonstration of social-ist municipalities to inaugurate avenues Jean Jaurès and Édouard Vaillant. One would not guess the toll that her disease had taken on her physical appearance by this point from the pace of her activity and the relative absence of comment about it in her diaries and correspondence. Her good friend and collaborator Henriette Sauret recalled Roussel's appearance at one of these last talks:

[Her] facial features were pointed, [her] skin of porcelain whiteness stretched over a skeleton . . . , [her] eyes unforgettable: brilliant and somber, a little sunken, wor-ried, burning, moving prodigiously, seeming to search incessantly for a connection, an echo, a fraternal fame. These eyes, this paleness, were all she was. The rest was almost a ghost. . . . a body of touching thinness, always taking refuge in the shadow of black fabric; [a body] becoming each day more immaterial, a delicate stem barely able to support the strange and impassioned face.

To see her so small, so weak broke one's heart. We thought she would not even be able to walk [to the stage] . . . [but] she moved forward, and she climbed up onto the unstable platforms . . . in the working class neighborhoods and suburbs. As soon as her light foot touched these humble springboards, an electric wave ran through her, an incredible force seized her and she spoke, her shoulders shaking, her head turned back a little, her arms widened into a full gesture of wings. And, in effect, she took flight: she was no longer only raised, frenetically, passionately; she was . . . an ascension into the light.[51]

This observation was echoed in another friend's description: "from 1918 to 1922, [Roussel] was tormented by the cruelest illness, but she never capitulated to it

. . . [always agreeing to speak when invited], she would come to gatherings and meetings already emaciated, short-winded, but more ardent and impassioned than ever."[52]

The energy she put into her political activity and the relatively few notations in her diary about her disease belied its progress. Because public activity fatigued her, which in turn sometimes reactivated symptoms, she and others often blamed her ill health on her activism itself, an attribution facilitated by the lack of any specific diagnosis ("neurasthenia" was no longer mentioned).[53] When in Fontainebleau in 1921, as autumn approached, her symptoms became acute. As in the past, she stopped eating dinner because her inability to digest kept her awake. "This perpetual fear of not digesting," she wrote to Henri, "of not sleeping! And the desperate battle of this poor soul breaking its wings against the walls of the miserable carcass that imprisons it!" The doctor she was then seeing proclaimed that the only thing wrong with her was a sore throat. He seemed to think her stomach ailment imaginary.[54] After returning to Paris, she began seeing yet another doctor, Pagnier, about twice a week, because her sore throat persisted.

Although Roussel never again spoke publicly, her disease did not yet silence her—she still had her pen. In January 1922, she wrote an article commemorating the anniversary of Louise Michel's death. Using much of the same language as in her presentation at the *Noël humaine*, her article read like a swan song. She repeated some of the most important themes of her career—with the notable exception of neo-Malthusianism—and passed the baton on to a younger generation, just as she had once envisioned herself taking it up from Louise Michel. Recalling the meeting of revolutionary workers on January 19, 1905, to raise funds for Michel's burial, Nelly wrote:

> I went, shaking with the enthusiasm of my twenty-five years, the only woman among all the speakers, in order to salute the great fighter who had just disappeared, in the name of young militants, in the name of the new ones who had come to battle, who dreamed of continuing her work, to raise again the flag, fallen in her dying hands, and be made the vestals of the purifying flames that had fired her love, her faith, her genius. . . . All the eyes were turned toward the setting sun, as one turns toward a dawn. And never as in this hour did I feel what the communion of an ideal among a crowd could be.

On that occasion in 1905, she had saluted "neophytes full of illusion"; this time, she was saluting those who had lived a life of "battle and suffering," who had taken backward steps and known defeat, but who had "never weakened, doubted or become discouraged." She went on to say that Louise Michel would have loved

La Voix des femmes, for its contributors were her intellectual daughters, and like her, rebelled against all "the tyrannies of race, class, and sex" and opposed everything that "created hierarchies, whether clericalism, capitalism, militarism, masculinism—inseparable and logically connected chapters."[55]

At the end of January 1922, just after completing this article, Nelly and Mireille left for the Midi, where they spent a month visiting friends and relatives in Toulon, Nice, and Monaco so that she could escape the Paris winter. She was absent from Paris when Marguerite Durand opened new offices for *La Fronde,* where she would not only relaunch the newspaper but planned to open a bookstore with a restaurant. Durand invited Nelly to the opening celebration of the offices and asked that she place her brochures in the bookstore. In Nelly's absence, Henri attended the reception. After taking tea and eating little cakes on delicate china, Godet quickly took his leave with the excuse that he had a meeting to attend. But before he escaped, Mmes Hammer and Harlor (Roussel's colleagues from the UFF, which she had abandoned) caught him. As he recounted to Nelly, they "tried their best to tell me how they regretted your poor state of health. Madame Hammer spoke to me of an invitation that she was proposing to send you, probably for a meeting at her home. Madame Raspail almost threw herself on my neck to beg me to tell you a bunch of things, and that certainly all these ladies admired you, that they were with you, even when you scandalized them—it's I who use this word, but I well understood the meaning of all their talk."[56] "Scandalized" was indeed Godet's word—perhaps it was he who had been scandalized—but this brief encounter emphasized how Roussel's path had diverged from that of the UFF women she had known for twenty years; it also showed that her feminist colleagues cared deeply about her, despite the more radical political turn she had taken.

Henri initially believed Nelly was doing well in the south, but within a month, she insisted on returning, despite his protests. She immediately resumed biweekly visits to Dr. Pagnier, and at the end of March, Henri took her to a Dr. Tapon for a radioscopic examination of her lungs and stomach. Two days later, he brought the x-rays to Pagnier. Nelly was told that Tapon saw "ganglions" on her right lung, but she was given no diagnosis. Pagnier knew that the x-rays revealed that Nelly had pulmonary tuberculosis. If he told Henri at that time—and subsequent events suggest that he did—they both concealed the true nature of her illness from her.[57]

In the early twentieth century, it was common to conceal certain diagnoses from patients and their families. A diagnosis of tuberculosis equaled a death sentence, and doctors believed patients would be better off in a state of ignorance. From this moment on, Henri and Pagnier participated in a conspiracy of concealment. Through April and the beginning of May, the doctor continued to treat Nelly, mostly at home, with shots "against bronchitis" and electric vibrator massages of her still ailing abdomen. She tried without result to have herself admitted to two different sanatoria, and Pagnier tried to send her to a Dr. Bon at the Chalet d'Arguel clinic, near Besançon (Doubs), which was run by nuns. He later told Henri, "I wanted above all to delude her about her hopeless case, knowing too well that she would only stay a short time [at the clinic] . . . at the present time, febrile tuberculosis is never completely cured."[58]

Nelly's home treatments continued, but on May 9, immediately after purging herself, a severe intestinal crisis set in. For the next month, she stayed in bed, and Pagnier administered shots of camphorated and cinnozyl oil. Her immediate family visited her, as did Mathilde and Charlotte Davy.[59] Even in her severely ill state, she continued editing Davy's autobiographical manuscript and worked on a letter to be read aloud at a demonstration sponsored by the *Voix des femmes* on May 20. In her letter, Roussel encouraged her "comrades" to form a single front, "not against men—of whom some, the best, are with us—but against *masculinism* and all the social monsters to which it gives birth." But she also spoke about what the journal had meant to her, knowing that she might not ever return: it had been an "oasis" to which she "gave her last combative forces" after her spirit and heart had been "too often wounded," and she gave it her warmest wishes.[60]

As in the past, severe family illnesses coincided. Mireille was recovering from a long bout of bronchitis just as Nelly's intestinal condition reached a point of crisis, and Henri succumbed to bronchitis as well. At the end of May, Mireille went to the Chalet d'Arguel clinic, to which Pagnier had wanted Nelly admitted. On June 9, Marcel and Nelly's mother took her to the Sanatorium des Pins in Lamotte Beuvron (Loir-et-Cher). Shortly afterward, Henri joined Mireille to complete his cure at Chalet d'Arguel, where he stayed for almost six weeks. Marcel was the only member of the family not confined to a sanatorium at this point.

At Lamotte Beuvron, Roussel began a monotonous routine: she stayed in bed, even for her meals, and wrote one letter a day to family and friends; she received a visit from one of three doctors—Hervé, Roussel, and Legourd—each morning and afternoon. But there she learned the truth. Eight days after her arrival, she wrote to Marcel, for the first time voicing her knowledge that she had pulmonary tuberculosis. As though to minimize the seriousness of the diagnosis, she mentioned it only after making numerous practical requests, such as asking him to bring her three Balzac novels, medications, and an umbrella of a color that would match her clothes, and telling him the good news that she received from "papa" and Mireille about the respective states of their health. She then wrote,

Dr. Hervé . . . told me how much better I am looking . . . he was shocked by the incoherent, inexplicable spiking of my temperature, which he attributes to my nervous
state. My stomach is not too bad, and my intestine is not too good. As for my lungs
. . . grandmother having asked for the results of the x-ray, I don't know whether I
should tell her the truth. (I have not yet told papa and Mireille, so as not to trouble
their rest cure.) It appears that I have, with a few "menaces" on the left, a serious
lesion at the top of my right lung—a recent one, since Dr. Tapon saw nothing other
than the "ganglions"; the consecutive weakening from my intestinal crisis must
have provoked it. Dr. Hervé, moreover, diagnosed "tuberculosis by denutrition,"
which means that my digestive apparatus is the great culprit; and if it is the cause
of the illness, it will also be an obstacle to the cure. Nonetheless, the doctor added,
"It's possible it will improve." You see I talk to you, *mon petit grand* Marcel, as a
serious man.[61]

In keeping with common practice, Dr. Hervé kept her hope alive by concealing the extent of her infection and by dismissing her fever as a matter of nerves.
When Dr. Lagourd, the throat specialist, later told her that the irritation had nothing to do with the pulmonary infection, and that it only resulted from a general
state of bad circulation, he too was probably trying to conceal the extent of her
disease. Their encouragement had positive effects. By the end of June, Nelly had
gained about three pounds; she began moving around, at first in a wheelchair,
then walking on her own. One of her most frequent destinations was the library,
where she not only borrowed many books but also deposited copies of her own
books of poetry, speeches, and articles. A tireless propagandist, she distributed
Ma forêt, Quelques lances rompus, and *La Voix des femmes* to those around her, including her doctors. Each day, she read, wrote letters, and doggedly continued to
edit Charlotte Davy's autobiographical manuscript.[62]

How Roussel, her family, and her friends understood her disease contributed
to a web of conspiracy, and a set of dissimulating family stratagems ensued.
Mireille had first been sent to the Chalet d'Arguel clinic because the bronchitis
she suffered in April had apparently caused a lung infection; when she entered
the clinic in May, she also had an irregular heartbeat, anemia, weight loss, and
gastrointestinal symptoms ominously similar to those her mother had long endured. Still ignorant of her mother's true condition, Mireille's symptoms produced in others a fear that she had inherited her mother's vulnerability to tuberculosis—and neurasthenia. She was prescribed complete, prolonged bed rest
and a diet heavy in butter. Mireille missed her mother and very much wanted her
to join her at the Chalet d'Arguel. But as Mireille's health improved, it became

clear that she was deliberately being kept away from Nelly out of fear that knowledge of her mother's true state would be deleterious for her health. Cost was not an issue, for Montupet was paying for Mireille's confinement.[63] Henri also told Mireille not to tell her mother about her own symptoms, and Nelly did not tell Mireille details about herself. When Marcel visited Mireille in August, he too remained silent about his mother. But while there, Nelly wrote a letter to them both, which should have suggested the gravity of her illness:

> My reveries turn to the past; because the future, for me, is too frightening—And I understand more than ever how everything is relative. I surprise myself in thinking tenderly, even with a kind of nostalgic regret (notably about the vacations in these last years), which, at the time, did not seem at all marvelous, filled with worry and suffering, but where, nonetheless, I was *living*, where I was doing a ton of things of which today I am deprived . . . our last trip to the Midi [just the previous February] especially comes to mind, like a vision already distant; the bad memories fade, the good ones become more vivid. Is it because I have suffered so much since? Because this was, for me, the last manifestation of normal life? Or is it simply because you were with me, my dear [Mireille], and your image is mixed with all that happened there? . . . Ah! My children, my dear little children! How happy I was to know that, despite everything, despite the lamentable state in which I have been for several years, since you were old enough to be aware, you as well kept a good memory of all that we saw together; and that you will remember later, with emotion, that your mama was a companion and friend for you, as long as she was able.[64]

Nelly also expressed remorse over the end of her career and her ability to perform. She wrote to Juliette Robin that her greatest deprivation, her greatest sorrow, was the loss of her voice and her ability to read poetry out loud. "I'll resign myself *perhaps* to never making any more speeches; but I'll never resign myself to not being able to sing with my lips the poetry that sings within me." She wanted desperately to write one more article for *La Voix des femmes* as it made its transition from a bimonthly journal to a daily newspaper. "I still have time . . . [but] this article will probably not be followed by many others." She had dreamed of having a newspaper like this at the peak of her career, when she was doing her lecture tours, "in the name of, and for the profit of which, she would have wanted to speak"—*La Fronde* had come (and gone, in its merger with *L'Action* in 1904) too soon, and *La Voix des femmes* had come too late. But, she said, "the essential thing is that it succeed with or without me." She did indeed finish the article, which was published on December 1.[65]

Henri also became increasingly emotional and sentimental. After his return from his bronchitis cure at the Chalet d'Arguel clinic on July 18, he began weekly visits to Nelly, a two-and-a-half hour train ride from Paris. In a memoir written some months later, he recalled his difficult routine: he would arrive at 11:00 a.m., often take Nelly to a restaurant despite her weakness, sit in the park with her, and then rush to catch the 4:00 p.m. train at the very last minute. After forcing himself to be cheerful with her, he would dissolve into tears on the train.[66]

Henri came to detest Lamotte Beuvron. He thought Dr. Hervé conducted his business "like a low-class profiteer," and that Dr. Lagourd was "immoral." Worse, Nelly hated the place as well. In September, she wrote, "My chronic insomnia is completely disastrous for me. It is making me ill. Today I am calmer and less sad because I slept. And I slept because I didn't eat last night. In the afternoon I had a dreadful stomachache. Really, I cannot endure this martyrdom any longer." The weather was cooling, and she complained the next day of how she continued to "freeze": "This morning I had a crisis of nerves caused by the cold. I'll never pardon those who have made me suffer so much." Henri then realized how out-dated and insufficient the heating system was in the sanatorium's old buildings. But he could not abide Nelly's earlier veiled threat that she would return home. For her to abandon this last effort at a cure would make him lose "his last hope of saving her."[67]

Henri's disgust over the conditions at Lamotte Beuvron drove him to find another sanatorium, that of Buzenval, just east of Paris. He and Marcel took her there on September 20. By this point Nelly weighed only 94 pounds and had been losing her hair, but she was still strong enough to distribute copies of *La Faute d'Eve* and *Ma forêt* to her doctor, other patients, and the sanatorium library. She found her surroundings pleasant, and Henri had great hope in the new doctor, Poussard. But when Poussard refused to turn on the central heating before November, Henri labeled him a "greedy shopkeeper" like the others. Henri then brought blankets and two electric heaters to Nelly's room, but the doctor protested that there would be no way of calculating how much she would owe for the extra electricity she consumed. Dr. Poussard's approach to medicine also disturbed Henri. He did not hide the fact that Nelly's state was "irremediably lost" and that both her lungs were badly infected. Henri nonetheless tried to talk the doctor into an (unnamed) experimental treatment that had elsewhere proved promising; Poussard had indeed heard of this treatment, but it required time— which, he bluntly told Henri, Nelly did not have. Godet then tried to persuade him to raise Nelly's morale by giving her some hope of recovery—they would share this role—Godet would "declare [his] confidence in [the doctor's] science, and recount stories of others' cures, and [Poussard] would show optimism based on scientific facts."[68]

In October, Roussel began having nightly injections of heroin, along with injections of other substances. She gained five pounds, but by the end of the month, she started requesting additional doses of heroin. She received visits from her mother and Montupet, as well as Marcel and two close friends, Louise Sauval and Germaine Lambert. She still managed to write a letter each week to Mireille, but it took her two days to pen them. As her throat condition worsened, the doctor gave her a vaporizer with cocaine, which she ingested for several days in addition to the heroin shots. By mid October, her left leg began to swell, symptomatic of a breakdown in her vital organs. Henri tried to remain optimistic. When he visited her, she would welcome him with a forced smile, and he would pretend to be "gay, full of hope." He talked about celebrating their twenty-fifth wedding anniversary the following June, and of how they would return to Italy and retrace the path they had taken on their honeymoon.[69] And then, recalling his routine, he described "the return home, this horrible return, with my eyes so full of tears that I no longer knew where I was stepping. I only succeeded in calming myself on the train." But even worse for him was seeing Nelly's mother and stepfather:

> I would arrive at her mother's; she waited anxiously for news, whatever news I could bring her—I threw myself in an armchair and allowed myself to go into a veritable crisis of despair—impossible to find any words—what could I say, other than that I found her worse, thinner. . . .
>
> This is the moment my father-in-law generally chose to subject me to his opinion about therapeutics—they were naturally as stupid as his opinions about everything else. This evil madman, this sadistic pseudo-moralist would expectorate a few judgments about politics, about ideas that he deemed subversive, and even about the reading of certain newspapers that brought illness and death to their subscribers . . . it was amid this sad ordeal that I was able to judge the abominable mentality of this horrible individual.[70]

Meanwhile, ignorant about her mother's true condition and her father's mental anguish, Mireille regularly corresponded with both. Forbidden to discuss her own illness with her mother, she sent lengthy, self-indulgent missives to Henri that detailed every symptom and aspect of her treatment. In the middle of September, when he was upset over the conditions at Lamotte Beuvron, Mireille wrote, "What has come over you? Are you sick?" To "punish" him for having written a letter she deemed "too serious," she wrote an "equally serious" letter in which she obsessed over the state of her health and where she would spend the winter. As though to penalize him further, she recounted to her atheist father the miracle of one young inmate of the clinic who, dying a horrible death in the last stages of tuberculosis, had gone to Lourdes and returned completely cured—which made Mireille "no longer doubt the reality of phenomena obtained at Lourdes." This story must have made Henri apoplectic.[71]

By November, so large was the gap between Mireille's understanding and the reality of Nelly's condition that Henri complained to her "politely" that the letters she was sending to her mother were full of "imbecilities." The final insult came during Mireille's pending departure from the clinic in November. Nelly had arranged for her to spend the winter with her friend Odette Laguerre, who lived in Don-par-Artemare (Ain), not far from Lyon. Mireille repeatedly begged her father to escort her to Don. Godet assigned Marcel that task, but he did comply with Mireille's wish that he purchase a statue of the Virgin Mary as a parting gift for a nun to whom she had become deeply attached.[72]

On November 24, Henri wrote the last letter his wife would read from him. He rose in the middle of the night to write of his "great grief to see you suffer without being able to relieve your pain." He deliberately wrote this letter with an uncharacteristically good hand, in the same style as "when we were engaged, and I applied myself, because, as I recall, not without pride, my handwriting pleased you." This thought led to reveries about their wedding anniversary and the persistent but decidedly unrealistic fantasy of a trip to Italy the following June. Ever optimistic, he said: "Something tells me that between now and then, we shall have triumphed over a bad destiny." The letter touched her deeply, and she said to him when he next saw her, "Anyone who writes such beautiful letters cannot call himself old."[73] Three days later, the cocaine caused a "crisis of poisoning" and further intestinal failure, which required that a nurse be with Nelly at all times. Her diary stops on Tuesday, December 12, with Henri's visit as the only entry. She died six days later, Monday, December 18, 1922, three weeks before she would have turned forty-five.

Henri wrote immediately to Odette Laguerre's family to inform them of Nelly's death, but he firmly instructed them to conceal the news from Mireille, because he so feared the impact it would have on her health. Instead, he sent their close friend Germaine Lambert to tell Mireille in person. Lambert arrived in Don on Thursday, December 21. "What sadness for me, and what effort I had to make in order to manage the poor little Mireille and hide the horrible facts until the next day," Odette Laguerre wrote after her arrival; "everything was done according to your intentions. Your poor child was filled in on the abominable news, only little by little, by transitions."[74] Henri joined his daughter in Don on Christmas, four days later—after Nelly's funeral had already taken place.

Remembering and Commemorating Roussel

Nelly Roussel was buried in the family vault in Père Lachaise cemetery on December 21, 1922, even before Germaine Lambert informed Mireille of her death. That day was, coincidentally, the winter solstice, which had held so much symbolism of pain, death, and rebirth for Roussel. After four days of stormy wind and rain, the sun "miraculously" shone as the funeral procession took off for the cemetery at noon. Close to 200 people attended. The scores of sympathy letters and cards sent to Godet in the days and weeks that followed indicate that many more people would have attended but for their absence from Paris during the holidays, ill health, or simply the very short notice of her death and of the funeral—indeed, many did not receive the news until after the funeral had taken place.[75]

In front of the family vault, numerous friends eulogized Roussel, among them Marguerite Martin, Marguerite Durand, Noëlie Drous, Marie-Thérèse Gil-Baer, Marbel, Amélie Hammer, Marianne Rauze, Charlotte Davy, and Colonel Converset, all friends and colleagues in feminism and feminist journalism. Noëlie Drous honored her for her perceptiveness, audacity, and courage, and for the risks she had taken in public meetings with her "advanced" ideas. Her "rare probity" had earned her "more than one enemy." Drous said that from the very beginning of her career, Roussel had "got to the bottom" of the feminist question, clearly defined its most basic principles, and "traced the path by which its goals could be achieved." Two speakers referred to the violent (verbal) attacks to which Roussel had been subjected, and how her talent had made others jealous. Repeated references were made to her profound generosity, loyalty, dedication in friendship, and humility. Several speakers called her an "apostle" of feminism and emphasized what a loss she would be to the movement. Colonel Converset and others acknowledged the important support she had received in her private life, especially from Henri. And several noted her extraordinary talent for public speaking.[76]

The effort to affix meaning to a deceased individual, just as with war commemorations and memorials, invariably evokes ambivalence and contradiction, as well as praise—especially around someone who has died before her time. Marbel had once said that Roussel embodied "a harmonious mixture of contrasts in intellectual virility, physical delicacy, and moral sensibility," which she put in

poetic terms: "And by a trait of her genius / Nature put all her splendor / into pro-
ducing so much contrast / In order to extract harmony from it." Another admirer
later noted that she had within her a "heroic mixture: *Tenderness and Virility*."[77]

But for others, Roussel's contrasts produced contradictions. One that emerged
in testimonies about her was the contradiction between her long-term illness
and her ability to continue propagandizing. In reference to her testimony in the
1918 legal defense of Hélène Brion, Drous recalled that Roussel's "emaciated
face contrasted with the energy of her words" and added, "From the moment it
was a matter of coming to the defense of a woman, or demanding freedom of
thought, or attacking an injustice, Nelly Roussel would overcome her illness and
respond: 'Present.'" Gil-Baer similarly noted how much Roussel wanted to continue working until the very end of her days, making reference to the last article
she had written for the *Voix des femmes*. But such dedication in the face of illness
incurred some confusion, even resentment. Marguerite Durand, in tears as she
spoke, said: "The disease that just took our friend was so courageously endured
by her, she was so habituated to her suffering that she . . . habituated us to it as
well. Many among us judged this disease almost imaginary on the part of this
pretty young woman who, so rapidly, so energetically, shook off her languor when
duty called. . . . We thus did not suspect that the intense flame that animated her
eloquence would consume her so soon!" A week after the funeral, Durand felt
compelled to explain herself further to Godet. Even after having received a letter
from him after one of his visits to the sanatorium—one she had intended to answer, but never did—she said that she "had never believed Nelly so sick. I judged
her very spoiled by all of you and a little removed . . . imagine how stunned I was
by this sad and, for me, sudden reality."[78]

That many individuals judged Roussel's illness imaginary, as Durand said
they did, is understandable, since for many years her disease was diagnosed as
"neurasthenia." Apart from fatigue and fluctuating weight, her symptoms were
largely invisible to others, especially those who had not seen much of her after
she became politically radicalized by the war. It took little further imagination,
then, to blame her illness on her work. Two obituaries listed her "brilliant" contributions to the feminist and freethinking movements at length, but then added,
"in her propaganda tours, in articles she gave to the militant press, in this incessant activity, she dangerously weakened her health"—as though tuberculosis had
nothing to do with her decline. Indeed, so prevalent was this view among those
who commemorated her that a recent biographical sketch of Roussel, although
noting that she had tuberculosis, concludes that she died of exhaustion during
her final political battles.[79]

Durand said something else that reflected collective perceptions: the "flame" that animated Roussel's eloquence also "consumed" her. Others used this metaphor as well. Roussel's colleague, Henriette Sauret, wrote eloquently that

> Nelly Roussel cried over the servitude of women, the death of children who were victims of misery or stupidity, over human beings corrupted by hatred. The pains of the world passed through her heart . . . [a heart] too big to be filled by egotistical pleasure. And that is what gave Nelly Roussel this beautiful, pale face, in which the large somber eyes sparkled like two sad jewels. And it is perhaps to this incoercible torment, to this dread of a soul consumed by an impossible dream of altruism, that must be attributed the premature death of our friend.

She later added: "She gave her entire self to each talk, each lecture. One can also say that she was consuming herself a little more each time that she spoke." Mireille also referred to Roussel's work of propaganda using the metaphor of a "flame" that "consumed her."[80]

The "consumption" metaphor used to describe Roussel's demise replicates the nineteenth-century understanding of tuberculosis as a consumptive disease that arose spontaneously from internal causes, an "inner fire of a soul" that destroyed the body. But by the time she contracted the disease, it was known to be caused by a germ. It is nonetheless noteworthy that her friends and family persisted in using the nineteenth-century language to describe not her disease but her devotion to her work. In their descriptions, her personal inspiration seems to substitute—becomes a metonym—for the disease, as though they could not accept the actual cause of her death. A persistent fear of tuberculosis—manifest in the silence about it and refusal even to use the word—partly explains these reactions.[81] Roussel's family and friends felt more comfortable believing that the source of her disease was the unusual flame within her, rather than a germ, especially since there was no cure.

Another cultural precept may have come into play here in the way her death was understood. David Barnes has argued that in Third Republic France, tuberculosis became a vehicle of moral and spiritual redemptive suffering for women. This redemptive function fitted in with the "dominant cultural perception of woman's nature as not only pathological but also dichotomous—irreconcilably torn between the poles of virtue and vice." The romantic discourse about Roussel's own dichotomous character and her "internal flame" reflected a sense of "eternal sacrifice" inherent in the need for female redemption. How ironic and sad that those who loved her said that her political struggle had killed her. Having devoted her life to denaturalizing the relationship between womanhood and self-sacrifice, this depiction of her last battle would have disturbed Nelly Roussel, especially as she struggled against her disease until the very end, never ceasing to believe that science could cure her.

Did her mourners think that Roussel somehow had to be "redeemed"? She had transgressed the boundaries of her class, of her gender, bourgeois feminism, and of revolutionary politics; for most of her auditors and readers, with the exception of people like Charlotte Davy, Nelly Roussel embodied dichotomies. A gaping silence in the testimonies at her funeral suggests another punishing ambivalence her memory evoked: no one said anything about her commitment to neo-Malthusianism, even though she had considered it the most important of all feminist issues. Although some of the eulogies made reference to "conscious motherhood," collectively, they downplayed this aspect of her career; no mention was made of the July 1920 law. No one, moreover, from the neo-Malthusian movement spoke at her funeral, and few of them attended, even though they too adored her. Eugène Humbert certainly would have wanted to speak, but he and his wife were both in prison.

Fortunately, consumption by her own flame and silence on the issue most important to her was not the only way Roussel was remembered in subsequent years. *La Voix des femmes* and *La Mère éducatrice* continued to commemorate her on the anniversaries of her death, and much more was said about her in the early 1930s when, thanks to Mireille and Henri, two more volumes of her lectures appeared. To this biographer, the most accurate remembrance appears in an article again by Noëlie Drous, who underscored Roussel's "feminine dignity, which was always at the base of her revolts and the secret of so many sympathetic ties she had with her most fervent disciples." Quoting from Marbel, Drous offered the essence of Roussel's work:

> In the development of [her various] subjects, she is the integral feminist for whom it is impossible to be indifferent to any side of a question, and who courageously demands all the emancipations: intellectual, economic, social, political, sexual. And this last question, too often neglected by more timid feminists, particularly had to solicit her daring and generous thought . . . no union without love, and no motherhood without consent, such is, in her eyes, the basis of the question.[82]

Even though Roussel herself did not use the word "sexual," and it rarely appeared in feminist writing, it was the one issue that so distinguished her, and the one that the July law of 1920 repressed.

Upon learning of her mother's death, Mireille lived up to her grandmother's injunction: "pauvre petite . . . in order to soften our pain a little, you will be courageous, won't you, for the memory of the one who showed us so much courage?" Many others also implored her to be courageous. Mireille then vowed to Marbel, "As you say it so well, the only possible consolation for us, her children, will be to follow her example. The idea to pursue her work in the measure of my means reattaches me to life, and I'll make every effort to be worthy of her."[83] Mireille devoted the rest of her life to keeping her mother's memory alive and assuring her legacy in the subsequent story of French feminism and its relationship to reproductive rights.

Epilogue

Mireille returned to Paris in March 1923, three months after her mother's death. She was twenty-three and uncertain about her future. Having decisively informed her father that she would not return to work as his secretary, she instead became a teacher with the educational program founded after the war by Roussel's close friend Germaine Lambert, L'Enfance heureuse (Happy Childhood). Every Thursday—a day when the schools were closed—as well as during other school vacations, the teachers in this coeducational program took children on field trips to museums, parks, gardens, zoos, monuments, and other sites. Mireille contributed articles about L'Enfance heureuse and about her mother to *La Mère éducatrice* and to Marguerite Durand's newly revived *La Fronde*, which she signed "Mireille-Nelly Roussel." Odette Laguerre and other friends encouraged Mireille's self-identification with her mother and compared her sincerity, idealism, and dedication to social causes to Roussel's. Laguerre praised Mireille for her "elegant and measured prose, simple and warm" in which one rediscovered her mother's "beautiful soul and eloquence." She even noted that she was beginning to confuse the two of them in her own "heart and thoughts," because Mireille was becoming so much like Nelly.[1]

But Mireille's persona and her life were very unlike her mother's; although she remained a pacifist and avid supporter of feminism and reproductive rights, she never became involved in political action. She worked with L'Enfance heureuse for many years and later earned a living at Père Castor, a publisher of children's books. She also presumably received a substantial inheritance from the Godet-Nel-Montupet family estates. Mireille never married or had children. She expressed no interest in marriage, nor any need for physical intimacy of any sort. Indeed, the thought apparently repelled her.[2] Such an outlook seems ironic, given her parents' happy marriage and Roussel's advocacy of an "integral" feminism that would allow women to be fulfilled as individuals and as mothers. Mireille was hardly unusual among women of her generation in remaining single, however: in the 1920s and 1930s, France had become a nation "of old men and single women" as a result of the enormous losses in the Great War.[3] Moreover, Roussel's feminism had left open the possibility that women could be happy without marriage. But although she had many close friends of both sexes, Mireille does not seem to have been happy—indeed, she replicated her mother's life in an unfortunate way: she was sickly throughout. In 1927, for example, she was back in the sanatorium of Chalet d'Arguel, suffering inexplicable weight loss. Doctors failed to come up with a diagnosis and concluded that it was "nerves." What were apparently psychosomatic maladies plagued Mireille most of her life. She died aged eighty-eight in 1987, having lived almost twice as long as her mother.[4]

Marcel had a briefer but apparently happier life than his sister. From being an enfant terrible, he matured into a "handsome and proud" young man, whose face, and especially his eyes, reminded everyone of Nelly. Eighteen at the time of his mother's death, he completed his education and ultimately became an engineer in the French branch of a British company, Wild-Barfield. In 1926, he married Simone Leymarie, whom the family warmly embraced. But within two years, tragedy again struck: Marcel contracted stomach cancer and, like his mother, died a painful death. His acute suffering lasted two months, during which Simone, Mireille, and Henri attended him. In the final moments Henri again shielded his daughter from the ravages of death and insisted she stay away.[5] Marcel died May 1, 1928, aged twenty-three.

Henri Godet, who was nearly sixty when his wife died, lived another fourteen years. He never remarried. Nelly's former feminist colleague Madeleine Vernet wrote that Nelly's death had been a "terrible ordeal for him. Suddenly, he aged, closed himself off in his pain and in a cult of death," which became all the worse, she said, when his son was "brutally removed from his affection." Thanks to his close network of family and friends, centered especially around his sister, Juliette Robin, Henri nonetheless carried on as an artist (fig. 17) and a socialist despite his tragic losses.[6]

One of Godet's preoccupations in his final years was the placement of his last large piece, the Clémence Royer statue, which he had sculpted not only in honor of Royer's work on Darwin but as a monument to the power of the female intellect. The statue had been completed prior to World War I, but the committee that had raised funds to pay for it turned it over to the city of Paris, where it remained in storage for seventeen years. Godet and other supporters suggested that it be placed outside the university residence halls, in the gardens of the Muséum national d'histoire naturelle, or at any of a number of other locations they considered appropriate. Shortly before his death, Godet even tried to have it placed in the Vincennes Zoo, but the director did not think the statue had a proper place "among the animals." Quite simply, apart from Joan of Arc, officials systematically resisted erecting public monuments to women.

Henri Godet died of undisclosed causes in October 1937, aged 74, agonizing over Hitler and Nazism. Shortly after his death, the Rudier foundry, which had never been paid for the bronze it supplied for the statue, repossessed it. The foundry melted down the statue, and turned into cannon what had been intended as a monument to women—a noteworthy sign of the times.[7]

Godet otherwise left a significant legacy in his sculpture. He had produced a large collection of objets d'art of bronze and marble in art nouveau and art deco styles—for example, an ink stand of a woman on a rock, female statues that served as electric lamp bases, and female heads emerging from flowers, pieces perhaps simultaneously representing Roussel's repeated references to women "blossoming" into their independence and Alexandre Dumas fils's *La Dame aux camélias,* a book whose symbolism had powerfully moved Godet. Many of these sculptures were sold through Sotheby's in the 1970s, 1980s, and 1990s, commanding prices in the range of £1,500 to £10,000.[8]

Nelly Roussel as a Mother

Nelly Roussel's treatment of her children, and particularly of Marcel, might offend modern American readers. It is worth emphasizing once again that not a negative word about Roussel's behavior as a mother emerges in all the private correspondence and all the public commentary about her—with the exception of Godet's single expression of frustration that she did not want to see her son in 1915 when she was feeling ill. Godet never commented on her maternal qualities other than to incorporate a positive image of her motherhood in his art and in his advice to her about how to present herself. Indeed, her reputation as a mother lived on among those who knew her in both her private and public personas. In her 1937 eulogy of Godet, Madeleine Vernet recalled her personal memories of Henri and Nelly's "domestic harmony, embellished by two children whom they adored."[9]

Roussel evidently did not easily mother infants and young children, but it was routine in her generation to employ nannies for their care, and upper-middle-class mothers who tended their own children were exceptional. That Nelly placed Marcel in a *pouponnière*—something highly unusual among mothers of her social class—for his first two years does seem bizarre, especially since she visited him so rarely. Today's child psychologists would no doubt point to his institutionalization during these formative years as a reason why he became a difficult child; he had no opportunity to bond with his parents at this key stage of childhood development. It was Henri, however, who proposed to Nelly that Marcel be handed over to his aunt Andrée when he was just four years old, within two years of his moving back in with his parents. Marcel's adolescence and young adulthood unfortunately coincided with the stresses of World War I and its aftermath, as well as with Roussel's declining health. But as he matured, Marcel became his mother's "little big man," and her final letters to him frankly express maternal love and tenderness. By the time of his premature death, Marcel had attained a measure of well-being and achievement that would have made his mother very proud.

Mireille had a different experience growing up, since although she lived with her grandparents, she usually saw her parents on a daily basis. Unlike her brother, Mireille was the "perfect child." We get a glimpse of her feelings from a letter she wrote in August 1923 in posthumous response to the letter Roussel had written to both children a year earlier, in which she had expressed the hope that they would remember her "with feeling, as a companion and friend." Perhaps Nelly had consciously chosen not to ask her children to remember her as a mother. But, more likely, it simply had not occurred to her, and the bonds of friendship she felt with her children were indeed strong. "Mama!" Mireille responded in a state of profound grief nine months after her mother's death, "How could you doubt for an instant that we would remember you and all the moments lived with you? . . . It's more than a good memory, it's *everything* that was good and beautiful in our childhood, [and] in my adolescence." Admitting that her state of denial about her mother's true condition had made it impossible for her to respond at the time, Mireille continued, "I want you to know, dear Mama, what you were, what you still *are* for me! In the most distant memories of my childhood, you appeared as a light, like a benevolent and beautiful fairy who consoles all the sorrows and opens the imagination to all the ideal visions. And you were this fairy until the last moment."[10]

Michel Robin recalls without the least hesitation or judgment that the whole Godet-Roussel-Nel-Robin family thought Roussel's absence from her children was a sacrifice she had to make for her work, and no one questioned it. His understanding of Roussel and her career comes primarily from Mireille, who held her mother in the highest esteem; but it also from his father and grandmother, Juliette Robin, also Nelly's sister-in-law.[11]

Roussel in Public Memory

In thanking Noëlie Drous for an article she had written about Roussel on the first anniversary of her death, Godet confessed: "One of [Nelly's] great preoccupations during her final days was to wonder whether her efforts had been in vain, and in my distress, I often posed the same question to myself. You have rid me of my doubts, and I now believe, like you, that Nelly Roussel will have an intellectual survival in the minds and hearts of all who knew her."[12]

La Mère éducatrice continued to publish commemorations through the 1920s on the anniversaries of Roussel's death, as did *La Fronde* and *La Voix des femmes*. With her father's help, Mireille had two more collections of her mother's articles and lectures published: *Trois conférences de Nelly Roussel* (Three Lectures of Nelly Roussel) in 1930, with a preface by Odette Laguerre, and *Derniers combats* (Last Battles) in 1932, with a preface by socialist and anarchist Han Ryner.

These collections received notice in nearly thirty articles and reviews in twenty-two newspapers and journals. But the way she was remembered was as tensely ambivalent as the reception of her rhetoric when she was alive. After announcing the appearance of *Trois conférences,* the editors of ever conservative *La Française* published a caveat in a subsequent issue: "we have reservations about [Roussel's] opinions, and particularly those that touch on the restriction of births." Other articles, however, supported her advocacy of birth control and stressed her "eugenics." One noted that Madeleine Vernet, Marcel Capy, and Jeanne Humbert pursued the same "apostolate" and inherited her "eloquence and courage"; it called for a biography to be written. But many of these articles also made indirect reference to the ephemeral nature of Roussel's campaign and lamented that no one had replaced her. One referred to her "hour of notoriety," implying that her influence had been short-lived. Yet another, written when Spanish women received the vote, wondered why there were no more militants like Roussel in France. In fact, she and her supporters had been silenced by a pronatalist political culture that continued to deny women the vote.[13]

Little else was published about Roussel between the wars. After World War II, Jeanne Humbert eulogized her at length in the neo-Malthusian journal *La Grande Réforme*. But she concluded her article pessimistically: "It is regrettable that the race of Nelly Roussels is extinguished." Another long article appeared in 1955, a printed version of a radio transmission that praised all of Roussel's feminist contributions, especially those concerning the issue of birth control.[14] In the long run, however, Godet was unfortunately correct in what he said in 1923: until 1978, the centenary of her birth, Roussel had a legacy only among those who had known her, not among the public at large—and given the legal history of birth control and of feminism in France, her efforts had indeed to some extent been in vain. Nelly Roussel, in short, was no Margaret Sanger. On the other hand, the birthrate in France remained stubbornly low until the post–World War II baby boom, despite the law of July 1920 and subsequent ones that reinforced it, suggesting that her message had hardly been irrelevant in practice.

Assessing the significance of Roussel's legacy—or lack thereof—raises a number of issues regarding the history of birth control movements, feminism, and the relationship between the two. Reactions to Roussel's feminist and free-dom-of-motherhood campaigns brought to the surface underlying attitudes that formed the base of French political culture. Like Marguerite Durand and others, Roussel's performance of femininity played a disruptive role. But her radicalism posed a more profound threat to the French moral order than did other forms of feminism. Her success and contemporary celebrity ultimately contributed to the legal silencing of the neo-Malthusian movement in 1920. Moreover, she laid bare the stubborn persistence of the "eternal feminine" and the notion of an eternally self-sacrificing womanhood in French imaginations across the political spectrum. Indeed, these notions endured beyond her life in at least two manifestations: the continued refusal to grant women political citizenship until 1944, and the familialist, pronatalist ideology that lay at the heart of Vichy regime politics (1940–44). The "eternal feminine" provided a foundational myth in Vichy France for policies about women's work, female education, family, and health. The rhetorical strategies of those who opposed her from both Right and Left reveal a concept of female self-sacrifice that French Catholicism in particular had employed, but that was secularized and perpetually reinvented with revolution and war. The gender component of Vichy's "National Revolution" had roots, not just in the 1930s, as historians have shown, but in the nineteenth century.[15]

The persistence of the eternal feminine in French political culture also left an indelible mark on feminism. Just as the feminist movement adapted itself to a nationalist rhetoric in the 1880s, it accommodated itself even further to pronatalist rhetoric during the interwar years. Rather than focusing on women's rights as individuals, mainstream feminists insisted that motherhood be recognized for its contributions to society, and therefore that mothers receive some sort of compensation. As Ann Cova has argued, the movement "often glorified motherhood in order to use it as a trump card in the acquisition of other powers."[16] To demand the right to birth control would have undermined their agenda. Rather than seeking rights as individual citizens, many feminists sought their individuality *through* motherhood. Roussel's former colleague Madeleine Vernet considered motherhood the "apogee of feminine individuality."[17] While tactics must not be confused with convictions, French feminists were forced to focus on motherhood as a social function worthy of government protection, rather than on political rights for women as individuals. The tactic paid off mightily, in that women did receive financial support in the form of family allowances—a twisted version of the paid maternity Roussel had advocated—and eventually state-supported childcare.

The 1920 law prohibiting birth control remained in effect until 1967. Ironically, however, couples continued to practice fertility control, and despite all the natalist propaganda and incentives, the birthrate in France remained very low until after World War II.[18] While some, mostly upper-middle-class, women used newer contraceptive devices such as the diaphragm, most French people continued to employ the same birth control methods as in the past: coitus interruptus, condoms, and abortion. Even after female contraceptive devices were legalized, many women continued to rely on traditional methods of family limitation. Until the 1970s, almost as many women (29 percent) reportedly continued to rely on coitus interruptus as took the pill (34 percent). Reliance on withdrawal was five times greater in France than it was in Britain, and ten times greater than in the United States. These statistics suggest that much of the French population retained traditional attitudes about contraception. The pattern changed at the end of the decade, with 18 percent relying on withdrawal, and by 1988, only 4.8 percent.[19]

The resistance to female contraceptive devices in France suggests that sexual practices and legal sanctions had as much to do with an abiding cultural precept about female nature as they did with a fear of population decline. Such is one of the lessons gleaned from studying Roussel's life and the opposition to her message. The durability of the "eternal feminine" also fits with the arguments of scholars such as Mona Ozouf and Elizabeth Badinter that Frenchwomen "accept nature's law" of sexual difference and accommodate themselves to it; relations between the sexes in France, in their view, are therefore more "civilized" than they are in the United States, where aggressive, "man-hating" feminism has poisoned gender relations.[20] Ozouf attributes the national differences to an inherent "exceptional" or "singular" French character. Though suggestive, this is an unprovable hypothesis. Perhaps the most important lesson to be learned from this study, moreover, is that the opposition Roussel experienced in her lifetime demonstrates how much work had to go into the efforts to preserve the notion of a "natural" womanhood. Public ridicule, court cases, journalistic polemics, and legislation were mobilized in the battle to sustain it.

That female-initiated contraception became officially accepted in France far more slowly than it did in the two other major democratic powers of the interwar period—England and the United States—bears further systematic comparison, particularly with regard to the relationship between national politics and the politics of reproduction. Not coincidentally, Great Britain and the United States had stronger feminist movements than did France, and their governments had also granted women the vote after World War I. While each of those countries had to grapple with the meaning of a lower birthrate—such as racist fears about the more prolific rate of reproduction among people of color and "race suicide" among the "better-bred" elements of their populations who had begun to have small families—their governments did not suppress public discussion of birth control the way the law of 1920 did in France. Ironically, Margaret Sanger returned from France (and the Netherlands) equipped with the latest forms of female contraceptives in 1915 and boldly established her first birth control clinic in New York in 1916.[21] Birth control clinics slowly became established in England after World War I. France would have to wait until 1961 for its first clinic.

A brief glimpse at the comparative history of birth control movements highlights another unique aspect of Nelly Roussel's career: her effort to integrate her advocacy of birth control into a broader feminist vision. While control over one's own reproductive potential has been a given in Western feminism since the 1970s, Roussel stood alone among the feminists of her own generation—and those of the next—in placing it at the center of female emancipation. Feminists such as Margaret Sanger, Emma Goldman, and Marie Stopes participated in and led birth control movements, but they never tried systematically to incorporate reproductive rights into an official feminist agenda.

In her initial campaign, Margaret Sanger had a great deal in common with Nelly Roussel. She too made speeches to workers and abhorred the pain and indignities working-class women suffered. Like Roussel (and Paul Robin), she originally argued that women's self-possession and the self-regulation of their bodies would form the basis of their political autonomy; she also said that the expression of sexual desire was central to women's development as individuals, as well as to social progress. But when Sanger returned from Europe, she had been convinced by the physician Alletta Jacobs in the Netherlands that the only way she could succeed would be to make birth control a medical rather than a feminist issue. At that point, Sanger pragmatically allied herself with eugenicists. But in the process, the rationale for birth control shifted from individual women's sexual and reproductive self-determination to family planning as a social and economic issue. The movement lost sight of women's interests. Sanger finally did succeed in establishing clinics between 1916 and 1937, but the initial vision of "voluntary motherhood" succumbed to a "gender-neutral (and nonfeminist) goal of 'planned parenthood.'"[22]

Nowhere did organized feminism embrace the cause of birth control. Moreover, as the histories of birth control movements in the Europe and the United States demonstrate, increased availability of female contraceptive methods did not necessarily equate with women's reproductive freedom, at least not initially. Instead, contraception became a social and medical concern intended to advance the health of families. Sanger had to operate within a specifically American constellation of gender, race, class, and medical politics, and the push for birth control in Britain took a similar path. Although less fettered by the legal system, birth control there became medicalized in the face of opposition from the Church and from doctors who not only feared race suicide and a decline of the Empire, but that contraception would cause sterility, fibroid tumors, and a number of other gynecological disorders. In 1930, the Ministry of Health finally approved the distribution of contraceptive devices—but only with the advice of local medical officers, and only to married mothers whose further pregnancies would be harmful to their physical health. Subsequently, opposition to birth control weakened, especially when it became a subject of scientific study for a younger generation of physicians and began to be discussed in the popular press and in women's magazines.[23]

Even with the relative openness of public discussion, female contraceptive devices were adopted haltingly everywhere, which testifies to both the historical rapidity and the short-term slowness with which the separation of sexuality from reproduction took place. Women everywhere in the 1920s and 1930s continued to associate female contraception with sexual emancipation outside marriage. Many feminists feared that birth control would lead to the sexual exploitation and objectification of women and would do nothing to counter male supremacy. Some argued that birth control would deprive married women of one of the few sources of power they held over men: the denial of sexual favors. Few considered female sexual pleasure an important component of female identity; birth control was thus irrelevant, if not contradictory to feminist goals. The rhetoric continued to reflect Victorian attitudes suspicious of sexuality: many believed the human race had simply become oversexed; that the pursuit of sexual pleasure was too individualistic and selfish; and that the separation of sex from reproduction deprived motherhood of dignity. In fact, recent histories provide convincing evidence that even in England and other countries where female contraception was available and public discussion far more open than in France, couples preferred the old-fashioned methods of coitus interruptus, abortion, and abstinence to pre-vent pregnancies, because they were more "natural" than the invasive mechani-cal devices.[24]

The situation in France offers a paradox in the comparatively lower birthrate despite legal sanctions against birth control—another testimony to the continued use of traditional methods of family limitation. The law of July 1920, reinforced by another law in 1923, repressed the possibility of open discussion about con-traception. Even if Roussel had lived longer, she would never have been able to wage a Sanger-style campaign. Jeanne and Eugène Humbert continued their efforts through the 1930s, but they exercised great caution in the language they used; both were repeatedly prosecuted and incarcerated, especially Eugène, who spent many years in prison and died there in 1944. Madeleine Pelletier contin-ued to advocate chastity and the right to abortion. As punishment for performing abortion, she was placed in a mental asylum in 1939, where she died within six months. The Vichy regime penalized abortionists with the death penalty.[25]

Public debate about birth control slowly resumed in France only after World War II, when the birthrate rose sharply. The relatively glacial progress toward the establishment of birth control clinics, even among a new generation, took the same medical path as it did in England and the United States. The debate also resurrected many of Roussel's arguments, although outside a feminist context. Jenny Leclerq, a Catholic doctor, published *Le Control des naissances et la malaise conjugal* (Birth Control and Conjugal Discomfort), in which she argued, as Rous-sel had, that male egotism caused men to ignore women's burdens; submitting to nature went against human intelligence and progress; couples needed to express sexual love. But her book was ignored until the 1950s. Finally, in 1955, a dramatic trial for infanticide became a case study illustrating the need for birth control, and a full-scale debate ensued. Jacques Derogy published a number of articles and a book highlighting the cases of female victims, for whom motherhood, as Roussel had said half a century earlier, was a kind of animal slavery rather than a source of human joy. Derogy's book generated at least 200 articles in the press about abortion and birth control and helped provoke another dialogue about the contradictory demands of motherhood and women in the workforce.[26]

The following year an organization known as the Mouvement français pour le planning familial (French Movement for Family Planning), originally Maternité heureuse (Happy Motherhood) formed; but it deliberately disassociated itself from the earlier, much maligned neo-Malthusian movement. This new organi-zation succeeded in operating within a loophole of the 1920 law as a private, non-profit-making association dedicated to research and providing information only to its members. It thus could not be accused of spreading propaganda, which, by definition, targeted an anonymous audience. The movement's founders overtly rejected the label "feminist" and shifted their focus from women to children: their goal was to make every child a wanted child, and—like their counterparts in England and the United States—they concerned themselves with the family, and not with female emancipation. In 1961, they opened a family planning center in Grenoble and began prescribing contraceptives to individual women, even though such devices remained technically illegal. The clinic received support and publicity from across the political spectrum and operated without persecution.[27]

In the mid 1960s, left-wing organizations (except for the Communist Party), the left-wing press, and women's organizations and magazines began to demand the revocation of articles in the 1920 and 1923 laws concerning information on contraceptives. The issue that most galvanized proponents of birth control was abortion, figures for which ranged from 150,000 to one million per year.[28] Finally, in 1967 the Gaullist Deputy Lucien Neuwirth submitted a proposal to legalize the Pill, the diaphragm, and the IUD. The committee that discussed the bill supported contraception to reduce abortion, but opposed the principle of birth control as a woman's right. The parliamentary debate that ensued focused on persistent fears about moral issues: prostitution, female sexual promiscuity, weakened male authority. The Neuwirth Law that finally passed in December 1967 legalized contraceptives by prescription only. They would be paid for privately and not be covered by social security. Publicity for birth control remained illegal.

The legalization of contraceptives did not result from feminism. Just after the passage of the Neuwirth Law, France was jolted by another political upheaval, one that gave impetus to its second-wave feminist movement—in which Roussel's message became relevant again. Women were involved in the 1968 student and worker rebellion, but they were not engaged in issues specific to their interests as women. It is telling how hard it was for them to assert themselves and speak publicly—harder, it seems, than it had been for Roussel sixty years earlier. Eventually women gained important experience with these events, and like their sisters elsewhere, rebelled at the menial chores to which they were relegated. Thus was born the Mouvement de liberation des femmes (Women's Liberation Movement, or MLF). Its members formed women's discussion groups, some of which focused on birth control. Although the Neuwirth law had legalized female contraceptives, restrictions remained. Women in the MLF began to include the private, as well as the public, and the relation between the two, in their concept of revolution—as Roussel had done. But doing so this time included a sexual revolution of the sort that Nelly Roussel's opponents had always feared, especially because of nonmonogamous sexuality and a focus on sexual pleasure.[29]

Mireille readily recognized that Roussel's original vision had been incorporated into modern feminism without acknowledgment. She also noted their differences: she protested the young feminists' use of obscenities, fearing, as she wrote to *Le Nouvel Observateur* and *Le Monde,* that "these women can only justify [with their language] a confusion between pornography and propaganda about contraception, [a confusion] that enemies of free motherhood made for a long time, and that was made official by the law of 1920." For this reason, she deplored Simone de Beauvoir's adhesion to the movement.[30] As the feminist movement became more visible, Mireille continued to write letters to newspapers and to their contributors in which she depicted her mother's feminist career at some length, again signing them "Mireille Nelly-Roussel." She became an active subscriber to *Choisir,* a pro-choice publication, and informed its editors that they were carrying on the work of her mother. She also wrote to public figures on the Left whose ignorance of feminism caused them to wonder whether it was reactionary.

Mireille then began a sustained effort to find scholars of feminism to incorporate her mother's work into their histories and to share with them the archive of her mother's papers, which she had preserved for more than fifty years. She recruited the feminist historians Daniel Armogathe and Maïté Albistur to organize an exhibition at the Marguerite Durand Library celebrating the centenary of Roussel's birth in February 1977, at which time she deposited her mother's private papers in the library. The exhibition displayed excerpts of Roussel's letters, her published collections of articles and speeches, personal items such as a lock of her hair, the stunning black shawl she wore to her lectures, and a small array of photographs. Albistur and Armogathe then published Roussel's speech "L'Éternelle sacrifiée," with detailed annotations based on their conversations with Mireille and on materials from the archive. The archive has since served numerous historians.

Until she died, Mireille Godet hoped that a biography would be written of her mother. This one might or might not have met her approval. My hope is that it has further illuminated ways in which concepts of gender influence culture, politics, and national identity. I also hope that it has done justice to feminism, to the history of birth control, and to Nelly Roussel.

Abbreviations

AN	Archives Nationales de France
APP	Archives de la Préfecture de Police de Paris
BMD	Bibliothèque Marguerite Durand
FR	Fonds Roussel
HG	Henri Godet
IISG	International Institute of Social History
MG	Mireille Godet
NR	Nelly Roussel

Introduction

Epigraph: Letourneau, *Évolution de la morale*, 463, quoted by Émile Darnaud to describe Roussel in his preface to her volume of speeches *Quelques lances rompues pour nos libertés* (1910), 3.

1. Cova, "Féminisme et natalité"; Armogathe and Albistur in Roussel, *Éternelle sacrifiée;* and Accampo, "Private Life, Public Image," focus on or include biographical information. Information about Roussel has also appeared in Albistur and Armogathe, *Histoire du féminisme français*, vol. 2; Klejman and Rochefort, *Égalité en marche;* Bard, *Filles de Marianne;* Waelti-Walters and Hause, eds., *Feminisms of the Belle Epoque;* McMillan, *Housewife or Harlot* and *France and Women;* and Offen, *European Feminisms.*

2. On the definition of the "new biography," as well as bibliographic suggestions and examples, see Margadant, "Constructing Selves in Historical Perspective," in *New Biography,* ed. id., 1–32, and other essays in the same volume.

3. Under the Civil Code of 1804, a Frenchwoman had few rights: she had to obey her husband, assume his nationality, and reside wherever he desired; she could not participate in a lawsuit or serve as a witness in court; she had no control over property or any income she generated; she had no control over her children. In 1893, single and separated women gained full legal status; in 1897, adult women gained the right to serve as witnesses to civil acts, and in 1907, married women were given the right to control their own wages. But another series of laws restricted their right to work.

4. McLaren, *History of Contraception,* 5; Linda Gordon, *Moral Property of Women;* Rid-

dle, *Eve's Herbs*, 6–8. See also Riddle, *Contraception and Abortion*, and Laqueur, *Making Sex*.

5. Steinbrugge, *Moral Sex*, 28; Laqueur, *Making Sex*; and Schiebinger, *Mind Has No Sex?* and *Nature's Body*.

6. On "republican motherhood," see Kerber, *Women of the Republic*, 11. The phrase is probably overused, however, and the underlying assumptions are being reexamined. Desan, *Family on Trial*, challenges the literature arguing that the Revolution relegated women to republican motherhood and shows that women in Normandy successfully used republican ideology to challenge domestic inferiority. See also Hesse, *Other Enlightenment*; Desan, "Constitutional Amazons," in *Recreating Authority in Revolutionary France*, ed. Ragan and Williams, 92; Godineau, *Women of Paris*; and Landes, *Women and the Public Sphere* and *Visualizing the Nation*.

7. McLaren, *Birth Control in Nineteenth-Century England*; id., *History of Contraception*, 181–82; Riddle, *Eve's Herbs*.

8. Hunt, *Family Romance* and "Unstable Boundaries"; Scott, *Only Paradoxes to Offer*; Thompson, "Creating Boundaries." On women's participation in the Revolution and the images and mythologies to which their participation gave rise, see Godineau, *Women of Paris*. But see also Desan's counterargument in *Family on Trial*.

9. Goethe, *Faust*, pt. 2 (Baltimore: Penguin Books, 1965), 288. The *éternel féminin* has been a frequent trope in France, to the point where *Le Robert Dictionnaire historique de la langue française*, 1: 1324, s.v. *éternel*, cites the phrase as exemplifying "ce qui semble ne pas évoluer" (that which seems not to evolve). On the use of the concept in literature, see Michaud, *Muse et madone* and "Artistic and Literary Idolatries." This argument about the pervasiveness of the concept is not, however, intended to dispute the fact that large numbers of women achieved some measure of liberation—at least ideologically, if not practically—with each revolution. Hesse, *Other Enlightenment*, and Margadant, ed., *New Biography*, are among many examples that show how unstable "femininity" was, and how individual women were able to negotiate identities beyond traditional definitions of womanhood.

10. Moses, *French Feminism in the Nineteenth Century*; McMillan, *France and Women*, 135. On the mythology surrounding women and the Commune, see esp. Gullickson, *Unruly Women*.

11. Jordanova, *Sexual Visions*, 79–83; Barthes, *Michelet*, 147–49; Stone, "Republican Brotherhood"; and see also Stone, *Sons of the Revolution*. For other works on the influence of Michelet on gender, see Jean Borie, "Une Gynocologie passionée," in *Misérable et glorieuse*, ed Aron, 153–89.

12. For examples of how this ideology became incorporated into the thinking of social reformers, see Le Play, *On Family, Work, and Social Change*; Coffey, *Léon Harmel*, 110–12; Simon, *Ouvrière*; Scott, "'L'Ouvrière! Mot impie, sordide . . . '"; Sanford Elwitt, *Third Republic Defended*, 73–75. Though this conception of womanhood dominated the male imagination, social reformers did not, indeed, could not, institute practical change based on a single conception of womanhood. See Accampo et al., *Gender and the Politics of Social Reform*.

13. Burton, *Holy Tears, Holy Blood*, 19.

14. Chesnais, *Demographic Transition*, table 11.1, p. 323.

15. As cited in Cova, *"Au service de l'église,"* 226.

16. Dupâquier, ed., *Histoire de la population française,* 3: 3, and *Annuaire statistique de la France, 1966,* 70–71, as cited in Cova, *"Au service de l'église,"* table 3, p. 226, and table 4, p. 227, respectively; Zeldin, *Anxiety and Hypocrisy,* 185, 70–71, and *Ambition and Love,* 186.

17. Cole, *Power of Large Numbers;* Nye, *Crime, Madness, and Politics,* and "Degeneration and the Medical Model"; Pick, *Faces of Degeneration.*

18. As paraphrased in Merriman, *History of Modern Europe,* 844.

19. McMillan, *France and Women,* 106; Adler, *Secrets d'alcôve;* Stewart, *For Health and Beauty,* 98–105.

20. See, e.g., Berlanstein, *Daughters of Eve,* esp. chaps. 7–9; Rearick, *Pleasures of the Belle Epoque;* Waldberg, *Eros in La Belle Époque;* for an alternative to woman as "Nature"—indeed as an erotic "machine," see Garelick, *Rising Star,* esp. 99–127; Michaud, "Artistic and Literary Idolatries," 128.

21. Roberts, *Disruptive Acts,* 4. This book is the most recent and fullest analysis of the New Woman in fin de siècle France. See also Tilburg, "Reimagining the Republican Ideal"; Mansker, "'Pistol Virgin.'"

22. A number of works have emphasized the massive impacts military defeat, fertility decline, and the Paris Commune had on the cultural and political self-image of the French, creating "crises" in both masculinity and femininity. In addition to works cited above (Nye; Gullickson; Accampo, Fuchs, and Stewart), see McLaren, *Sexuality and Social Order;* Offen, "Depopulation, Nationalism, and Feminism"; Berenson, *Trial of Madame Caillaux.* Burton, *Holy Tears, Holy Blood,* argues that political upheaval helped contribute to a culture of female self-sacrifice.

23. Sontag, *Illness as Metaphor;* Barnes, *Making of a Social Disease.*

24. NR to HG, Apr. 8, 1905. Roussel's archive, the Fonds Roussel, is in nine cartons, plus two or three separated dossiers, in the Bibliothèque Marguerite Durand. The Roussel-Godet correspondence is mostly in carton 6, but the FR list does not always accurately represent the somewhat haphazard contents of the cartons.

25. NR, "Encore le 'droit de la chair,'" *L'Action,* Apr. 24, 1908, reprinted in Roussel, *Quelques lances rompues,* 141–42. Unless otherwise indicated, all newspaper articles by or about Roussel cited in this book come from her press clippings in FR, cartons 5 and (mostly) 7.

26. Philinte, "Causerie de la semaine," *Express* (Mulhouse), Apr. 21 and 22, 1907.

27. Davy, *Une Femme,* 242–43. "As a young woman . . . Beauvoir was certainly aware of the work of the birth-control, or neo-Malthusian, movement in France. She particularly admired Nelly Roussel," Felicia Gordon writes (*Integral Feminist,* 243n13).

One • Conversion Experiences

Epigraph: BMD, FR, carton 7, "Cahiers d'écolière."

1. Gemie, *Women and Schooling in France,* 60–61.

2. Gullickson, *Unruly Women,* 223.

3. Ibid., esp. 176–83; Przyblyski, "Between Seeing and Believing"; Christiansen, *Paris Babylon;* Eichner, *Surmounting the Barricades.*

4. Berenson, *Trial of Madame Caillaux;* Pick, *Faces of Degeneration;* Nye, *Crime, Madness, and Politics,* 119–70.

5. Williams, *Dream Worlds;* Miller, *Bon Marché;* Rearick, *Pleasures of the Belle Epoque;* Schwartz, *Spectacular Realities;* Tiersten, *Marianne in the Market.*

6. BMD, FR, carton 7, "Cahiers d'écolière." See also Clark, *Schooling the Daughters,* 64. Recording *morale* maxims in notebooks was a typical practice. On the inculcation of a gendered moral system, see also Margadant, *Madame Le Professeur,* 32–37.

7. BMD, "Correspondance MG," MG, Oct. 13, 1980; interview with Michel Robin, June 7, 1997; Armogathe and Albistur, preface in Roussel, *Éternelle sacrifiée,* 8.

8. NR, "Aux libres-penseurs," *Almanach de la libre-pensée,* 1903.

9. *The New Oxford Companion to French Literature* (Oxford: Clarendon Press, 1995), ed. Peter France, 666; FR, carton 7, "Confidences," 1889 and 1898.

10. FR, carton 4, dossiers "Théâtre" and "Jeux."

11. FR, carton 4, Nelly Roussel "La Soeur de Comte Jean: Drame en quatre actes et cinq tableaux, en prose."

12. FR, carton 4, NR, "La Passion du jeu."

13. Roussel's tropes imitate those in the domestic novels Bonnie Smith analyzes in *Ladies of the Leisure Class,* 187–213. The themes of "metaphorical incest" and antipatriarchal sentiment are also similar to those analyzed in Hunt, *Family Romance,* 127–31.

14. FR, carton 7, "Confidences."

15. Clark, *Schooling the Daughters,* 9, 14, 25, 31–32, 34, 46–47, 68.

16. Ibid.; Martin-Fugier, *Bourgeoise;* Armogathe and Albistur, preface in Roussel, *Éternelle sacrifiée.*

17. Clark, *Schooling the Daughters,* 52; Winock, "Jeanne d'Arc"; Darrow, *French Women and the First World War,* 27; Warner, *Joan of Arc.*

18. Pope, "Immaculate and Powerful"; Bellanger et al., eds., *Histoire générale de la presse française,* 3: 335.

19. Clark, *Schooling the Daughters,* 32, 37, 39

20. Pope, "Immaculate and Powerful."

21. Agulhon, *Marianne au pouvoir.* On Marie-Antoinette, see Goodman, ed., *Marie-Antoinette.*

22. Armogathe and Albistur, preface in Roussel, *Éternelle sacrifiée,* 8–9; FR, carton 5, 1893 agenda; carton 6, correspondence, NR to Thomas Nel; carton 4, manuscript biography of Roussel, written by her husband, Henri Godet c. 1903 and, in the third person, biography by Roussel herself c. 1911.

23. Berlanstein, *Daughters of Eve;* FR, carton 4, Roussel, manuscript biography of herself.

24. Roberts, "Acting Up," 1110–11.

25. NR to Thomas Nel, Aug. 2, 1896; for another example, NR to Thomas Nel, Mar. 1, 1897.

26. Armogathe and Albistur, preface to Roussel, *L'Éternelle sacrifiée,* 9.

27. FR, carton 4, HG, manuscript biography of Roussel.

28. Bellanger et al., eds., *Histoire générale de la presse française,* 3: 344.

29. Agulhon, *French Republic,* 89.

30. FR, carton 4, HG, manuscript biography of Roussel.

31. I thank Christiane Demeulenaere-Douyère for the photograph of *La Maternité*.

32. FR, carton 4, HG, manuscript biography of Roussel.

33. FR, carton 7, HG, "Nelly Roussel, 5 Janvier 1878–18 Décembre 1922: Souvenirs," *Mère éducatrice*, no. 11 (November 1923): 147–48.

34. FR, carton 4, HG, manuscript biography of Roussel.

35. Interview with Michel Robin, June 7, 1997; HG, "Nelly Roussel."

36. FR, carton 7, "Confidences," Feb. 7, 1889.

37. HG, "Nelly Roussel."

38. HG, manuscript biography.

39. HG, "Nelly Roussel."

40. APP, Ba 1651 dossier 59480, police report, Dec. 25, 1901.

41. Réquillard, *Initiation des femmes*, 144–47.

42. Mercier, *Universités populaires*; Weisz, *Emergence of Modern Universities in France*, 311–14; Rebérioux, *République radicale?* 47–49; Elwitt, *Third Republic Defended*, 226–47. For an example of right-wing criticism, see A. de Boisandré, "L'Enseignement laïque: Les Universités populaires," *Libre Parole*, Oct. 30, 1903; see also Chapter 2 in this volume.

43. APP, Ba 1651, dossier 59480, report of police agent "Foureur," Dec. 6, 1901; FR, carton 4, HG, manuscript biography of Roussel.

44. FR, carton 4, *manuscrits divers*, NR, "Impressions d'un jour de mélancolie," June 1899.

45. The "fear, mystery, and even secrecy surrounding sexual and physical life among all women in the nineteenth century can never be overemphasized," Bonnie Smith writes (*Ladies of the Leisure Class*, 82). On childbirth, see Stewart, *For Health and Beauty*, 112–29.

46. Valici-Bosio, *Mère et l'enfant*, 63. Thebaud, *Quand nos grand-mères donnaient la vie*, 178.

47. Loudon, *Death in Childbirth*, 84–106, and "Childbirth." The three commonest causes of death from childbirth were puerperal fever (33 to 50 percent), pregnancy-induced hypertension (20 percent), and hemorrhage (15–20 percent).

48. Rich, *Of Woman Born*, 166; Villani, with Ryan, *Motherhood at the Crossroads*.

49. Stewart, *For Health and Beauty*, 126; Thebaud, *Quand nos grand-mères donnaient la vie*, 254; Knibiehler and Fouquet, *Histoire des mères*, 210.

50. Yvonne and Fouquet, *Histoire des mères*, 212.

51. Bonnie Smith, *Ladies of the Leisure Class*, 107.

52. Finney, *Story of Motherhood*, 156. See also Rich, *Of Woman Born*, 156.

53. Bossuet, *XIe Élévation sur les mystères*, quoted in McMillan, *France and Women*, 4 (originally quoted in P. Hoffman, *La Femme dans la pensée des lumières* [Paris: Orphys, 1977], 18).

54. Gélis, *History of Childbirth*, 155.

55. Finney, *Story of Motherhood*, 175.

56. Knibiehler and Fouquet, 212. For some of the realities of motherhood, particularly with regard to social policies, see Fuchs, *Abandoned Children* and *Poor and Pregnant in Paris*.

57. Nye, *Masculinity and Male Codes of Honor*, 218–19.

58. Thebaud, *Quand nos grands-mères donnaient la vie*, 253–62.

59. Ibid.; Stewart, *For Health and Beauty*, 129.

60. Scarry, *Body in Pain*, 18–19; Porter, "Pain and Suffering."

Two • Mother and Missionary

Epigraph: Antoine Godeau, *Instructions et prières chrestiennes pour toutes sortes de personnes* (Paris: Vve Camusat et P. Le Petit, 1646), cited in Gélis, *History of Childbirth,* 155.

1. Cova, *Maternité et droits des femmes,* 29–30. The censuses of 1890, 1891, and 1892 showed a drop in the number of births. In 1895, births numbered 834,000 and deaths 852,000.

2. Ibid., 31; Cole, *Power of Large Numbers,* 191–94.

3. Cole, *Power of Large Numbers,* 193–202.

4. Jacques Bertillon, "Le Problème de la population: Le Programme de l'Alliance nationale pour l'accroissement de la population française," *Revue politique et parlementaire* 12 (1897): 531–74; Offen, "Depopulation, Nationalism, and Feminism." Withdrawal remained the primary contraceptive method, giving men control over the process; the second most common method to prevent births was abortion, clearly the woman's domain. See Sohn, *Chrysalides,* 2: 803–46; id., *Du premier baiser à l'alcôve,* 126–35; Adler, *Secrets d'alcôve,* 116–17; Payer, *Medicine and Culture,* 50; McLaren, *History of Contraception* and *Sexuality and Social Order,* 136–53.

5. FR, dossier 07.

6. FR, carton 4, HG, manuscript biography of Roussel; Noëlie Drous, "Nos pierres noires," *Voix des femmes,* Dec. 13, 1923.

7. Offen, "Depopulation, Nationalism, and Feminism."

8. H. Thulié, "Variétés: La Femme. Fonctions sociales," *Harmonie sociale,* no. 26 (Apr. 8, 1893); "Hygiène: L'Allaitement," *Fronde,* Apr. 14, 1899; Harlor, "Maternité totale," ibid., Feb. 20, 1901, all cited in Cova, *Maternité et droits des femmes,* 35–37, 130.

9. Klejman and Rochefort, *Égalité en marche,* 138

10. Offen, "Depopulation, Nationalism, Feminism," 634.

11. Scott, *Only Paradoxes to Offer.*

12. NR, "Sur l'éducation des jeunes filles," *Paris qui passe,* Oct. 29, 1899.

13. Ibid.

14. Klejman and Rochefort, *Égalité en marche,* 102.

15. Roberts, "Acting Up," "Feminist Journalism," and *Disruptive Acts;* Klejman and Rochefort, *Égalité en marche,* 129–30. On breast-feeding, see citations in n. 8 above.

16. NR, *Derniers combats,* 198.

17. APP Ba 1244, dossier on Paul Robin; Demeulenaere-Douyère, *Paul Robin,* 334, and "Être néo-malthusien"; Giroud, *Paul Robin,* 10, 111.

18. Giroud, *Paul Robin,* 36; Demeulenaere-Douyère, *Paul Robin,* 133–56. See also McLaren, "Revolution and Education."

19. Demeulenaere-Doyère, *Paul Robin,* 319.

20. APP Ba 1244. The accusations were apparently based on his stated opinion that older men should sexually initiate young girls, because boys and young men were not up to the task. I have read nothing, either in police reports, newspapers, or secondary sources that specified what exactly Robin did to merit his expulsion, other than promote coeducation.

21. "Notre programme," *Régénération,* December 1896.

22. Nye, *Crime, Madness, and Politics* and "Degeneration and the Medical Model"; Pick, *Faces of Degeneration.*

23. Ronsin, *Grève des ventres*, 55.

24. APP, Ba 1244, extract from police report, Apr. 11, 1896.

25. APP, Ba 1244, "Le Congrès féminist," *Débats*, Apr. 13, 1896; "Encore Robin," *Grand Journal*, Apr. 12, 1896.

26. Klejman and Rochefort, *Égalité en marche*, 164.

27. APP Ba 381 prov, L.G., "Abominable Propagande," *Peuple française*, Jan. 1, 1897; police report, Jan. 16, 1897; *Petite République*, Jan. 27, 1897; report to prefect, Mar. 5, 1897.

28. Ibid., *Moyens d'éviter les grandes familles*, January 1896.

29. See esp. Devaldès, *Individualité féminine*, and Accampo, "Rhetoric of Reproduction."

30. Armengaud, *Les Français et Malthus*, 44–47. Dupaquier, "Combiens d'avortements en France avant 1914," *Communications* 44 (1986): 87–105, cited in McLaren, *History of Contraception*, 189n43; McLaren points out that many people in the nineteenth century viewed abortion "as simply one more step on the continuum of fertility-controlling practices" (89). Some women preferred abortion to contraception and believed it to be less immoral. See also McLaren, *Sexuality and Social Order*, 136–53. Sohn, *Du premier baiser à l'alcôve*, 133, and *Chrysalides*, 2: 803–46.

31. APP Ba 381 prov, police report, Apr. 6, 1902. The agent also reported on the growth of the League: in the spring of 1902, it was meeting every first Saturday and third Sunday of each month. Although that attendance was small (only fifteen people), it organized lectures that drew much larger audiences, and subscriptions to the journal rapidly increased.

32. Paul Robin, "Aux gens mariés!" quoted in Ronsin, *Grève des ventres*, 54.

33. *Régénération*, December 1896, quoted in Demeulenaere-Doyère, *Paul Robin*, 346.

34. FR, carton 4, manuscripts 05, NR, "Causerie sur le féminisme."

35. See, e.g., NR, "Correspondance," *Républicain de Veron*, Dec. 19, 1903.

36. Pateman, "Equality, Difference, Subordination"; Cova, *Maternité et droits des femmes*, 13–14; Scott, *Only Paradoxes to Offer*.

37. Scott notes this relationship between law and "nature" in *Only Paradoxes to Offer*, ix.

38. Colonel Jean Converset, *Voix des femmes*, Dec. 18, 1924.

39. Godet was cautious about neo-Malthusianism. FR, correspondance from HG to NR, Sept. 1, 1903.

40. See Cole, *Power of Large Numbers*, 195n40.

41. NR, "Féminisme et fécondité," *Rappel*, Oct. 19, 1900.

42. Noëlie Drous, "Nos pierres noires," *Voix des femmes*, Dec. 13, 1923.

43. André's death notice indicates where he died. She put her third child, Marcel, in a *pouponnière*, and given her attitude toward motherhood revealed in her "Impressions d'un jour de mélancolie" (FR, carton 4, *manuscrits divers*, Nelly Roussel, June 1899), as well as in her subsequent correspondence and behavior, I suspect that she did not breast-feed Mireille either—a family friend recalled to Godet years later having run the errand of procuring bottles of sterilized milk for her (E. Maccarin to HG, Jan. 17, 1923).

44. Correspondence between Henri Godet and Nelly Roussel, 1903, passim. The correspondence between them, and with other family members, is found in FR, cartons 6 and 8.

45. Ibid., HG to NR, Aug. 26 and Sept. 11, 1902. Just two weeks earlier, he had refused to attend the wedding of a close friend because he would not be able to tolerate the celebra-

tion of the mass, and provided a false excuse (his spleen). His letters do not indicate which sculptures he was trying to sell.

46. Ibid., HG to NR, July 28, 1902.

47. Ibid., HG to NR, July 13, 1902.

48. Ibid., HG to NR, July 31 and Aug. 6, 1902.

49. Ibid., HG to NR, Aug. 22, 23, 24, and 25, 1902.

50. Ibid., HG to NR, July 28 and 31, Aug. 20, 22, 23, and 25, 1902.

51. Ibid., HG to NR, Aug. 22, 24, and 26, 1902.

52. *Fronde*, Mar. 22, 1903; *L'Action*, May 22, 1903, *Rappel*, Oct. 13, 1903.

53. L. Gallot, "Andromaque à l'université populaire," *Independent de Seine-et-Oise*, Dec. 28, 1902.

54. Humbert, *Eugène Humbert*, 11–12; Ronsin, *Grève des ventres*, 74.

55. Humbert, *Eugène Humbert*, 11–12; Ronsin, *Grève des ventres*, 58–61. About 20 or 30 people attended the bimonthly meetings in Paris.

56. NR, "L'Amour fécond, l'amour stérile," *Régénération*, January 1903.

57. "Un Manifest Malthusien," *La Patrie*, Mar. 20, 1903; "Les Malthusiennes," *Rappel*, Mar. 20, 1903, in APP Ba 381 prov.

58. International Institute of Social History (IISG), Amsterdam, Humbert archives, # 323 (correspondence to *Régénération*), letter from HG to Paul Robin, Feb. 13, 1903.

59. FR, carton 5, "Discours et conferences," 1901–21.

60. Roussel, "Discours sur la liberté de la maternité à l'initiative de P. Robin fondateur de la ligue de Régénération Humain," FR, carton 5, *manuscrits*. This speech is listed in her agenda as having been delivered Mar. 5, 1903, with the title "Discours d'ouverture sur la grève des mères."

61. APP Ba 381 prov; report, Prefecture of Police, 3d Brigade, Mar. 6, 1903; see also report of same date from the 2d Brigade.

62. "Le Féminisme," *Journal de Mantes*, Feb. 11, 1903.

63. NR, *Par la révolte*, 4th ed., with speech by Sébastian Faure. This was originally published c. 1903. Roussel often referred to women's "flanks," no doubt to emphasize her contention that repeated, uncontrolled, unwanted pregnancies made women animal-like.

64. She was assisted by three other actresses and accompanied by an organist, M. Gavioli, who played one of his own compositions. The performance was "warmly applauded" and the play, according to *La Fronde*, was a "beautiful work of great stature." *Le Jour* reported less enthusiastically that the play obtained "a very legitimate success." But when she performed it the following month for the Syndicat des femmes de lettres, *L'Ouvrière* called it a dramatic scene of great force, whose author "is a true tragic actress." Roussel's diaries and agendas indicate who participated in the play, and her letters refer to the number of copies she sold while on tour. See, e.g., her diary entry of Jan. 3, 1904. The announcement of the sale of the brochure appeared in *Régénération*, April 1904.

65. HG to NR, Sept. 2, 1903.

66. HG to NR, Sept. 1 and 2, 1903.

67. A. de Boisandré, "L'Enseignement laïque: Les Universités populaires," *Libre Parole*, Oct. 30, 1903; reprinted in the *Nouvelliste d'Amiens; Patriot orléannis; Journal de Redon; Indépendence bretonne; Anjou; Journal de Belfort;* and *Journal de Bolbec.*

68. A. de Boisandré, "L'Enseignement laïque: Les Universités populaires," *Libre Parole*, Nov. 8, 1903. Again the controversy spread far outside Paris. The *Revue de l'Ouest* (Niort) reprinted part of Roussel's letter and copied, word for word, as its own, de Boisandré's query about whether these theories might not be misunderstood and lead ultimately to the right to abortion ("Enseignement laïque et universités populaires," *Revue de l'Ouest*, Nov. 12, 1903).

69. FR, carton 4, *manuscrits*, Roussel, speech honoring President Magnaud.

70. "Glanes du matin," *Gazette de France*, Nov. 1, 1903 (reproduced in *Journal de Saint Quentin*); "L'Apothéose du bon juge," *Journal de Chartres*, Nov. 8, 1903. Favorable coverage of the event appeared in *L'Action*, Oct. 31, 1903; *Gil Blas*, Oct. 31, 1903; *Fronde*, Nov. 1, 1903; *Rappel*, Nov. 1, 1903 (article reproduced in *Progrès de la Somme*); *Temps*, November 1903 (article reproduced in *Tribune républicaine* of Saint-Etienne and *Journal de Bayeux*); *Pensée libre* (Algeria), Nov. 22, 1903. Jeanne Humbert, "Nelly Roussel, 1878–1922," *Libre Pensée autonome des Bouches-du-Rhône*, April 1980.

71. "Féminisme!" *L'Avenir du XIIème*, Nov. 7, 1903.

72. On Faure, see Maitron, ed., *Dictionnaire biographique du mouvement ouvrier français*, pt. 3: *1871–1914: De la Commune à la Grande Guerre*, 12: 174–76; Humbert, *Eugène Humbert*, 55–58. APP Ba 381, report by Finot, Nov. 17, 1903. *Régénération*, December 1903.

73. "Conférence Sébastian Faure 'Le Problème de la population' présidée par Mme. Nelly Roussel, Salle des Sociétés savantes, 16 novembre 1903: Allocution de la présidente," in Roussel, *Quelques discours*, 7–10.

74. *Fronde*, Dec. 1, 1903.

75. Roussel recorded having given twenty-three public talks in 1903, mostly in Paris and its environs, at popular universities and meetings of anarchists, neo-Malthusians, feminists, anticlericals, socialists, and freethinkers, which received plenty of press coverage; their titles included "On Feminism," "On Feminism and Free Thinking," "The Admission of Women into Freemasonry," "Motherhood and the Revolt of Mothers," "The Strike of Mothers," and "The Persecution of the Feminine Mind." FR, carton 5, "Discours et conferences," agenda, 1903.

76. Lalouette, *Libre Pensée en France*, 63.

77. Ibid., 64.

78. Ibid., 93.

79. Rebérioux, *République radicale?* 45–47.

80. See Offen, "Depopulation, Nationalism, and Feminism," and Klejman and Rochefort, *Égalité en marche*, as well as Chapters 4 and 5 in this volume.

81. Roussel must have had the same reaction to Freemasons. Although she belonged to a mixed lodge, with many feminists, and Freemasons varied a great deal in their attitudes, the majority opposed neo-Malthusianism and generally embraced the concept of the *éternel féminin*, as Réquillard has pointed out in *Initiation des femmes*, 199–200, 219. It is unclear to me how long Roussel remained in her lodge, because she never explicitly mentions it in her correspondence or her diary. On women and Freemasonry, see also Allen, "Sisters of Another Sort."

82. "Conférence Sébastian Faure" (cited n. 74 above).

83. HG to NR, Aug. 28 and 30, 1903.

84. "Conference de Mme Nelly Roussel," *Fronde*, Jan. 1, 1904.

85. *Fronde*, Jan. 1, 1904, and *Pour la République* (a republican and socialist monthly), no. 2 (January 1904), published her address at the National Congress of Free Thought, and it also received coverage and responses in the *Nouvelliste* (Rouen), *Petit Bleu* (Brussels), *Petit Provençal*, and *Petit Troyen*, all Dec. 28, 1903; *Correspondencia España* (Madrid), *Étoile belge*, *France* (Bordeaux), *Petit Phare* (Nantes), *Petite République* (two articles), *Phare de la Loire*, and *Rappel*, all Dec. 29, 1903; as well as in *L'Action*, Dec. 31, 1903, which called it "one of the best talks given at the Congress."

86. Henri Duchmann, *Libertaire*, Feb. 13, 1904.

87. NR, *Libertaire*, Feb. 20, 1904.

88. Henri Duchmann, *Libertaire*, Feb. 27, 1904.

89. See Tilburg, "Reimagining the Republican Ideal."

90. Nye, *Masculinity and Male Codes of Honor*, writes: "a journalist had to expect occasional visits from the seconds of a man who imagined himself outraged by something he had written. As the seasoned polemicist and dueler Edouard Drumont said in 1886, 'Behind every signature everyone expects to find a chest.' . . . The sort of bravado this assumption inspired discouraged editors from printing anonymously written articles when they might contain something controversial. As dueling manuals made clear, the editor himself must assume responsibility for an unsigned article unless the author voluntarily revealed himself. Besides, there was something suspect, even feminine, in anonymity" (187). See also Nye, "Medicine and Science as Masculine 'Fields of Honor,'" and Reddy, *Invisible Code*. Both Madeleine Pelletier and Aria Ly overtly challenged male codes of honor. Pelletier dressed as a man and carried a gun, as she thought all women should. Ly challenged a man to a duel for having accused her of being a lesbian. See Sowerwine and Maignien, *Madeleine Pelletier;* Felicia Gordon, *Integral Feminist;* and Mansker, "'Pistol Virgin.'"

91. Godet apparently had other motives for entering this fray as well, for to the dismay of "revolutionaries" such as Duchmann, he was deeply involved in electoral politics in the twelfth arrondissement. For this reason, according to police, "he prohibited his wife from having relations with anarchists," for they would undermine his efforts. APP Ba 1651, dossier 59480, police report, Mar. 9, 1904. The police believed Godet was actually running for office himself, but I have found no evidence that he did.

92. See, e.g., Fassin, "Purloined Gender."

93. Henri Duchmann, "La Réaction féministe," *Libertaire*, Mar. 12, 1904.

94. Henri Duchman, "Ne touchez pas à la Reine," *Libertaire*, Apr. 9, 1904.

95. "Réponse à M. Cambensy de Chicago," *Libertaire*, Apr. 16, 1904.

96. Rochefort, "Antiféminisme."

97. See Linda Gordon, *Woman's Body, Woman's Right*, 93–113.

98. NR to Thomas Nel, Apr. 9, 1904.

99. NR, "Lettre ouverte à Monsieur le docteur Toulouse," *Régénération*, no. 22 (March 1903).

100. FR, dossier 091 ROU, NR to Marguerite Durand, June 28, 1904.

Three • The Making and Marketing of a Spectacular Apostle

1. FR, carton 7, "Une Heureuse initiative," *L'Action*, Feb. 27, 1904; carton 5, diary (daily agenda), 1904. Roussel resumed her diary in 1904, though as noted in the Introduction above, it only amounted to perfunctory daily listings of what she had done and whom she had seen.

2. The living arrangement was permanent when Roussel resumed her diary in 1904. It is possible that the Godets' apartment lacked sufficient space for three people to live comfortably, especially since Nelly required work space; or that they were too busy to care for Mireille themselves as Nelly's career developed, and—as suggested in her memoir of 1899—she had little patience with the demands of small children.

3. Maitron, ed., *Dictionnaire biographique du mouvement ouvrier française*, pt. 3: *1871–1914: De la Commune à la Grande Guerre*, 11: 307. The bulk of information about Émile Darnaud is from his copious correspondence to Roussel in FR, carton 5; the quoted words and phrases are from Darnaud to NR, July 27, 1904; Oct. 15, 1904; Mar. 15, 1905, and passim.

4. BMD, "Correspondance Mireille Godet," letter from Charles Darnaud, Dec. 5, 1977.

5. FR, carton 5, Darnaud to NR, Aug. 29, 1904, quoting from his personal journal, Jan. 26, 1903.

6. Émile Darnaud to NR, n.d. (1904). His "feminism" at this point was hardly edifying. He recounted discussions at the meetings of the "feminist committee" in which he had pointed out that women could hardly serve in a civil capacity—i.e., as witnesses—because they always lied about their age.

7. FR, Correspondance Darnaud, 1904–5, passim.

8. Roberts, *Disruptive Acts*, 105–6. Originally, it had not been Durand's intent to make *La Fronde* explicitly feminist; but by the time she had made the decision to abandon it, it had become so. Roberts suggests that in addition to bad management, financial difficulties, and personal problems with other activists, Durand decided to leave *La Fronde* precisely because, having become feminist, it was more conventional, predictable, and less "disruptive." She may have thought the feminist message would be more disruptive if it appeared in *L'Action*.

9. Although records about speaking fees do not exist for this first tour, beginning in 1905, Roussel kept separate agendas in which she recorded the fees and the proceeds from selling *Par la révolte*. See FR, carton 5, agendas.

10. FR, carton 7, 1905 press clippings. Sowerwine notes that *La Fronde* offended socialist feminists because of its attitude toward working-class women and quotes Marguerite Durand: "Working women . . . will make the revolution for their bourgeois sisters, but what good are arms which flail about when there are no brains to guide them?" (Sowerwine, *Sisters or Citizens?* 75).

11. NR to HG, Apr. 15, 1904; May 10, 1905.

12. FR, carton 6, Thomas Nel to NR, Apr. 13, 1904.

13. NR to HG, Apr. 16, 1904.

14. HG to NR, Apr. 18, 1904.

15. On a tour three years later, Nelly freely recounted to Henri the fervent admiration of a "bizarre" Mr. Feller, who wouldn't leave her side the entire evening; and about dining with

a Mr. Coffin, who was single and took his meals at her hotel. Mr. Coffin then took her on a *vivifiante* (bracing) walk. And she wrote of yet another admirer: "Ah! This Fulpuis! Do you know what he did? Well! My dear, he kissed me, last evening, after the lecture, and kissed me backstage! But don't get indignant. He is a good grandfather. I have plenty of them, these older worshippers." NR to HG, Feb. 26 and 27, Apr. 10, 1907, and another example, Apr. 27, 1907.

16. NR to HG, Apr. 16, 1904. "Barnum" was used in France to mean someone who "exhibits sensational phenomena amid much publicity" (*Le Robert Dictionnaire historique de la langue française*, 1: 333).

17. *Pétit Méridional*, Apr. 17, 1904.

18. "La Conférence Nelly-Roussel," *Union républicaine*, Apr. 16, 1904, reproduced in *L'Avenir Cazoulin*.

19. NR to HG, Apr. 16, 1904.

20. Bellanger et al., eds., *Histoire générale de la presse française*, 2: 399–400.

21. NR to HG, Apr. 18, 1904.

22. Ibid.

23. NR to HG, Apr. 21, 1904.

24. NR to HG, Apr. 26, 1904; Roussel, "Impressions de militante," *L'Action*, June 8, 1904.

25. *Vérité* (Cannes), Apr. 28, 1904.

26. Laguerre (1860–1956) was the highly intelligent and cultivated daughter of a diplomat who undertook "brilliant" literary studies in Paris. She was known for her work with rural school teachers. Klejman and Rochefort, *Égalité en marche*, 176–77.

27. Léonie Talsans, "Chronique lyonnaise: Un Leçon," *Travail de la femme et de la jeune fille*, June 1904.

28. Ibid.

29. According to Mireille Godet, as she recounted in the 1970s, Roussel believed in free unions and admired those who contracted successful ones. But she did not personally encourage young women to engage in them, because they too often ended badly for women. See Roussel, *Éternelle sacrifiée*, ed. Armogathe and Albistur, 72n22.

30. Le Bon's best-selling *Psychology of Crowds* had an extraordinary influence on the French imagination, and specifically on Darnaud and others who commented on the impact Roussel had on crowds (see Chapter 4). On Le Bon, see Nye, *Origins of Crowd Psychology;* Barrows, *Distorted Mirrors;* and Pick, *Faces of Degeneration*.

31. Jules Burty, "Morale laïque et indépendante," *L'Éclair comtois*, June 28, 1904; Eugène Tavernier, "Libres-Penseuses," *Univers*, June 29, 1904; "Leur morale," *Avenir de Luxembourg d'Arlon*, July 3, 1904; "Lycées des Filles," *Nouvelliste*, July 6, 1904; "La Logique des faits," *Journal de Colmar*, July 3, 1904; favorable articles included "La Main aux Dames!" *Républicain de Granville*, June 16, 1904; "Attaques cléricale," *Régénération*, July 1904; and "Maternité & misère," *Lyon républicain*, July 14, 1904.

32. Burty, "Morale laïque et indépendante."

33. This estimate is based on the audience sizes that either she or newspapers reported.

34. NR to Eugène Humbert, May 2, 1904; HG to NR, May 4, 1904. Godet wrote to

Humbert, "Madame Godet will not be in Paris before the 22d, and her lecture tour and her itinerary have stopped definitively. I must even tell you that she will do no further lecturing this year for reasons of her health. When I add that she can hardly talk about this subject without causing facile jokes, you will have understood the cause of this unforeseen difficulty." IISG, Humbert Archives, # 139.

35. HG to NR, Apr. 30, May 9 and 15, 1904; NR to HG. May 3, 1904.

36. NR to HG, May 9, 1904; *Paris qui passe*, May 22, 1904; HG to NR, Apr. 30, 1904.

37. When taking a break from her tour to visit her grandfather in Monaco, she wrote to Henri: "I was thinking again that in exactly three weeks we'll be reunited, and this thought did me much good; for, in spite of everything, I am bored; neither my oratory successes nor the delights of this marvelous region succeed in replacing you. You don't doubt it, I hope?" (NR to HG, May 1, 1904).

38. NR to HG, Apr. 29 and May 18, 1904. Roussel normally weighed about 105–112 lbs.

39. NR to HG, Apr. 21 and May 18, 1904.

40. NR to HG, May 9, 1904.

41. NR to HG, May 11, 1904.

42. HG to NR, May 14 and 15, 1904; "Le Féminisme et la libre-pensée," *L'Action*, May 14, 1904; *Figaro*, May 14, 1904 (reproduced in *Nouvelliste* [Rouen]). On Pelletan, see Stone, *Sons of the Revolution*, 282–86; Agulhon, *French Republic*, 102.

43. See FR, carton 7, 1907, press clippings regarding the collaboration between freethinkers and feminists.

44. HG to NR, Sept. 11, 1902.

45. On "Barnum," see n. 16 above.

46. Correspondence NR to HG, HG to NR, Apr.–May 1904, passim.

47. FR, dossier 091 ROU, letter from NR dated June 28, 1904. The irony here is that having another child actually helped advance Roussel's cause.

48. NR, "Impressions d'une militante," *L'Action*, June 8, 1904.

49. NR, "Un Exemple," *L'Action*, Aug. 3, 1904.

50. Darnaud to NR, Aug. 31, 1904.

51. NR diary, 1904

52. NR, "Un Bienfaiteur de l'humanité," *L'Action*, Oct. 5, 1904; reprinted in id., *Quelques lances rompues*, 165–69.

53. HG to NR, Sept. 20, 1909. This cryptic comment suggests that Lucas's formula was problematic, but nothing else in the archives indicates that he "killed many women."

54. FR, carton 8, correspondence from Dr. Lucas; Roussel, "Bienfaiteur de l'humanité."

55. Sussman, "Wet-Nursing Business" and "End of the Wet-Nursing Business," 237–58; Fuchs, *Abandoned Children*.

56. Flammeche, "Une Grande Oeuvre," *L'Action*, May 24, 1909. The article also declared that the infant mortality was as high as 70 percent among infants placed in nurseries or with wet nurses.

57. Sohn, *Chrysalides*, 1: 274.

58. Harlor, "Maternité totale," *Fronde*, Feb. 20, 1901, cited in Cova, *Maternité et droits des femmes*, 130.

59. Fuchs, *Abandoned Children*, 51.

60. See NR, "Un Bienfaiteur de l'humanité," *L'Action*, Oct. 5, 1904.

61. Darnaud to NR, n.d. (1904).

62. Darnaud to NR, n.d. (1904).

63. Nelly Roussel, "Qu'est-ce que le féminisme?" *Petit almanach féministe illustré* . . . , 1906. The Union fraternelle des femmes enlisted Roussel to define feminism in the first of three almanacs that appeared in 1906, 1907, and 1908, and she did so succinctly: feminism was "a doctrine of individual happiness and general interest . . . of justice and harmony [that] proclaims natural equivalence and demands social equality between the two elements of the human gender." This definition not only reflected the core of Roussel's doctrine but reveals it as a very bourgeois acclamation of the pursuit of individual happiness. For the other two almanacs, Roussel provided theoretical articles on recognition of motherhood as a social function, on neo-Malthusianism, and on the right to work.

64. Summaries of the meeting were published in *Parti ouvrier*, Oct. 30 (reprinted in *Femme affranchie*, November); *Petite République*, Oct. 30; *Rappel républicain* (Lyon), Oct. 30 (an exceedingly negative commentary); *L'Action*, Oct. 31; *Eclaireur de l'Est* (Reims), Oct. 31; *Temps*, Oct. 31; *Bulletin des Halles*, Oct. 31; and *Jura* (Porrentruy), Nov. 1; all 1904.

65. FR, carton 5, speaking agenda. This lecture was first published in Roussel, *Éternelle sacrifiée*, ed. Armogathe and Albistur.

66. NR to HG, Apr. 8, 1905.

67. NR to HG, April 1905.

68. *Tribune républicaine* (Saint-Etienne), Apr. 11; *Action républicaine* (Haute-Loire), Apr. 12; *L'Action*, Apr. 13; and *Haute-Loire*, Apr. 16; all 1905.

69. *Tribune de Saint-Etienne*, *Progrès de Lyon*, and *Lyon républicain*, all Apr. 14, 1905.

70. NR to HG, Apr. 21 and May 19, 1905.

71. FR, carton 5, speaking agenda; NR to HG, May 13, 1905.

72. Darnaud to NR, May 29, 1905.

73. Darnaud to NR, June 17 and 19, 1905. He also told Roussel that his wife had lost their first infant, and nearly died herself. "Ah, the pains of Motherhood!" he said. The occasion of meeting Roussel, and for the first time hearing her speak, of course deepened Darnaud's affection for her. Even before her visit, he expressed himself very emotionally; he always referred to her qualities as a mother and mentioned her children (indeed, a good deal more than she did.) Typical of his letters is the following, written to both Nelly and Henri: "And I who has the joy of feeling myself not only the disciple but the friend of your Nelly, of this mama of the charming Mireille, of the admirable woman who wrote me six pages with an open heart just two weeks after the birth of your big Marcel; . . . I write this to you at a triple gallop of the pen, with a full heart, almost with tears in my eyes" (May 25 1905).

74. See, e.g., NR to HG, May 7, 1905.

75. NR to HG, Apr. 21, 22, and 24, and May 7, 1905. HG to NR, Apr. 21, 1905.

76. NR to HG, May 10 and 19, 1905; HG to NR, Apr. 23 and May 19, 1905.

77. HG to NR, Apr. 17, 18 and 30, 1905.

78. *L'Action*, Jan. 19, 1906. HG to NR Oct. 25 and 26, 1906. Henri continued to express pleasure at his wife's success and took his own role in shaping her career seriously, though he did so with undisguised irony, particularly in his always playful salutations, such as "Henri Godet, mari de Mme Nelly Roussel." He continued to express obsessive concern

about her health and gave her detailed advice. In nearly every letter, she requested his services: errands, correspondence, and phone calls. He arranged for all her train tickets, which required detailed information about her itinerary, train schedules, and the fluctuating ticket prices. Roussel used her speaking fees—apparently about 45 francs—and the sale of her brochures at 50 centimes each to finance her travel. On this particular tour, she sold 400–500 brochures. There were admission charges for most of her lectures, up to 50 centimes. A second-class train fare between Bordeaux and Paris was about 45 francs; hotels, usually covered by the organizers, cost 3–5 francs. Roussel traveled second class, while Godet traveled third, "studying psychology and art," as he put it. See HG-NR correspondence, April–May 1905.

79. NR to HG, Apr. 14, 1905; "Les Conférences de Nelly Roussel," *L'Action*, Apr. 24, 1905.

80. "Nelly Roussel," *Idée socialiste* (Lyon), Apr. 8, 1905.

81. NR to HG, May 10, 1905.

Four • *The Public and Private Politics of Female Self-Sacrifice*

Epigraph: Lucien Leduc (Ledont), "Une Conference de Nelly Roussel au cirque," *Jeune Champagne* (Reims), March 1905. The newspaper erroneously attributed the article to Lucien Leduc; Lucien Ledont to NR, Nov. 27, 1905.

1. Press coverage, *Réveil normand,* Jan. 26–Feb. 2; *Journal du Caen,* Jan. 22, 23, and 31; *Impartial* (Caen), Feb. 3; all 1906.

2. That "real" women—those true to their feminine nature—could not be held responsible for their actions and words constituted the defense and ultimate reason for the acquittal of Madame Caillaux in her murder trial. See Berenson, *Trial of Madame Caillaux.* Marguerite Durand and the other *frondeuses* likewise had considerable difficulty attaining legitimacy, even through the printed word, because women were thought incapable of reason, as Roberts, *Disruptive Acts,* 91–93, has demonstrated.

3. FR, carton 8, correspondence related to Roussel's lectures. Marguerite Wolf to HG (translated article from Budapest newspaper), May 23, 1908; undated letter with an illegible signature from a man living at 27 rue de Berri; carton 7, *Petit Niçois* and *Dépêche* (Nice), both May 1, 1911; "La Conférence Nelly Roussel à Gray," *Indépendant de la H^{te}-Saône* (Gray), Mar. 8, 1911.

4. Ivimy, *Woman's Guide to Paris,* 107. I thank Margo Bistis for bringing this guidebook to my attention.

5. De Giorgio, "Catholic Model," in *History of Women,* ed. Fraisse and Perrot, 4: 166–97.

6. FR, carton 5, speaking agenda and Roussel manuscripts 03/639. NR to HG, Feb. 24, 1907; NR to HG, Apr. 27, 1907. Roussel recorded having received 3,860 francs in speaking fees from 1905 to 1907. On *Par la révolte,* see Pederson, *Legislating the French Family,* 166–70.

7. FR, carton 8, A. B. de Liptay, (with the letterhead) Publicité Médico-Mondaine de Paris, Mar. 8, 1906; Isabelle Gatti de Gamond to NR, n.d.; M. Pailhé, Lisbon, Feb. 25, 1906, to NR; Victor Ragosine to NR, Oct. 3 and November (?) 1905. For reaction to an earlier performance in Paris, see Melanie Demoulin to NR, May 10, 1903, who wrote from the eighteenth arrondissement indicating that she could guarantee an audience of 300 or

400 and she was certain these women would be transformed if Roussel could repeat her performance.

8. Roussel often noted the anniversary of her first communion, when she was 11; e.g., NR to HG, May 9, 1907, and May 9, 1911.

9. The roots of this model lay not just in their own Christianity of the past, but in the early forms of worker organization in "brotherhoods" that practiced rituals similar to the celebration of the mass. Perrot, "On the Formation of the French Working Class," in *Working-Class Formation*, ed. Katznelson and Zolberg, 94.

10. NR, "La Liberté de maternité," in id., *Trois conférences*, 42.

11. Valentine Valette to NR, Apr. 10, 1905. Many men and women who wrote to Roussel called her an "apostle of feminism." See, e.g., letters to Roussel of H. Piens (a midwife), Feb. 27, 1907; "Pearl," Mar. 3 1907; T. Moraud, Apr. 15, 1909, and others in FR, carton 8.

12. NR to HG, Apr. 13, 1905.

13. NR to HG, May 9 and 10, 1907. Her description in the second letter gives an idea of some of the difficulties she had to face, with poor acoustics, dust, and smoke that wore her down.

14. Sewell, *Work and Revolution in France;* Katznelson and Zolbert, eds., *Working-Class Formation*, 45–154; and Magraw, *History of the French Working Class*.

15. Roussel, *Éternelle sacrifiée*, ed. Armogathe and Albistur, 55, 59.

16. Ibid., 57.

17. Ibid., 57–59. For a good example of changing aspirations among provincial women, see Emilie Carles, *A Life of Her Own: The Transformation of a Countrywoman in Twentieth-Century France*, trans. Auriel A. Goldberger (New York: Penguin Books, 1992).

18. Roussel, *Éternelle sacrifiée*, ed. Armogathe and Albistur, 59.

19. NR to HG, Apr. 3, 1906. Rebérioux, *République radicale?* 90–98; for the Lyon region, see Lequin, *Ouvriers de la région lyonnaise*, 2: 297–366.

20. NR to HG, Apr. 9 and 12, 1906; HG to NR, Mar. 29 and July 26, 1906.

21. NR to HG, Apr. 13, 1905.

22. NR, "Liberté de maternité," in id., *Trois conférences*, 37–38.

23. Ibid., 39.

24. FR, carton 8, B. Cremnitz, Feb. 16, 1907. On Roussel provoking tears, see also Mlle Guy to NR, Apr. 14, 1907; NR to HG, Oct. 26, 1906.

25. See, e.g., *Libre Pensée* (Lausanne), Jan. 17, 1906; Louise Olline to NR, Feb. 16, 1907; Pearl to NR, Mar. 3, 1907; G. Mazade to NR, Nov. 29, 1907.

26. Jeanne Bans, Aspiran (Hérault) to NR, Nov. 8, 1905.

27. Roussel, "Liberté de maternité," in id., *Trois conferences*, 39.

28. NR, "Décadence ou progrès?" *L'Action*, Jan. 18, 1907.

29. Roussel, "La Liberté de maternité," in id., *Trois conferences*, 43–44.

30. Roussel described her observation of this pattern during her 1904 tour in an article published in *L'Action*, June 8, 1094, quoted in Chapter 3 above. On her 1906 tour, she described an organizer's wife as "insignificant and indolent." NR to HG, Apr. 6, 1906.

31. E.E., "Conférence à St. Lô," *Journal de la Manche*, Jan. 24, 1906; George Gat, "Une Conference féministe," *Journal du Caen*, Jan. 22 and 23, 1906; "La Femme et la libre pen-

sée," *Briard*, Apr. 5 and 6, 1907; "Conférence de Madame Nelly Roussel," *Progrès de la Haute Savoie* (Annemasse), Apr. 20, 1907.

32. See, e.g., "La Libre Pensée de Saint Lô," *Courrier de la Manche*, Jan. 28, 1906; Aimée Reboux, Nîmes, to NR, Aug. 28, 1906; Marthe Jacob, Chaux-de-Fonds, Switzerland, to NR, Oct. 17, 1906; anonymous letter from Chaux-de-Fonds, Switzerland, to NR, Oct. 16, 1906; an "unknown who very much appreciated your lecture," Yvendon, Switzerland, to NR in Lausanne, Oct. 23, 1906; W. Brosch, Lausanne, Oct. 27, 1906; and letter from a woman in Geneva, Apr. 17, 1907, all in carton 8.

33. NR to "Monsieur," Mar. 13, 1909. The letter criticizes Kergomard for her close-mindedness after she had written a letter, probably published, about freedom of expression and ideas. Roussel begins her own letter by saying that she is not in the habit of attacking her colleagues in feminism (and she rarely did), and for that reason perhaps she never sent the letter. On Kergomard, see Klejman and Rochefort, *Égalité en marche*, 132, 145, 154, and 156–57.

34. Augusta Moll-Weiss, "Maternité," *Siècle*, Jan. 12, 1908.

35. Aria Ly to Caroline Kauffman, n.d. (sometime in 1911). I thank Andrea Mansker for sharing this letter. Aria Ly to NR, May 15, 1912.

36. "Conférence féministe," *Journal de St. Lô*, Jan. 17, 1906. Other articles made similar points, such as J.D., "Conférence à St. Lô," *Gars normand*, Jan. 28, 1906, which claimed women would not be able to resist giving away a vote "before the fear of a refusal of absolution" and complained that they already had too much influence over the electorate because of the power they had over their husbands.

37. Favorable articles described Roussel's appearance, oratory, charisma, and audience opposition and reaction in detail, as well as giving summaries of her message. Much of the opposition came in response to these articles. This was only the second lecture free-thinkers in St. Lô had ever organized. The author of one five-page article refuting all of Roussel's points thought that choosing her as a speaker reflected badly on the freethinking movement, especially because she was associated with neo-Malthusians; he cited the lecture in Paris (Nov. 20, 1905) that had instigated the Cassagnac affair, discussed later in this chapter. E.E., "Conférence à St. Lô," *Journal de la Manche*, Jan. 24, 1906. See "Le Public de la conférence," *Gars normand*, Jan. 28, 1906.

38. FR, carton 8, letter from Camille Guesmere (or Guesmierce) to Henry Bérenger, July 14, 1904. Bérenger ironically considered the press as a whole, despite his prominent role in it, "an insidious female force seducing and enslaving its readers and, thus, eating away at democracy," according to Roberts, *Disruptive Acts*, 80.

39. Camille Guesmere to NR, Dec. 8, 1904.

40. Jean-Jacques Rousseau, *Émile* (1762), trans. Barbara Foxley (London: Everyman's Library, 1989), 323.

41. Monsieur Celérier to NR, Paris, n.d. (c. 1907).

42. David Halperin, *One Hundred Years of Homosexuality and Other Essays on Greek Love* (New York: Routledge, 1990), 29–33, quoted in Nye, ed., *Sexuality*, 23, 25. Aria Ly argued for celibacy. See also MacKinnon, "Does Sexuality Have a History?" in *Discourses of Sexuality*, ed. Stanton.

43. Flammèche, "À la terrasse: Dénouements," *L'Action*, Sept. 9, 1905; NR, "Eclaircissements," *L'Action*, Sept. 16, 1905. See also Pedersen, *Legislating the French Family*, 170

44. "Ligue pour la Dépopulation," *Eclair*, Nov. 17, 1905, reprinted in *Verité française*, *Républicaine* (Melun), and *Mémorial des Vosges* (Epinal).

45. Le Liseur, "Carnet du Liseur: Joseph de Maistre malthusien," *Avenir de la Vienne* (Poitiers), Dec. 6, 1905; "Dépopulation et Répopulation," *Matin*, Nov. 18, 1905. The comment about Piot's newly published statistics appeared in "Chronique parisienne," *Petit Provençal*, Nov. 19, 1905. See also "Malthus et M. Piot," *Petite République*, Nov. 19, 1905. *Régénération* thanked *L'Action*, *Libertaire*, *Humanité*, *Petite République*, *Temps nouveau*, and *Anarchie*, as well as the "reactionary" press, for either helping announce the lecture or helping advertise it by opposing it (December 1905).

46. APP Ba 381, report of the 2d Police Brigade, Nov. 21, 1905. G. Hardy, "La Conférence de Nelly Roussel," *Régénération*, December 1905. FR, carton 7, notebook of "articles sur Nelly Roussel" indicates at least eleven Paris and provincial newspapers produced twelve articles about her lecture.

47. "Pour la dépopulation," *Eclair*, Nov. 21, 1905.

48. Guy de Cassagnac, "Morale des temps presents," *Authorité*, Jan. 23, 1906. Théroigne de Méricourt became active in revolutionary activities in 1789 and attempted to found a women's society; she ardently advocated forming an armed battalion of women. She went insane and was committed to the Salpetrière hospital where she died in 1817. Louise Michel participated in the Paris Commune of 1871 and did what de Méricourt advocated in wearing a National Guard uniform, and carrying and using a rifle. She was the "great female warrior" of the Commune and became known as the "Red Virgin." Among the critics of the Commune, she was called a "virago." She was exiled to New Caledonia. De Cassagnac probably did not know that Louise Michel was Roussel's greatest heroine.

49. G.C., "Papier timbré," *Autorité*, Feb. 10, 1906.

50. "La Citoyenne Roussel à Fontenay-Trésigny," *Tribune briarde*, Mar. 27, 1907, and "Cour d'appel de Paris," *Gazette du Palais*, Apr. 10, 1907; André Pique, "En Police correctionnelle," *Autorité*, June 29, 1906.

51. *Gazette de Tribunaux*, July 5, 1906; G.C., "À la neuvième chambre," *Autorité*, July 6, 1906.

52. G.C., "À la neuvième chambre," *Autorité*, July 6, 1906.

53. "Cour d'appel de Paris," *Gazette du Palais*, Apr. 10, 1907.

54. FR, carton 7, notebook of press clippings "de Nelly Roussel." Louis Roya, "Escarmouches . . . épistolaires," *Rénovation*, Dec. 15, 1911.

55. Darnaud to NR, n.d. (January 1907); Apr. 21, 1908, and Feb. 27, Mar. 23, Oct. 21, and Dec. 8, 1909.

56. Darnaud to Roussel, Apr. 6, 1906; Oct. 27, 1908.

57. V. Hamelin to Darnaud, as copied in Darnaud to NR, Aug. 12, 1905. Nelly had made this claim to Hamelin.

58. Darnaud to NR, July 21, 1907.

59. Darnaud to NR, Apr. 28, 1909. The father-in-law of Darnaud's son, Jean, had met Jane Misme at the home of the well-known author Octave Mirabeau. The father-in-law claimed that Mirabeau gave Misme 40,000 francs a year. But Misme was then, alleg-

edly, ravished by one Coquelin *aîné*, who gave her 30,000 francs per month. Darnaud frequently and repeatedly brought up the subject of the duchesse d'Uzès as an example of why women should not be granted the vote, even though he thought elite women (but only the elite) should have it. See for example, Darnaud, postcard to NR, June 1, 1910.

60. Darnaud to NR, Mar. 16, 1906, and Mar. 17, 1910. In the latter, he shares a letter from an 18-year-old mother of two who found neo-Malthusian methods disgusting. She said women should either love their children or remain chaste, but then—as though to affirm Roussel's point—she complained bitterly of the poor workers who gave birth every year, and of how pitiless the men were.

61. NR to HG, Oct. 23, 1906.

62. NR to HG, Apr. 3, 1906.

63. Klejman and Rochefort, *Egalité en marche*, 218. On women neo-Malthusianists, see McLaren, *Sexuality and Social Order*, 161–66; Ronsin, *Grève des ventres*, 158–63; Bard, *Filles de Marianne*, 209–15. On Madeleine Pelletier, see Sowerwine and Maignien, *Madeleine Pelletier;* Felicia Gordon, *Integral Feminist;* Bard, ed., *Madeleine Pelletier*, esp. Marie-Victoire Louis, "Sexualité et prostitution," 109–25; Scott, *Only Paradoxes to Offer*, 125–60.

64. NR to HG, Mar. 30 and 31 and Apr. 12 and 21, 1906; HG to NR, Apr. 22 1906. Roussel's diaries note the growing list of names of friends and family, often followed by "etc."

65. HG to NR, Apr. 5, 6, and 12, 1906.

66. NR to HG, Apr. 9, 1906. Other examples of other stickers, see Guerrand, *Libre maternité*, 61–62.

67. NR to HG, Apr. 29, 1906; HG to NR, May 4 and 8, 1906.

68. HG to NR, Mar. 31, 1906.

69. HG to NR, Mar. 31, Apr. 20 and 29, May 3, 4, and 7, and July 27, 1906; May 4, 1907; NR to HG, May 4, Aug. 6, and Oct. 23, 1906. For example, Nelly wrote Henri from Clermont during her 1906 tour regarding her future lecture in Toulon, venting her frustration as well as a measure of Parisian snobbery: "I wrote this morning to Runel de Gallargues (what a noble name!), and I am going to write to What's-his-name of Toulon, . . . since the letter where you announce that I accept the date of April 29 does not seem sufficiently explicit to these southern *libre-poires* [suckers, and a play on *libres penseurs*]. Send him, this . . . what's-his-name, whose address you have, some documents on your phenomenon" (NR to HG, Apr. 5, 1906).

70. HG to NR, May 8, Oct. 21 and 24, 1906; Bellanger et al., *Histoire générale de la presse française*, 3: 375.

71. NR to HG, n.d.; NR to HG, July 26, 1906.

72. NR to HG, Aug. 5, 1906.

73. According to Roussel's 1906 diary, she saw Marcel five times—on Jan. 18, Feb. 15, Mar. 4, May 17, and June 21—before they brought him home in September. HG to NR, May 7 and July 28, 1906; NR to HG, Aug. 5, 1906.

74. NR diary entries, October 1906.

75. HG to NR, Oct. 17, 18, 19, 21, 23, 24, 25, 27, 30, and 31, 1906. Andrée Nel was known in her family as a *gourde*—what we would call an airhead today. She talked incessantly and said nothing. Conversation with Michel Robin, June 20, 2004.

76. HG to NR and NR to HG, May 2, 1907; in response to his "zut" letter, Nelly wrote in anger that she was "too well brought up" to respond in kind (NR to HG, May 9, 1907).

77. HG to NR, Apr. 23, 1907

78. NR to HG, Apr. 27 and 30, 1907; HG to NR, May 4–5, 1907.

79. Darnaud to NR, n.d. (1907); *Liberté*, Sept. 28, 1907; *Liberté d'opinion*, July–August, appearing in October 1907. Aria Ly to NR, May 15, 1912.

80. J. Hellé, preface, Roussel, *Quelques discours*, 6; *Société nouvelle*, October 1907, quoted this passage with effusive praise for Roussel, and *Liberté d'opinion*, October 1907, found the introduction "deliciously feminine."

81. She did experience hardship as well as glory. During her 1907 tour, after a twelve-hour train trip and two lectures in as many days, she complained of insomnia and not having closed her eyes once during the night; "left to battle bedbugs, to pass my time in crushing them, and to put compresses on the blisters they gave me, I decided to flee the enemy that I could not vanquish, and get dressed to pack my trunk, and leave on the first train" (NR to HG, May 14, 1907).

82. This is not to say that the romantic affection had by any means gone out of their marriage; see, e.g., NR to HG, Mar. 3, 1907. But tense moments prevailed. Roussel complained of his forgetfulness and the lack of decorum in his correspondence; he complained of her slowness in sending him information about her speaking and travel schedules and was so confused by the information she did send that he called her letters "Chinese." See NR to HG, Apr. 24 and 27 and May 9, 1907; HG to NR, May 4 and 6, 1907.

83. HG to NR, May 15, 1907; Henri also complained about Andrée and Paul fighting, and about her spending habits on Feb. 27, Apr. 12 and 19, and May 7, 1907.

84. HG to NR, Mar. 2, Apr. 2, 14, 22, and 23, 1907; NR to HG, Mar. 1, 1907.

85. HG to NR Apr. 19 and 26, 1907; NR to HG, Apr. 30, 1907; HG to NR, July 24, 1907.

86. Marcel, dressed in feminine clothing as was standard at the time for male babies and young boys, is younger than two years old in Fig. 12, so it is safe to assume that the photograph was taken during one of her visits to Versailles.

87. NR diaries, 1904–22. The friendship networks have persisted to this day (conversations with Michel Robin, Martine Robin, and Marc Giron, June 13 and 20, 2004).

88. Davidoff and Hall, *Family Fortunes*, 338, make the point that this transition was long, uneven, and contested. In their historical anthropology of Swedish middle-class life in nineteenth and early twentieth century, Frykman and Lofgren, *Culture Builders*, 123–24, describe the actual practices of motherhood, as opposed to the prescribed role, in terms that make Roussel's relationship with her children appear "normal." They note that mothers were "all too rarely at the children's side," especially among the upper strata of the bourgeoisie, where women's social obligations left them little time for children. They instead transferred maternal tasks to hired labor. Sociological studies indicate a huge diversity of family structure and practices in France that varied by region. Different systems of authority influenced relations between parents and children, each giving rise to "specific tensions and pathologies" (Michelle Perrot, "The Family Triumphant," in *From the Fires of Revolution to the Great War*, ed. id., 127). Literary representations of motherhood such as Gustave Flaubert's *Madame Bovary* and studies of domestic service, such as Martin-Fugier, *Place*

des bonnes suggest a rather large gap between the prescribed maternal role and maternal practices.

89. Among the people she saw with great regularity were Marguerite Durand, Marbel, Mme Hammer, Hellé, Eugène Humbert, Liard-Courtois (anarchist, neo-Malthusian, ex-convict, and former neighbor), Salomon Reinach (neo-Malthusian), Paul Robin, Georges Yvetôt (head of the CGT), Alfred Naquet (member of the Chamber of Deputies and author of the 1884 divorce law), and the deputy Albert Cremieux. NR diaries, 1904–14.

90. See NR diaries.

91. HG to NR, May 4, 6, and 7, 1906, Aug. 20, 1907.

92. HG to NR, Feb. 23, 1907; diary entries 1908.

93. HG to NR, Oct. 30, 1906.

Five • Pathologies and Persecutions

1. Maïté Albistur, introduction, Bouglé Collection, Bibliothèque historique de la Ville de Paris.

2. Émile Darnaud to NR, Mar. 23, 1909.

3. Jean-Marie Mayeur, *Vie politique*, 223; Rebérioux, *République radicale?* 148–56; Agulhon, *French Republic*, 137–39; Stora-Lamarre, *Enfer de la IIIe République*, 206.

4. Jean Luy, "Poison révolutionnaire," *Accord social*, Dec. 12, 1909.

5. FR, carton 7, press release on the UFF, Feb. 25, 1911; Klejman and Rochefort, *Égalité en marche*, 170–72.

6. IISG, Humbert Archives, # 323, HG to Paul Robin, Feb. 13, 1903, correspondence to *Régéneration*. Some neo-Malthusian activities assumed a bawdy tone. Humbert received a dinner invitation featuring a mostly nude woman dangling a female contraceptive device in front of her groin. The banquet was a *diner des joyeux condoms*, and the menu included such dishes as *Sage femme aux mousses de vagin*. IISG, Hubert Archives, # 339.

7. Roussel's diary entries, 1908; Eugène Humbert had already made clear to both Henri and Nelly in 1907 that he would be leaving the League. HG to NR, Feb. 22, 1907. On the schism, see Ronsin, *Grève des ventres*, 66–70; Humbert, *Eugène Humbert*, 64–70.

8. See notebooks of press clippings; in a letter written October 1910, probably to Gabriel Giroud, she noted that she had not been in contact with the Bérengers since ceasing to write for *L'Action*. IISG, Humbert Archives, # 275, correspondence from Roussel to Humbert, October 1910.

9. HG to NR, Apr. 12 and 19, 1907. Added to his sense of humiliation was that the famous liberal judge Paul Magnaud, whose bust he had sculpted, didn't even recognize him on passing him in the street, after having sat for him for hours.

10. Harvey, *Almost a Man of Genius;* Wright, "Clémence Royer: Polymath out of Season," in id., *Notable or Notorious?* 43–56. Wright notes: "Charles Darwin . . . called her 'one of the cleverest and oddest women in Europe.' Ernest Renan is said to have described her as 'almost a man of genius.'" Darwin took her to task because she ignored revisions he made to *Origin of Species*, and he sought another translator. Royer helped organize France's first mixed Masonic lodge in 1893 and contributed to Marguerite Durand's *La Fronde*.

11. With this money, Godet hoped to repay Montupet 1,200 francs (HG to NR, May 30

and June 10, 1910); he did complete the statue of Royer but found nowhere to put it on display. For its eventual fate, see Epilogue.

12. See HG to NR, Feb. 12, 13, 14, 16, 24, and 28, and Mar. 14, 16, 20, and 25, 1908.

13. See Roussel and Godet correspondence, February and March 1908.

14. NR to HG, Mar. 1, 1908; NR to Thomas Nel, Mar. 2, 1908.

15. NR to HG, Mar. 25, 1908.

16. Diary entries June, July, and August 1908. NR to HG, Sept. 1, 1908.

17. NR to HG, Sept. 8, 1908.

18. "You could put your dressing table in front of the window of your bedroom," he noted (HG to NR, Sept. 8, 1908). Having separate bedrooms followed the aristocratic tradition and did not indicate any lack of passion between them. On the contrary, separate bedrooms among the upper classes provided a form of birth control. See McLaren, *History of Contraception*, 186–87.

19. HG to NR, Sept. 8, 1908. HG made further complaints to NR, Feb. 20 and 28, 1908.

20. NR to HG, Sept. 10, 1908.

21. HG to NR, June 18, 1909. Roussel's diary entries indicate her spending habits.

22. Diary entries and speaking agenda, 1908–9.

23. *Avenir* (Tournai), Feb. 8 and 9, 1909. Her brochures sold out in "the blink of an eye," according to *Pensée* (Brussels), Feb. 14, 1909; see also ibid., Mar. 7, 1909; *Nouvelles,* Mar. 5, 1909. Taudière quoted in *Soleil,* June 6, 1909, reprinted in *Courier des Deux-Sèvres,* June 15, 1909, and *Croix de Belfort,* June 20, 1909. *Croix de Belfort,* Oct. 12, 1909, deplored her influence.

24. Jeanne Tilquin to HG, Feb. 14, 1909 (in envelope with the HG-NR 1909 correspondence).

25. Stora-Lamarre, *Enfer de la IIIe République,* 179–206. Stora-Lamarre notes that the censorship laws were so vague that they could easily be used for political purposes, and were.

26. Elosu, *Amour infécond;* Guerrand, *Libre maternité,* 68–69.

27. APP Ba 381, Direction générale des recherches, and separate report, May 27, 1908; report to the prefect of police, "Conférence organisée par le groupe 'Génération consciente,'" Oct. 27, 1908.

28. Humbert, *Eugène Humbert,* 90. According to the law, the publisher of "affronts to indecency" was responsible, not the author.

29. Ibid., 91.

30. AN F^7 13955, Commissaire de Police de Sottevile-lès-Rouen, Feb. 8, 1908.

31. IISG, Humbert Archives, # 337, Proceedings of the trial of Humbert and Liard Courtois before the Rouen court of appeal, 1909–10.

32. Ibid. See also Humbert, *Eugène Humbert,* 85–89.

33. Montupet to HG, Aug. 1, 1904. See NR diaries, passim.

34. NR to HG, June 21, 1909.

35. NR to HG, June 21 and 28, 1909.

36. HG to NR, September 1909; Roussel, *Quelques lances rompues,* 3.

37. NR to HG, Aug. 12, 1909.

38. Mireille to Louise Nel, n.d. and Aug. 13, 1909; HG to NR, Sept. 18, 1909.

39. Roussel appears as witness for Humbert: *Paris-Journal*, reprinted in *Radical*, *Intransigeant*, *Petite République*, *Peuple français*, and *Libre Parole*, all Dec. 1, 1909. Darnaud to NR, Dec. 2, 1909. Roussel responded Dec. 7, 1909: "Why do you expect that I am so less well informed about this subject [of childbirth] than you are?" This time she lambasted him for his refusal to understand: "Many men are in agreement with [me], and since they can't share our suffering, let them have at least the loyalty to recognize it, to salute it, to deplore it, and above all to admit that we would sometimes like to shield ourselves from it. Apart from this suffering, there are many other reasons not to want to have a lot of children."

40. IISG, Humbert Archives, # 139, letter from HG to Humbert, Feb. 7, 1910; letter from NR to Darnaud, *République de l'Ariège*, Mar. 10, 1910. Articles regarding this meeting appeared in the *Radical*, Feb. 11, 1910; *Siècle*, Feb. 12, 1910; *Nouvelles*, Feb. 14, 1910; *Féministe* (Nice), Feb. 17, 1910; *République de l'Ariège* (by Darnaud), Feb. 27, 1910; *Travailleuses* (St. Quentin), March 1910; and *Journal des Femmes*, March 1910.

41. "Nos Suffragettes: Elles sont trois qui affronteront la lutte électorale," *Matin*, Feb. 14, picked up in the *Intransigeant*, Feb. 15; *Est républicain*, Feb. 17; *Journal d'Alençon*, Feb. 17; *Bessin* (Isigny), Feb. 20; *Gil Blas*, Feb. 16; *Gazette de Bruxelles*, Feb. 18; *Indépendance roumaine* (Bucharest), Mar. 6; and *World* (New York), Mar. 13; all 1910. Roussel also marked in her notebook of press clippings that there had been announcements of her candidacy in the *Journal* (Havre), *Patriote normand*, *Petit Béthunois*, *Avenir de l'Orne*, and *Journal* (Condé), "etc., etc., etc."

42. NR to HG, Mar. 12, 1910. In this same letter she also relished the fact that people had surrounded her at a funeral she had attended that afternoon. "Nelly Roussel," she wrote, "has become someone." The meeting at which she spoke was important not only because it was the first large feminist meeting on the question of suffrage—with particular attention to municipal elections—but deputies and senators spoke in support as well. Articles about the meeting appeared in thirteen provincial papers—most of them in departments to which she had traveled—as well as in *Nouvelles*; *Gil Blas*; *Figaro*; *Petite République*; and *Paris-Journal*, all Mar. 12; *Temps*, Mar. 13; *L'Action*, Mar. 16; *Siècle*, Apr. 5; and *Journal de Femmes*, April 1910.

43. "Meeting de protestation des neo-malthusiens," *Radical*, Apr. 1, 1910; "Un Meeting neo-malthusien," *Paris Journal*, Apr. 1, 1910;

44. "Le Carnet du jour," *Autorité*, Apr. 4, 1910. Information about the meeting, and announcement of the publication of all the speeches in a volume *Défendons-nous* appeared in the *Ouvrier-syndicqué* (Marseille); *Voix du peuple*, *Libertaire*, and *Éclaireur* between June 16 and 26, 1910.

45. Darnaud to HG, Feb. 22, 1907; HG to NR, Mar. 12 and May 25, 1910; NR to HG, May 24 and 25, 1910.

46. NR to HG, May 24 and 25, 1910; Elosu to HG, May 24, 1910; HG to NR, May 25 and 27, 1910.

47. HG to NR, May 29 and 31, June 2 and 4, 1910; NR to HG, June 10, 1910.

48. When Roussel's symptoms became more acute during World War I, she referred to herself as having neurasthenia. See Chapter 6.

49. Ballet, *Neurasthenia*, 46. Dubois, *Psychic Treatment of Nervous Disorders*, 18, quoted

in Shorter, *From Paralysis to Fatigue*, 221. Charcot introduced the diagnosis in France at least by 1897 and probably earlier.

50. Ballet, *Neurasthenia*, 17–18. In the third edition, the authors noted the widespread abuse of the term they had helped popularize in France: "Everybody knows it and makes use of it and, as in the case of all technical terms that have become public property, it has been applied at random."

51. Ibid., 94–95.

52. The patient was to stay in bed, in a state of "total inactivity" and silence. "She must neither get up nor make use of her own hands under any pretext." Ibid., 352. Weir Mitchell's well-known rest cure is terrifyingly described in Charlotte Perkins Gilman's *The Yellow Wallpaper* (Boston: Small, Maynard, 1899).

53. Diary entries June 13–Oct. 3, 1910; NR to HG, Sept. 9 and 12, 1910; Mireille to HG, Sept. 12, 1910. Her diary notes that she received several hundred francs from her mother and grandfather over the course of several months.

54. Roussel, *Pourquoi elles vont à l'église*. This play is published as a pamphlet, though without date or publisher. Roussel's diary first mentions it when she records reading it to the UFF on Nov. 26, 1910.

55. Roberts, *Disruptive Acts*, 38.

56. HG to NR, Feb. 19, 1911.

57. "La Conférence Nelly Roussel à Gray," *Indépendant de la H^{te}-Saône* (Gray), Mar. 8, 1911.

58. NR to HG, Apr. 2, 5, 6, and 10, May, 7 and 9, 1911.

59. Ronsin, *Grève des ventres*, 92–115. See also AN F^7 13955 and APP Ba 381.

60. "Notre Propagande," *Rénovation*, June 15, 1911. When Nelly received the invitation, her grandfather became impassioned with interest, encouraged her, and wanted her to send newspaper accounts of the event immediately afterward. NR to HG, May 9, 1911.

61. NR to HG, May 9 and 24, 1911. "Les Théories néo-malthusiennes: Une Conférence-contradictoire à Auxerre," *Indépendant auxerrois*, May 25 and 26, 1911.

62. "Théories néo-malthusiennes," *Indépendant auxerrois*, May 25 and 26, 1911.

63. AN F^7 13955, report of the prefect of the Yonne to the president of the Council of the Minister of the Interior, Nov. 2, 1911.

64. Ibid., passim.

65. AN F^7 13955, "La Propagande neo-malthusienne," report of Nov. 29, 1911 (Paris).

66. HG to NR, Feb. 11, Apr. 1, May 8 and 16, 1911; NR to HG, Feb. 1 and 3, Apr. 10 and 27, May 9 and 19, 1911.

67. MG to her grandparents, July 25, 1911.

68. NR diary, July 1911–February 1912.

69. Paul Bureau, "La Propagande néo-malthusienne et sa répression" (report to the 2e Congrès national contre la pornographie), in FR, carton 2, *Periodiques divers*; see also Ronsin and Guerrand, *Sexe apprivoisé*, 68.

70. Bureau, "Propagande néo-malthusienne," 1–2. Robin did make the point about "older men and young girls" in his pamphlet *Le Secret du bonheur*.

71. Bureau, "Propagande néo-malthusienne," 5–8.

72. Ibid., 10.

73. Ibid., 17.

74. The meeting was summarized in Mauricius, "Une Conférence anti-malthusienne," *Rénovation*, Jan. 15, 1913.

75. On natalist discourse and the 1920 law prohibiting neo-Malthusian propaganda, see Roberts, *Civilization Without Sexes*, 93–119.

76. Giroud, *Paul Robin*, 291, quoted in Demeulenaere-Douyère, *Paul Robin*, 387.

77. Demeulenaere-Douyère, *Paul Robin*, 387–88; NR, *Derniers combats*, 198.

78. Diary entries, Feb. 17 to Apr. 9, 1913; NR to HG, Mar. 3 1913; HG to NR, Mar. 14, 1913. See Roberts's insightful analysis in *Disruptive Acts*, 37–47. Marguerite Durand to NR, Feb. 25, 1913.

79. To emphasize the link between the "real" *éclaireuses* and the play's fictional ones, the panel spoke from the actual stage set of the climactic act 3. Coverage of this event and of the lunch that followed appeared in *Excelsior*, Mar. 21; *Nouvelles* and *Palais*, Mar. 15; *Loire républicaine*, Mar. 17; *Comedia*, Mar. 14 and 19; *Petite République*, *Havre-Éclair*, *République de Travailleurs*, *Tribune républicain* (Saint-Étienne), *Moniteur de Puy-de-Dôme*, and *Liberté*, Mar. 20; all 1913. NR to HG, Mar. 16, 1913.

80. Roberts, *Disruptive Acts*, 38.

81. HG to NR May–June, 1913. Unfortunately, her letters from the sanatorium are not in her archive.

82. For example, Henri wrote: "How I would have loved to share this bedroom with you . . . [where we would] commit a thousand follies. . . . I love you so much and our separation makes me judge our love still more, which gives me the proof that you alone know how to give me the illusion of youth" (Sept. 4, 1913). In two other letters, he mentions how he "does not look at other women" and says: "All this makes me think that there is only one whose kisses I would eat, the others make me sick, they are always something which is not my dream, and my own dream is not finished, it is a beautiful dream that I already lived for fifteen years and that I continue and that I will begin again. . . . I prefer to continue because the longer it lasts, the more it becomes delicious, the more my love adapts in the most complete way, more perfect to my ideal and to myself, the better we know each other, the better our forms and our characters marry each other more intimately, this is perhaps a little stupid, but it is very true" (Sept. 25, 1913). Henri had never before made any reference to other women—and those here indirectly suggest that he might have at least been tempted by some extramarital encounters, which would not have been the least unusual in his bohemian milieu. More explicit, however, is his reavowed commitment to her—perhaps more pronounced because he feared losing her.

83. NR to HG, Dec. 23 and 28, 1913; Jan. 1, 4, 11, and 16, 1914.

84. Réné Théophil Hyacinth Laennec (1781–1826) discovered nonpulmonary tuberculosis in his autopsy studies at the beginning of the nineteenth century (Iseman, *Clinician's Guide to Tuberculosis*, 5–6, 181–83). The various forms of abdominal tuberculosis include peritoneal, ileocecal, anorectal, and mesenteric lymph node infections. Roussel might have had either of the first two forms, given the symptoms she described: abdominal pain, anorexia, diarrhea/constipation, weight loss—but symptoms of abdominal TB vary widely. The "protean" presentation of the disease also lends itself to frequent diagnostic errors. See Humphries and Lam, "Non-Respiratory Tuberculosis," in *Clinical Tuberculosis*, ed. Davies,

187. I thank Michael D. Iseman for his response to my inquiry about Roussel's symptoms, in which he affirms that they conform to those of abdominal TB. Although there is no way of ascertaining this, it was probably common among Europeans in her day, because of its bovine origins, he notes. "In that era clinicians did not quibble about regular TB or bovine TB; only in recent times have we come to readily distinguish them (primarily because of differences in routes of transmission and prevention)" (email, Apr. 12, 2004).

85. *La Faute d'Eve* was first published in *Mouvement féminin*, Sept. 15, 1913.

Six • *The Great War*

1. Humbert, *Eugène Humbert*, 152.

2. Bard, *Filles de Marianne*, 64. See also Darrow, *French Women and the First World War*, 58, and Grayzel, *Women's Identities at War*.

3. Studies of war correspondence have mostly focused on exchanges between the home front and the front line. But France "became a nation of letter writers" during the Great War, Hanna, "Republic of Letters," notes. Indeed, we learn from one of Mireille's letters that one of the baccalaureate exam questions in 1918 asked, "Do you think the current tragic events will renew the importance of correspondence, of interest in beauty, and why?" (Mireille to HG June 28, 1918).

4. HG to NR, Aug. 13, 1915, July 24, 1916, Sept. 18, 1917.

5. Note added by NR to letter from MG to Andrée Nel, Aug. 4, 1914.

6. MG to Andrée Nel, August 1914. NR diary, Aug. 11, 1914.

7. Émile Darnaud to NR, n.d. On reactions to the outbreak of war in France, see Darrow, *French Women and the First World War*, 53–56.

8. NR diary, August–September, 1914. Hausser, *Paris au jour le jour*, 542.

9. Leonard V. Smith et al., *France and the Great War*, 40.

10. Ibid., 39; Becker, *Great War*, 48–49; Bard, *Filles de Marianne*, 58.

11. Bard, *Filles de Marianne*, 51–52. Amélie Hammer, president of the UFF—the one feminist association in which Roussel most consistently participated—was firmly anti-pacifist. Darrow, *French Women in the First World War*, 66, 78–86; Thébaud, *Femme au temps de la guerre de 14*, 112–18. For Mireille's soldier, see FR, carton 5, "Guerre 1914–1918." Her "fileul de guerre" was Arthur Loriette, husband and father of two little girls. He sent Mireille pictures of himself and his wife and daughters; his correspondence from the trenches was generally fairly upbeat and devoid of detail.

12. Caroline Kauffmann to NR, Dec. 14, 1914.

13. NR diary, August 1914; Bard, *Filles de Marianne*, 58–59.

14. Letter from NR quoted in "Pour la jeunesse féminine," *Humanité*, Nov. 30, 1914.

15. FR, carton 3, dossier 4, L. Frier to NR, Jan. 11, Jan. 25, Feb. 12, and Apr. 13, 1915. Hers was not the only article to be suppressed, and the editors concluded that the censors were not just acting in the interests of national defense but using their power to suppress feminism.

16. Nelly-Roussel, "Notre idéal," *Équité*, Apr. 15, 1915.

17. FR, carton 2, Urbain Gohier, "Les Gardiennes du foyer," *Journal*, Nov. 15, 1915.

18. FR, carton 2, "Coupures de la presse, les femmes et la guerre."

19. NR, "Quelques réflexions sur la guerre," *Libre Pensée internationale*, Dec. 12, 1914.

20. See NR, "Atrocités," *Libre Pensée internationale*, Feb. 6, 1915; letter from the editor to NR, Feb. 9, 1915, as well as other letters regarding censorship of her articles in FR, carton 5, "Guerre de 1914–18," and carton 8, "Correspondence." The editor wrote, "The police commissioner of Evian believed it necessary to hold our journal because of your article. We live in a very difficult moment; in Switzerland we have been subjected to censorship for the past six months, and now in France we have been sequestered. Your article is very good, very well thought out; it caught the attention of our friends in Lausanne. . . . We do not wish to give up the fight, we believe ourselves on the right path, and shall continue to make the voice of reason heard. I like to think that you, too, will remain faithful. Give me the address of the person to whom you desire the journal to be sent in Germany; up to this point the issues are very successful among our subscribers." Marianne Rauze, the founder of *L'Équité*, bitterly complained about what the censors had done to Roussel's article. "I'll publish either everything or nothing," she proclaimed, and she asked Roussel to go with her to the minister of the interior to protest the censorship. Rauze to NR, Feb. 8, 1915; see also L. Frier to NR, Apr. 13, 1915.

21. FR, carton 5, manuscripts; NR, "Pour le salut de nos blessés" (MS).

22. Ibid.

23. Ibid.; Nelly-Roussel, "Notre idéal," *Équité*, Apr. 15, 1915.

24. Bard, *Filles de Marianne*, 94–99. One thousand delegates came from the Netherlands, 47 from the United States, 28 from Germany, 16 from Sweden, 16 from Austria-Hungary, 12 from Norway, 6 from Denmark, 5 from Belgium, 3 from England, 2 from Canada, and 1 from Italy. The Congress formulated resolutions for peace, justice, and democracy that inspired Wilson's Fourteen Points.

25. NR, "Mégères austro-boches," *Libre Pensée internationale*, May 15. Marianne Rauze, editor of *L'Équité*, read this article at her freethinkers' meeting and at that of the Socialist Women of the L'Eure and Loir Federation to great audience appreciation; she invited Roussel to speak again and complimented her on her courageous attitude in the face of current blindness; history, she said, would recognize Roussel as an admirable pioneer. FR, carton 8, Marianne Rauze to NR, n.d.

26. NR diary, Mar. 14, 1915; speaking agenda, 1915 and 1916; *Française d'aujourd'hui*, March 1916.

27. NR diaries, passim. She marked the first day of her period with an "x," and often indicated nothing else but "repos" or "repos au lit." "Colcotar" refers to ferric oxide. See Mireille to HG, Sept. 19; NR to HG, July 9, Aug. 17, Oct. 11, and Oct. 23, 1917, and June 28, 1918.

28. HG to NR, 1915 correspondence.

29. Roussel recorded in her diary, and sometimes kept an account of, money that her mother gave her, usually 250–300 francs at a time, and sometimes 600 francs. Several times in 1918, Montupet sent them money orders for 500 or 600 francs. See Montupet to HG, Sept. 15 and 17, 1917; HG to Montupet, Sept. 15, 1917; HG to NR, Sept. 7, 1915. Godet noted: "Pépé, to whom I wanted to talk to about oil and steel responded to me with [a lecture about] Vichy pastilles and morning enemas on an empty stomach. He again took out these old claptrap speeches in a lecture that wouldn't end until nightfall." Godet called him "sontupet." HG to NR, Sept. 15 and 16, 1917; Oct. 19, 1917.

30. HG to NR, May 11 and 13, 1915.

31. HG to NR, May 11, 12, 13, 15, and 17, 1915; NR diary, May 1915; NR to HG, May 14, 1915.

32. NR to HG, July 26; Montupet to HG, July 19, 1915.

33. Roussel also had to conceal from her stepfather the newspapers she was reading, saying she had read an article in the *Petit Parisien* and then the principle news in *Matin:* "Don't tell Pépé." Ironically, Jeanne and her family "agree completely with Pépé on all questions concerning the war. I avoid discussing it with them. But all the same, I read *Humanité* every day." NR to HG, May 14 and 18, 1915.

34. Henri to Montupet, May 18, 1915.

35. NR to HG, July 1, 22, and 26, 1915; HG to NR, July 24 and 27, 1915.

36. HG to NR, July 24 and 29 and Aug. 3, 1915. NR to HG, Aug. 1, 1915.

37. NR to HG, Aug. 2 and 6, Sept. 1 and 11, 1915; HG to NR, Aug. 29, 1915. Efforts to evoke the dead in such a manner became more common during World War I. See Winter, *Sites of Memory, Sites of Mourning,* 54–77.

38. Mireille visited in mid August and wrote to her father: "I found Mama on the milk cure and tired. She tried your remedy before you advised her to, she didn't take lacto-lacine for two days, which caused an intense crisis of intoxication and obliged her to put herself on milk yesterday. Today she is a little better, but still being a bit tired, she is very happy to have me as her secretary." Mireille to HG, Aug. 15, 1915.

39. HG to NR, Aug. 25; NR to HG, Sept. 11, 1915.

40. HG to NR, Aug. 16, Sept. 3 and 12, 1915.

41. HG to NR 23, June 28, 1915; copies of the cards are in the Musée d'Orsay, Documentation, Sculptors, Henri Godet. The content of these cards offers another sign of Godet's ability to overcome his principles in his desperate attempt to earn money. These fascinating images include "Victory" (a woman with two young girls standing atop dead German soldiers), "Justice Pursuing Crime" (crime represented by a German soldier), "Judgment of History" (German soldier being judged for war crimes); "Belgium Liberated" (French soldiers rescuing a woman from German soldiers), and "Glory" (victorious French soldiers).

42. For Fritz Robin, NR's diary Oct. 5, 11, and 12, Nov. 15, 1914. Paul Nel was called up immediately, and it was apparently Montupet who succeeded in getting him a deferment. HG to NR, Aug. 5, 1915.

43. NR to HG, Aug. 2, HG to NR, Aug. 3, NR to HG, Aug. 6, 1915.

44. HG to NR, Sept. 13, 15 and 30, 1915; HG to NR Aug. 14, Oct. 8, 1916, Sept. 24, 1917. In 1917, Godet listed "sculptor" as his occupation on the *carnet du pain* (bread ration coupon).

45. "Yesterday Mireille was joyous about leaving for the front—she is going to hear cannons—happily she will still be far away from them," Henri wrote Nelly (HG to NR, June 28, 1915).

46. Mireille to NR, July 25, 1915, and subsequent correspondence; Mireille to HG, two postcards, July 5 and 12, 1915; postcard to NR, July 12, 1915. Among items censored were "All postcards depicting scenes or bearing legends likely to have a bad influence on the morale of the army or the population" (Becker, *Great War,* 49). Carton 5, correspondence, 1914–1918, Marcel Noble to HG Dec. 14, 1914, and June 15, 1915. Noble asked Montupet

and Godet to keep the news of his amputation absolutely secret. The correspondence from friends contains much news of this sort. Particularly difficult for Mireille was the death of the boyfriend of a teacher with whom she was very close. See Mireille to NR and HG, Sept. 18, 1917; to NR, October, n.d. (1917).

47. Mireille to NR, July 9, 1916; July 3–4, 5, 8–12, 1917; HG to NR, July 9, 1917. Mireille to HG and NR, Apr. 6 and 8, 1914. Reform of the baccalaureate program in 1902 made it an easier option for girls to pursue, and teachers began to encourage them to do so as a means of creating more opportunities for respectable careers. See Margadant, *Madame le Professeur*, 217; Francoise Mayeur, *Éducation des filles*, 149–79, and *Enseignement secondaire*, 377–98.

48. HG to NR, Sept. 16, 1916; Mireille to NR, Oct. 21, 1916.

49. Mireille to NR, June 20 and July 25, 1915. For more examples of Mireille's protective stance toward Nelly, see Mireille to HG and NR, July 12, 1915; to HG, July 25 and Aug. 15, 1915, Sept. 5, 1916, Sept. 13 and 19, 1917; to NR, Sept. 27 and Oct. 15, 1916, Sept. 27, Oct. n.d., and Oct. 13–14, 1917. Mireille and Nelly also shared intellectual and feminist interests. Mireille read a novel by the feminist Hellé (a.k.a. Marguerite Dreyfus), Nelly's friend, that scandalized Louise Nel, and translated feminist articles in English for her. Mireille to NR, June 23 and Aug. 28, 1915, June 25, 1916.

50. Typical were the following instructions Mireille sent to her father when he was in Paris with Marcel: "What he is he becoming! My devil of a brother! Tell him that he has to redo everything that he has done up to now in English and that he has to repeat orally the homework he already finished. Without this, he will forget everything. Hug him for me (if he has worked hard) and keep for yourself lots of good kisses from Mama and me." HG to NR, July 26, 1915; Mireille to HG, Aug. 15, 1915, and to NR, May 16, 1915.

51. HG to NR, June 23, Aug. 29, and Sept. 3, 1915; Mireille to HG, Sept. 12 and 15, 1915. When Marcel went off for a month in September 1915 to a children's program in Agon (Manche), aged 11, Henri wrote that he felt lonely without him, saying, "this kid is a little tiresome, but he has that in common with all kids." While away, Marcel continued to infuriate his grandparents, parents, and sister, only this time by his silence; he rarely wrote to any of them.

52. HG to NR, July 9, 1915. Roussel expressed the same concerns about Marcel disrupting her silence and tranquility the following summer as well, but he nonetheless joined her, Louise Nel, and Mireille for a water and rest cure in Bourbon l'Archambault; he infuriated her when he put tadpoles into the thermal baths and made so much noise playing tennis that he annoyed other guests. NR to HG, July 3, 6, and 28, Aug. 14 and 21, 1916. On the other hand, Marcel was very bright and able to do well in school if he applied himself, which he did occasionally. Henri wrote proudly of Marcel's academic success, and said to Nelly: "Glory to Marcel, celebrate his genius." HG to NR, July 23 and Aug 22, 1916.

53. NR diary, Feb. 27, 1912.

54. The correspondence from Mathilde is located in FR, carton 6, and dates mostly from 1918 and 1919. Mireille to HG, July 8, 1918; HG to NR, July 12, 1917; NR to HG, Sept. 30, 1916. Roussel referred to a letter from Mathilde in which the latter wrote of her boredom and impatience with Roussel's absence. For the leverage Mathilde exercised, see especially the family correspondence of 1918.

55. Roussel, "Ivresse," *Ma forêt*, 12: "Heure d'exaltation trop brève, / À ma souffrance exquise trêve, / Sublime bonheur d'un moment, / Réalité plus belle que le rêve, / Je viens, dans l'été qui s'achève, / Chercher votre éblouissement. / Je viens, vibrant comme une lyre, / Clamer ma joie et mon délire / Me plonger, ivre, en ta splendeur, / Qui tour à tour m'enchante et me déchire, / Automne, héroique sourire / De la Nature qui se meurt."

56. Roussel, *Ma forêt*, 6. NR to HG, June 27, 1916. She was particularly happy in this letter because she had been able to "digest white beans with their skin," an indication of how difficult digestion had become for her.

57. See correspondence from Mireille, Marcel, and NR to HG, summer 1916 and 1917. Montupet had bought the children cameras and bicycles, and Marcel built and attached a cart to his bicycle so that he could give Nelly rides through the forest. HG to NR, Sept. 3, 1916; NR to HG, Sept. 7, 1916.

58. NR to HG, July 3 and 28, Aug. 21, 1916; Oct. 3, 1917. For her falling out with Andrée, NR to HG, Oct. 10, 1916; Aug. 15, Oct. 3 and 11, 1917. The letter of October 3 indicates that Andrée discussed her sister's behavior with Mathilde, another sign of the relative intimacy that the family had with this domestic servant. The sisters' fight deeply troubled Montupet, and it renewed his anger at Henri for not having told him about it immediately (Montupet to HG, Sept. 15, 1917).

59. HG to NR, Oct. 17, 1917.

60. She sent her poems to Mme Hammer, Marie-Thérèse Gil-Baer, and Mmes Bien-aimé and Beal. See diary, Nov. 13 and 17, and NR to HG, Oct. 10, 1916. Mireille gave them to her teachers (Mireille to NR, Oct. 3–4, 1917). Roussel also sent poems to the wife of Henri's business partner, Del Pozo. The Del Pozos had visited the Godets in Barbizon and named their baby girl after Nelly.

61. NR to HG, Oct. 18 and 23, 1917. Ballet, *Neurasthenia*, 272–73; see NR diary entries for November and December 1917.

62. NR diary, 1918; Great Britain, Ministry of Information, *Chronology of the [Great] War*, ed. Gleichen et al., vol. 3: *1918*, table, p. 14; Fierro, *Histoire et dictionnaire de Paris*, 221; Hauser, *Paris au jour le jour*. On the night of March 11–12, sirens caused such panic at a metro station serving as a refuge that sixty-two people were trampled to death by a crowd. For the exodus, see Becker, *Great War*, 310–12.

63. Mireille and HG to Louise Montupet, Apr. 2, 1918.

64. Mireille and NR to Louise Montupet, Apr. 13 and 26 and June 19, 1918.

65. HG to the Montupets, n.d., May 1918.

66. NR to Louise Nel, Apr. 13 and 18, May 1, 1918; HG to the Montupets, Apr. 26, 1918.

67. NR to HG, June 23, 1918

68. Mireille to the Montupets, June 29–30, 1918; Marcel to the Montupets, July 4, 1918; Marcel to HG, July 8, 1918.

69. NR to Louise Nel, July 7, 1918.

70. HG to NR, July 5, 1918.

71. HG to NR, June 30 and July 14, 1918. The reference to what "everyone" thought once again provoked comments about the theories regarding crowd behavior. It reminded Henri of a book he had found in their library about "the soul of the crowd," which Darnaud had probably given to Nelly. In it, he read that the "crowd is more stupid than the individ-

ual," leading him to think that public opinion must therefore be distrusted. Unlike most other people, Henri remained convinced that the bombardment and the war itself would continue indefinitely. "The soul [*âme*] of the crowd always turns a man into the ass [*âne*] of the crowd," he wrote, indulging in the wordplay he so loved. Nearly four years after his death, Darnaud continued to influence both Henri and Nelly, as did the crowd psychology theory of Gustave Le Bon.

72. NR to HG, July 17, 1918; Mireille to HG, July 22, 1918.

73. Mireille to HG, July 16, Aug. 7, 1918; NR to HG, July 18 and 20, 1918; Mireille and NR to HG, July 30, 1918; NR to HG, Aug. 3 and 6, 1918. Roussel quoted the proverb, "Often the fear of something bad drives us to something worse." In this case, "fleeing the Gothas and Berthas, we have jumped into the throat of a wolf, represented in the occurrence of flu, bronchitis, and other horrible maladies." She begged him to locate his headquarters in Grenoble instead of Lyon. Henri responded that her attitude toward the Lyonnais climate was "laughable. One would think that we're talking about going to the Congo" (n.d., August 1918). Mireille also pressured her father on Nelly's behalf; she argued that wood and coal would be more expensive in Lyon, and that milk would be impossible to obtain for Nelly.

74. NR, Mireille, and Marcel to HG, July 8, 1918; NR to HG, July 17 and 18, 1918; Mireille to HG, Aug. 7, 1918. Against his mother's instructions, Marcel went swimming in a river on a very hot day after having eaten. At the same time, Marcel seemed to be doing constructive things. Henri asked him to run errands for his business, which he had apparently done effectively, and he was learning how to be a baker in the local *boulangerie*. Overall, he seems to have contributed to the family's well-being (e.g., finding the La Balme residence) but does not seem to have got much credit for the positive things he accomplished. Marcel apologized to his mother and made promises to improve his behavior, but Nelly had little faith that he would change.

75. NR to HG, Aug. 20, 1918; NR diary, August and September 1918.

76. Kolata, *Flu*, 3–14.

77. Zylberman, "Holocaust," 193–94. In Paris alone, 10,281 flu deaths occurred from June 1918 through April 1919. Determining the exact mortality rate is extremely difficult, because many cases went unreported, or symptoms were not properly diagnosed; often victims died of secondary infections, especially pneumonia; Fierro, *Histoire et dictionnaire*, 222; Iezzoni, *Influenza 1918*, 201; Hausser, *Paris au jour le jour*, 685.

78. Delumeau and Lequin, eds., *Malheurs des temps*, 419; Hausser, *Paris au jour le jour*, 693; Fierro, *Histoire et dictionnaire*, 222; Zylberman, "Holocaust in a Holocaust," 194.

79. NR to HG, Sept. 15, Oct. 21, 28, and 29, 1918; Hausser, *Paris au jour le jour*, 694.

80. NR to Louise Nel, Nov. 29, 1918; NR, diary, Nov. 25, 1918. Madeleine Vernet was a feminist who extolled motherhood; her journal focused on its social function. Roussel privately dismissed Vernet, whose feminism was far more conservative than hers.

81. NR, diary, Dec. 12, 15, 21, and 22, 1918; NR to Louise Nel, Dec. 31, 1918.

82. NR to Louise Nel, Dec. 16, 1918. Mireille to Louise Nel, Dec. 18, 1918.

83. HG to the Montupets, Dec. 22, 23, 24, and 25, 1918.

84. HG, correspondence cited in the preceding note.

85. Roussel, "Invincible Croyance," *Ma forêt*, 15.

Seven • Last Battles

1. NR to HG, July 15 and 18, 1919.

2. Leonard V. Smith et al., *France and the Great War*, 158–59.

3. Of those mobilized, 63 percent either died or were mutilated, a percentage that exceeded that of any other country. France mobilized 8,410,000 men, of whom 1,358,000 died, 1,040,000 became permanent invalids, and 3,000,000 became semi-invalids. Sowerwine, *France since 1870*, 117. Precise figures for World War I are impossible to determine, and these differ somewhat from those given by Winter, *Great War*, 75, who cites 7,891,000 Frenchmen mobilized, and 1,327,800 killed. Another source, citing the same statistics as Sowerwine for mobilized, killed, and wounded adds 537,000 missing among French troops, with an overall casualty rate of as high as 76.3 percent (www.spartacus.schoolnet. co.uk/FWWdeaths.htm [accessed December 15, 2005]). This rate was the highest among all the sixteen countries listed; the rate was 52.3 percent for the Allied powers, 62.7 percent for the Central Powers, and 57.6 percent overall. On other losses, see Sowerwine: the number of marriages that took place in 1915 was only 30 percent of the number in 1913; the 1921 census counted 6,216,000 women in the 20–39 age group and only 5,178,000 men. France lost around 900,000 buildings, 9,000 factories, 200 coal mines, 6,000 bridges, and 2,400 kilometers of rail lines.

4. Harris, "'Child of the Barbarian.'" Several public figures—and purportedly even a Catholic priest—suggested that women should abort the fetuses of German fatherhood. A journalistic debate ensued, and in March 1915, a ministerial directive sought to prevent abortion by allowing women to give their children up for public care, with falsified birth certificates. See also Bard, *Filles de Marianne*, 61–64.

5. Horne, "Soldiers, Civilians and the Warfare of Attrition," and Leonard V. Smith, "Masculinity, Memory, and the French First World War Novel." Jay Winter and Blaine Baggett's documentary *The Great War and the Shaping of the Twentieth Century* (1996) shows poignant footage of soldiers who came out of the war with shell shock, lost limbs, and deformed faces.

6. Perrot, "New Eve and the Old Adam"; Leonard V. Smith, "Masculinity, Memory and the French First World War Novel"; Roberts, *Civilization Without Sexes*, 37–41.

7. Audoin-Rouzeau, *Men at War*, 129–33.

8. Daniel Sherman further notes the discomfort after 1918 with women's wartime agricultural activities: "For if women could generate life on their own, in the absence of able-bodied men, what could compel them to resume their subordinate roles once the men returned? The many references to men's 'seed' in other dedication speeches can plausibly be read as an attempt to shut down such potentially subversive meanings, to restore to the phallus its preponderant role in procreation, making women, as it were, once again safe for insemination" (Sherman, *Construction of Memory*, 303–5). Leonard V. Smith et al., *France and the Great War*, 162–63; Harris, "'Child of the Barbarian'"; Darrow, *French Women and the First World War*, 5. See also Urbain Gohier quoted on p. 177 above.

9. Roberts, *Civilization Without Sexes*, 91.

10. NR speaking agenda, 1919.

11. Klejman and Rochefort, *Égalité en marche*, 196–97. Bard, *Filles de Marianne*, 118. For a fascinating analysis of Céline Renooz (and other French women writers), see Allen, *Poignant Relations*.

12. One such attack concerned bourgeois women's use of household domestics, which sparked a debate in *L'Humanité*, May 23 and June 1, 5, 14, 18, and 26, 1919. Roussel participated; she foresaw a time when all women would have professions, and would need "household workers"—a term she preferred to "maid." Such workers, she hoped, would be unionized and their work would become a *métier* (trade).

13. Bard, *Filles de Marianne*, 122; Klejman and Rochefort, *Égalité en marche*, 197–98, 206.

14. FR, carton 2. This masthead, drawn by Marie-Thérèse Gil-Baer, only appeared in 1922. Bard, *Filles de Marianne*, 262; Hause, with Kenney, *Women's Suffrage and Social Politics*, 216–17; Klejman and Rochefort, *Égalité en marche*, 197.

15. Louise Bodin to NR, June 18, 1919 (two letters). Bodin shared her contempt for the moderate Union française pour la suffrage des femmes (French Union for Women's Suffrage) and its leader Cécile Bruschvicg (1877–1946), the recipient of a 100,000-franc annuity, who thought that having a child was easy and that feminists should persuade working-class women to have more.

16. NR, "Les Femmes et la guerre," *Voix des femmes*, Oct. 9, 1919; Magdeleine Marx, "Les Femmes et la guerre: Réponse à Madame Nelly Roussel," ibid., Oct. 19, 1919; ibid., NR, "Les Femmes et la guerre: Réplique à Mme Magdeleine Marx," Nov. 6, 1919.

17. NR, "La Règne de l'homme," *Voix des femmes*, Apr. 22, 1920; "Les Vrais Assassins," *Mère éducatrice*, April 1920.

18. FR, carton 8, Colonel Jean Converset to NR, Dec. 31, 1919, Feb. 5, 1920, Mar. 12, 1920, Apr. 22, 1920. He died in November 1924; articles about him appeared in *Mère éducatrice*, Dec. 18, 1924, and November 1925.

19. Jean-Marie Mayeur, *Vie politique*, 254–58; Wright, *France in Modern Times*, 322–23.

20. "Scrutin de folie: Après les elections legislatives," *Voix des femmes*, Dec. 4, 1919, and *Libre Pensée internationale*, Dec. 3, 1919.

21. APP F⁷ 13955. To evade censorship and police surveillance, Giroud wrote under the pseudonym "Georges Hardy"; after the third issue, the paper was shut down. Giroud then changed its name to *La Grande Question*. Letter from NR, Jan. 18, 1917, published in *Neo-Malthusien*, June 1917. Eugène Humbert remained in Spain until July 1919, fearing prosecution if he returned (he was 44 when the war broke out, but men up to age 47 were subject to the draft.) Shortly after his return, an anonymous letter, signed by a "mother who lost her son during the war," alerted the police about the "draft dodger," and two agents came to find him. He was not home at the time, and they did not return. Shortly thereafter, he rejoined Giroud in neo-Malthusian propaganda. APP F⁷ 13955, police reports of Feb. 2 and May 31, 1916. See also Jeanne Humbert's recollections in *Eugène Humbert*, 173.

22. NR, "Sotise et impudeur," *Neo-Malthusien*, March 1919; "Posons nos conditions!" *République intégral*, December 1919.

23. NR, "Le Tocsin," *Voix des femmes*, Jan. 8, 1920; reprinted in *Neo-Malthusien*.

24. NR, "La Médaille des mères," *Voix des femmes*, June 3, 1920. See n. 8 above and sources cited there. Roussel would never have supported eugenics because of her strong belief in individual liberty. Her preference for the terms "conscious motherhood" or "lib-

erty of motherhood" over "neo-Malthusianism" distinguished her from those in the movement who were eugenicists.

25. NR, "La 'Journée des Mères de Familles nombreuses'" *Voix des femmes*, May 9, 1920, and "La Médaille des mères," ibid., June 3, 1920.

26. Guerrand and Ronsin, *Sexe apprivoisé*, 69.

27. AN F⁷ 13955; "Un Scandal: Qu'attend le gouvernment?" *Democratie nouvelle*, Dec. 18, 1919; APP Ba 381, letter to Maurice Barrès from M. Pelissier, 106 rue Monge, May 29, 1919; police report of Sept. 18, 1919.

28. APP Ba 381 prov. The police had an abiding fear of the neo-Malthusian influence on working-class women. See, e.g., report of prefect of police to the minister of the interior, June 21, 1913, and AN f/7/13955, report from the Central Commissary of Police in Tourcoing to the general controller of administrative police services (the minister of the interior), May 19, 1914.

29. AN F⁷ 13955, F. Blanc, ingenieur des mines, president du Groupement économique des industries françaises, "Congrès de Nancy: Le Problème de la natalité et les manoeuvres allemandes" (1919); report of E. Laurent, prefect of police, to the minister of interior, May 31, 1916; a report dated Feb. 28, 1916, from the Paris Prefecture of Police, noted how many children Humbert had "lost for France."

30. AN F⁷ 13955, "Le Problème de la natalité: Le Gouvernement et les manoeuvres allemandes."

31. "Contre les ennemis de la race française," *Action française*, May 10, 1920.

32. A.B., "Le Meeting de St-Ouen," *Voix de femmes*, May 13, 1920.

33. NR, "De lâcheté au cynisme," *Voix des femmes*, June 24, 1920.

34. Ibid.

35. Humbert, *Eugène Humbert*, 175–78; Guerrand and Ronsin, *Sexe apprivoisé*, 69–70; Roberts, *Civilization Without Sexes*, 93–119, and Pedersen, *Legislating the French Family*, 162–91.

36. Guerrand and Ronsin, *Sexe apprivoisé*, 71, 72. They refer to Professor Balthazard, whose lecture on December 13, 1920, at the Faculty of Medicine was published the following year in *Progrès medical*, but they offer no further citation. Ironically, the "pornographic" element in the propaganda he cited (which had nothing to do with Roussel) was not instruction on contraceptive devices but advice on the commonly practiced coitus interruptus followed by mutual masturbation.

37. Roberts, *Society Without Sexes*, 111; Ronsin, *Grève des ventres*, Pedersen, *Feminism, Theater, and Republican Politics*, 164–66 and passim.

38. Huss, "Pronatalism and the Popular Ideology of the Child." These cards were the sort of kitsch against which Godet's more artistic, allegorical postcards could not compete (see Chapter 6 above). NR, "Notes de la semaine," *Voix des femmes*, Dec. 8, 1921. Roussel said she was not surprised that, after having suffered so many births, the mother of nine would not be able to think rationally. But she also suspected that the words came, not from the woman, but from the bourgeois newspaper.

39. NR, "La 'Totale liberté,'" *Voix des femmes*, Nov. 4, 1920.

40. Humbert, *Eugène Humbert*, 181–84; AN F⁷ 13955, police report on Marie Aline Blanc (Jeanne Humbert's mother), Jeanne (Humbert) Rigaudin, and Eugène Humbert, Nov. 19, 1920.

41. Sonn, *Anarchism and Cultural Politics*, 19–20.

42. NR, "La 'Totale liberté,'" *Voix des femmes*, Nov. 4, 1920; "La Loi 'super-scélérate'?" ibid., June 23, 1921; "Inconscience? . . . ou hypocrisie?" ibid., July 7, 1921; "La Loi super-scélérate," *Lutte féministe pour le communisme*, June 25, 1921. Roussel's belief in the rights of *all* human beings was genuine and deeply committed.

43. NR, letter in *Voix des femmes*, June 29, 1921.

44. NR, "Education," *Mère éducatrice*, March; "Education," *Voix des femmes*, July 14, Dec. 22; "Programme 'bourgeois'?" ibid., Aug. 11; "Féminisme et révolution," ibid., Dec. 22; all 1921.

45. NR, "'Masculinisme' inconscient," *Voix des femmes*, Sept. 29; "Nécessité du féminisme," ibid., Nov. 17; "Glanes," ibid., Jan. 5; all 1922.

46. Davy, *Une Femme.*

47. The meeting took place, according to Roussel's agenda, on Apr. 10, 1920, and was summarized in "Le Meeting de *La Voix de femmes*," *Populaire*, Apr. 12, 1920, and *Voix des femmes*, Apr. 15, 1920.

48. Davy, *Une Femme*, 242–43; "Lettre ouverte à Madame Nelly Roussel," *Voix des femmes*, July 8, 1920. Charlotte Davy to NR, Apr. 13, 1922; id. to HG, Dec. 25, 1922. Her other books were *Le Roman de mon oncle; Lettres; Judith la Juive;* and *Savoir pardonner.*

49. NR, "L'Ecole des propagandists," *Voix des femmes*, Dec. 2, 1920; and NR diaries 1920–22. There is no record of how many students took these classes.

50. "La 'Noël humaine': Allocution de Nelly-Roussel," *Voix des femmes*, Dec. 30, 1920.

51. Henriette Sauret, "In Memoriam: Nelly-Roussel la généreuse," *Voix des femmes*, Jan. 15, 1933.

52. André Lorulot, "Nelly Roussel," national radio address, published in *Idée libre*, August–September 1955, 184. Lorulot had been her colleague in anticlericalism, anarchism, and freethinking.

53. When regretting that she would not be able to participate in a pro-Russian demonstration in December 1919, she wrote privately that "the fatigues of propaganda" had put her in a state of "fragile" health. Her retreat was "momentary" and had not in any way "cooled or weakened the ardor of her convictions." NR to "Madame," Dec. 13, 1919. For other such examples, see NR, "La Nécessité du féminisme," *Voix des femmes*, Nov. 17, 1921; *Ce qu'il faut dire*, Jan. 27, 1917.

54. NR to HG, Sept. 8, Oct. 10 1921.

55. NR, "Anniversaire," *Voix des femmes*, Feb. 2, 1922.

56. HG to NR, Feb. 24, 1922.

57. HG to NR, Jan. 28; Feb. 2, 4, 7, 12, 13, 17, 19, 21, and 24, 1922. Diary entries, Mar. 27–29, 1922. The results of the x-rays are only referred to later, in NR to Marcel, June 17, 1922. For evidence that Pagnier knew she had pulmonary tuberculosis at this time and told Henri, see Dr. Pagnier to HG, Jan. 11, 1923.

58. Pagnier to HG, Jan. 11, 1923. On conspiracies of concealment around TB, see Sontag, *Illness as Metaphor*, 6–7.

59. Diary entries Apr. 14–May 20, 1922. Charlotte Davy learned the true nature of Roussel's illness from others. Roussel welcomed her as a confidante, which testified to her genuine ability to cross class boundaries in her emotional commitments. Davy urged

Roussel to take care of herself, and then proclaimed a truth that others did not realize, "Yes, I understand how inaction must weigh you down, you who are so combative and so active, but you must give in to the force of things . . . you must take it upon yourself to turn your mind away from everything that can make you sad" (Davy to NR, Apr. 13, 1922). Roussel wrote to Davy on Apr. 23 and 26, and Davy visited her on May 17 in the midst of her severe intestinal crisis—when she saw almost no one else beyond family.

60. NR, "Le Front unique des femmes," *Voix des femmes*, May 25, 1922.

61. NR to Marcel, June 17, 1922.

62. NR to HG, postcard, n.d., June or July 1920. She also worried more over practical matters, particularly the price of her "cure," which was much steeper than Dr. Pagnier had led her and Godet to believe it would be. Though her mother gave her 1,000 francs when she entered Lamotte Beuvron, that was not sufficient, and Nelly was irritated that Henri wanted her to discuss the details of bills with her doctors; she feared that she would be considered unreasonably demanding and "eccentric." She threatened to return home. Diary entries, June 28–July 18; NR to HG, postcards (of Lamotte Beuvron), n.d., June–July 1922.

63. Mireille to HG, Aug. 28, 1922. Mireille quoted the clinic director to the effect that "all the precautions I shall have to take will be inspired by the fear of heredity far more than my current state of health." Henri insisted she have chest x-rays even when her symptoms improved. Despite the discovery of the TB bacillus in 1882, the belief that it was hereditary persisted. See Herzlich and Pierret, *Illness and Self in Society*, 28; Barnes, *Making of a Social Disease*, 51.

64. NR to Mireille and Marcel, Aug. 24, 1922. Although she could barely find the energy to write, she continued to remark on Marcel's letter-writing skills, telling him how much she appreciated the quantity and quality of his correspondence. "These are real letters, alive and not taxing homework." But she then criticized him for the wrong date in his letter, for a contradiction in his narrative, and for mistakes in typing her poetry (NR to Marcel, Sept. 6, 1922).

65. NR to Juliette Robin, Sept. 2–3, 1922.

66. FR, carton 4, HG, memoir "Lamotte Beuvron."

67. NR to HG, Sept. 10, 11 (postcard), 1922. HG, carton 4, memoir, "Buzenval."

68. HG, "Buzenval." The experimental treatment he mentioned was "caleophare."

69. Ibid. HG to NR, Nov. 24, 1922.

70. HG, "Buzenval."

71. Mireille to HG, Sept. 15, 1922. Mireille's ignorance about Nelly's state is further indicated in letters to Henri (Sept. 27, Oct. 17, 1922) in which she expresses her happiness at the "good news" about her mother.

72. Mireille to HG, Nov. 10, 14, and 19, Dec. 12, 1922.

73. HG to NR, Nov. 24, 1922. He added her response to this letter.

74. Hélène Raymonol (Laguerre's daughter) to HG, Dec. 20, 1922; Odette Laguerre to HG, Dec. 21, 1922. Juliette Robin also promised to conceal the news from Mireille, and did not write to her until January 17, "apprehensive about discussing the subject that preoccupied them both." She said Nelly "illuminated her existence." Juliette Robin to HG, Dec. 20, 1922; id. to Mireille, Jan. 17, 1922.

75. Louise Nel to Mireille, Dec. 22, 1922.This estimated attendance is based on the signatures of the guest book. Marguerite Durand, who did attend, was deeply upset that she had only found out only the night before, and by accident, because she was staying at different address and had been very ill. Marguerite Durand to HG, Dec. 31, 1922; see other correspondence to Henri in FR, carton 6.

76. *Voix des femmes* devoted the first two pages of its Jan. 4, 1923, issue to many of these eulogies, with a large portrait of Roussel and excerpts of her speeches and articles on the front page.

77. "X" (Marbel), "Mme Nelly Roussel, écrivain et conférencière," *Paris—Notabilités étrangères,* December 1911; Noëlie Drous quoted Marbel in "Nos pierrres noires," *Voix des femmes,* Dec. 13, 1923. A. Bailly, "Les Livres," *Voix libertaire,* Dec. 24, 1932.

78. Durand's eulogy in *Voix des femmes,* Jan. 4, 1923. Marguerite Durand to HG, Dec. 31, 1922. Durand declared herself both guilty and remorseful in this very moving and candid letter. She apologized for not having spoken the way she had wanted to at the funeral, explaining that she had learned of Roussel's death only at the last minute and by chance. "I suffered both morally and physically at the cemetery. You must have perceived it. Never has my regret been more profound for being in such a state, without voice, without eloquence. To speak about Nelly suitably would require speaking like she herself spoke . . . lacking words my very sincere tears must have indicated my emotion and my sadness—my remorse as well. . . . You are right that there were between Nelly Roussel and myself many affinities. We only saw one another rarely and, nonetheless, I always felt her present."

79. "Nécrologie: Nelly Roussel," *L'Ère nouvelle,* Dec. 21, 1922; "Nécrologie: Nelly Roussel," *Petite Provençal,* Dec. 23, 1922. *Dictionnaire des intellectuels français,* 1008–9.

80. Henriette Sauret, "Un Apôtre du feminism: Nelly Roussel," *Française,* Mar. 14, 1931; "In Memorium: Nelly-Roussel La Généreuse," *Voix de femmes,* Jan. 15, 1933. Commemorating her mother in 1927, for example, Mireille referred to the "memory of her life of ardent and generous battle, where her delicate nature was too quickly consumed" ("Une Voix de l'au delà," *Mère éducatrice,* October 1927). Crediting his own internationalism to a 1919 lecture by Roussel, Louis Martin, senator from the Var, similarly said that she had been "consumed by the internal flame that set her on fire" ("Politique extérieur," *Petit Var,* Sept. 10, 1932; Martin repeated the metaphor in "La Protection des forêts," ibid., Aug. 12, 1934).

81. Sontag, *Illness as Metaphor;* Herzlich and Pierret, *Illness and Self in Society,* 28; Barnes, *Making of a Social Disease,* 51; Porter, "Case of Consumption."

82. Noëlie Drous, "Nos pierrres noires," *Voix des femmes,* Dec. 13, 1923.

83. FR, carton 8, Louise Nel to MG, Dec. 22, 1922; Mireille to Marbel, Jan. 9, 1923.

Epilogue

1. FR, carton 8, Odette Laguerre to MG, Aug. 20, 1923, Dec. 31, 1923, Aug. 30, 1926, Sept. 9, 1926; Mireille Nelly-Roussel, "L'Enfance heureuse," *Fronde,* Aug. 25, 1926; "Combien furent-elles?" ibid., June 4, 1927; "Au voix de l'au delà," *Mère éducatrice,* October 1927.

2. Michel Robin, interview, June 7, 1997.

3. Popkin, *History of Modern France,* 202.

4. FR, carton 8, Mireille to HG, September–October 1927; interview with Michel Robin, June 7, 1997.

5. FR, carton 6, HG to "Mon cher maître," Mar. 15, 1928, and carton 5, Godet manuscript, May 1, 1928.

6. Madeleine Vernet, "À la mémoire d'Henri Godet," *Mère éducatrice,* November–December 1937; interview, Michel Robin, June 7, 1997, and subsequent conversations 1997–2004.

7. FR, carton 5, HG to Monsieur Faure, Feb. 4, 1937; Achille Urbain, director of the Vincennes Zoo, to Senator Fleurot, Dec. 12, 1937; Hargrove, *Statues de Paris,* 989; Roussel, *Éternelle sacrifiée,* ed. Armogathe and Albistur, 84n24. See also Musée d'Orsay, Documentation, Sculpture, Godet.

8. Musée d'Orsay, Documentation, Godet. Sotheby's catalogue and *Gazette,* Nov. 1, 1991. See HG to NR, Sept. 27, 1921, in which Henri says he is rereading *La Dame aux camélias* and seeing the symbolic function of the flowers for the first time.

9. Madeleine Vernet, "À la mémoire d'Henri Godet," *Mère éducatrice,* November–December 1937.

10. Mireille to NR, September 1923; recopied, February 1966. For Roussel's letter, see Chapter 7 above.

11. Interview with Michel Robin, June 7, 1997.

12. HG to Noëlie Drous, Dec. 13, 1923.

13. *Mère éducatrice,* Apr. 24, 1924, November 1925, December 1926, October 1927, November 1930, November–December 1932; *Voix des femmes,* Apr. 24, Dec. 18, 1924, Jan. 15, 1925, November 1930, Jan. 15 and 31, 1933; *Petit Var,* Sept. 10, 1932, Aug. 21, 1934; *Eveil de la femme,* Nov. 3 and 10, 1932; *Revue bibliographique,* May–June 1930; *Amitié française,* July 13, 1930; *Pages féminines: Maternité,* August–September 1930; *Française,* Mar. 14, 1931; *Droit des femmes,* February 1931; *Grande Réforme,* July and August 1931, November 1932, July 1933; *Révue du droit public et de la science politique,* December 1931; *Voix libertaire,* Dec. 24, 1932; *Solidarité* (Nice), Dec. 5, 1932; *Flambeau,* Jan. 5, 1933; *Idée libre,* December 1932; *Pensée libre,* December 1932; *Griffe,* Jan. 25, 1934; *Patrie humaine,* Jan. 28, Feb. 4, 1933; *Ère nouvelle,* Mar. 3, 1933; *Voix libertaire de Limoges,* Apr. 8, 1933; *Carnet de la semaine,* Jan. 22, 1933; *Contre-poison,* July 1933. *Française,* Mar. 14, 1931. Manuel Devaldès, "Nelly Roussel," *Grande Réforme,* July 1933. Victor Margueritte, "Au fil de l'heure," *Volonté,* Jan. 8, 1933. "La femme conservatrice," *Griffe,* Jan. 25, 1934.

14. Jeanne Humbert, "Les Précurseurs," *Grande Réforme,* March 1946. See also Humbert's article in *Réfractaire,* January 1976. *Idée libre,* August–September 1955.

15. See Koos, "Fascism, Fatherhood, and the Family"; id., "'On les aura!'"; id., "Gender, Anti-Individualism, and Nationalism"; Muel-Dreyfus, *Vichy et l'éternel feminin;* Pollard, *Reign of Virtue;* Burton, *Holy Tears, Holy Blood.*

16. Cova, *Maternité et droits des femmes,* 116.

17. Ibid., 282.

18. The birthrate spiked just after the war and then gradually fell to near prewar levels by 1980; see graph in Ronsin, *Grève des ventres,* 241

19. Payer, *Medicine and Culture,* 50. According to this survey, 6 percent of British

women and 3 percent of American women relied on withdrawal. Payer points out that by the time the ban was lifted, the Pill was already available, which at least partly explains why mechanical means, such as the diaphragm, never became popular in France. See more statistics provided by the Institut national d'études démographiques at www.ined.fr/population-en-chiffres/france/index.html (accessed December 14, 2005).

20. A debate about American and French feminism that began with the publication of Mona Ozouf's *Mots des femmes* (1995) was published in *Débat*, November–December 1995; excerpts have been reproduced in Célestin et al., *Beyond French Feminisms*, 225–38.

21. Margaret Sanger lived in Paris for several months in 1915, where she sought information about birth control, but her inability to understand French limited her contacts to the working-class friends of one English-speaking neo-Malthusian. Sanger, *Autobiography*, 103; Reed, *Birth Control Movement*, 89–96.

22. Reed, *Birth Control Movement*, 89–96; McCann, *Birth Control Politics*, 1.

23. Soloway, *Birth Control*, 312.

24. Linda Gordon, *Woman's Body, Woman's Right*, 231–42; Offen, *European Feminisms*, 336–39; Soloway, *Birth Control*, 134–36, 152–53. See also Fisher and Szreter, "'They Prefer Withdrawal'"; Cook, *Long Sexual Revolution*, 91–142.

25. Ronsin, *Grève des ventres;* Humbert, *Eugène Humbert;* Guerrand and Ronsin, *Sexe apprivoisé;* Sowerwine and Maignien, *Madeleine Pelletier;* Felicia Gordon, *Integral Feminist.*

26. Duchen, *Women's Rights and Women's Lives*, 120–27.

27. Ibid., 173.

28. Ibid., 120–81. The Communist Party believed birth control diverted the working class from its true socialist goals; like the socialists of Roussel's day, it claimed that numerous children would not be a burden for women after the fall of capitalism, a stance that led many women to leave the Party. The communists subsequently changed their position because of high abortion rates.

29. Duchen, *Women's Rights and Women's Lives*, 207–9.

30. FR, carton 7, correspondence of Mireille Godet, 1956–85, MG to *Nouvel Observateur*, Feb. 17 and 21, 1972.

Primary Archival Sources

Archives nationales de France (AN)
  F^7 13955
Archives de la Préfecture de Police de Paris (APP)
Bibliothèque historique de la Ville de Paris
  Bouglé Collection
Bibliothèque Marguerite Durand (BMD)
  Fonds Roussel (FR)
  Correspondance Mireille Godet, 1956–1985
International Institute of Social History (IISG), Amsterdam
  Archives of Eugène Jean-Baptiste Humbert (1870–1944)
Musée d'Orsay
  Documentation. Sculpture. Henri Godet

Writings by Nelly Roussel

Par la révolte: Scène symbolique. 4th ed., with speech by Sébastian Faure. Originally published 1903.
Quelques discours de Nelly Roussel. Paris, 1907.
Quelques lances rompues pour nos libertés. Paris: V. Giard & E. Brière, 1910.
Pourquoi elles vont à l'église. N.p.: n.d. [c. 1910?].
Paroles de combat et d'espoir. Épône: Éditions de l'Avenir Social, 1919. An expanded version of *Quelques discours de Nelly Roussel.*
Ma forêt. Épône: Éditions de l'Avenir Social, 1921.
Trois conférences. Paris: Marcel Giard, 1930.
Derniers combats: Recueil d'articles et de discours. Paris: L'Émancipatrice, 1932.
L'Éternelle sacrifiée. Collection Mémoire des femmes. Edited by Daniel Armogathe and Maïté Albistur. Paris: Syros, 1979.
"Freedom of Motherhood." In *Feminisms of the Belle Époque: A Historical and Literary An-*

thology, ed. Jennifer Waelti-Walters and Steven C. Hause, trans. Jette Kjaer, Lydia Willis, and Jennifer Waelti-Walters, 242–50. Lincoln: University of Nebraska Press, 1994.

Other Published Sources

Accampo, Elinor A. "The Rhetoric of Reproduction and the Reconfiguration of Womanhood in the French Birth Control Movement, 1890–1920." *Journal of Family History: Studies in Family, Kinship, and Demography* 21, 3 (July 1996).

———. "Private Life, Public Image: Motherhood and Militancy in the Self-Construction of Nelly Roussel, 1900–1922." In *The New Biography: Performing Femininity in Nineteenth-Century France*, ed. Jo Burr Margadant, 218–61. Berkeley: University of California Press, 2000.

Accampo, Elinor A., Rachel G. Fuchs, and Mary Lynn Stewart. *Gender and the Politics of Social Reform in France, 1870–1914*. Baltimore: Johns Hopkins University Press, 1995.

Adler, Laure. *Secrets d'alcôve: Histoire du couple, 1830–1930*. Paris: Plachette, 1983.

Agulhon, Maurice. *Marianne au pouvoir: L'Imagerie et la symbolique républicaine de 1880 à 1914*. Paris: Flammarion, 1989.

———. *The French Republic, 1879–1992*. Translated by Antonia Neville. Oxford: Blackwell, 1990.

Albistur, Maïté, and Daniel Armogathe. *Histoire du féminisme français*. Vol. 2: *De l'Empire napoléonien à nos jours*. Paris: Des Femmes, 1978.

Allen, James Smith. *Poignant Relations: Three Modern French Women*. Baltimore: Johns Hopkins University Press, 2000.

———. "Sisters of Another Sort: Freemason Women in Modern France, 1725–1940." *Journal of Modern History* 75 (December 2003): 783–835.

Armengaud, André. *Les Français et Malthus*. Paris: Presses universitaires de France, 1975.

Armogathe, Daniel, and Maïté Albistur. "Préface, notes et commentaires." In Nelly Roussel, *L'Éternelle sacrifiée*, passim. Paris: Syros, 1979.

Aron, Jean, ed. *Misérable et glorieuse: La Femme du XIXe siècle*. Paris: Fayard, 1980.

Audoin-Rouzeau, Stéphan. *Men at War, 1914–1918: National Sentiment and Trench Journalism in France During the First World War*. Oxford: Berg, 1992.

Ballet, Gilbert. *Neurasthenia*. Translated by P. Campbell Smith, M.D. New York, 1909.

Bard, Christine, ed. *Madeleine Pelletier: Logique et infortunes d'un combat pour l'égalité*. Paris: Côté-Femmes, 1992.

———. *Les Filles de Marianne: Histoire des féminismes 1914–1940*. Paris: Fayard, 1995.

———, ed. *Un Siècle d'antiféminisme*. Paris: Fayard, 1999.

Barrows, Susanna. *Distorted Mirrors: Visions of the Crowd in Late Nineteenth-Century France*. New Haven: Yale University Press, 1981.

Barthes, Roland. *Michelet*. New York: Hill & Wang, 1987.

Barnes, David S. *The Making of a Social Disease: Tuberculosis in Nineteenth Century France*. Berkeley: University of California Press, 1995.

Beauvoir, Simone de. *Le Deuxième Sexe*. Paris: Gallimard, 1949. Translated by H. M. Parshley as *The Second Sex* (New York: Knopf, 1952).

Becker, Jean-Jacques. *The Great War and the French People*. Oxford: Berg, 1985.

Bellanger, Claude, Jacques Godechot, Pierre Guiral, and Fernand Terrou, eds. *Histoire générale de la presse française*. Vol. 3: *De 1871 à 1940*. Paris: Presses universitaires de France, 1972.

Berenson, Edward. *The Trial of Madame Caillaux*. Berkeley: University of California Press, 1992.

Berlanstein, Lenard R. *Daughters of Eve: A Cultural History of French Theater Women from the Old Regime to the Fin-de-Siècle*. Cambridge, Mass.: Harvard University Press, 2001.

Blanc de Saint-Bonnet, Antoine. *De la douleur*. Lyon: Giberton & Brun, 1849.

Burton, Richard D. E. *Holy Tears, Holy Blood: Women, Catholicism, and the Culture of Suffering in France, 1840–1870*. Ithaca, N.Y.: Cornell University Press, 2004.

Carlile, Richard. *Every Woman's book, or, What is Love?* London: R. Carlile, 1826.

Célestin, Roger, Eliane DalMolin, and Isabelle de Courtivron, eds. *Beyond French Feminisms: Debates on Women, Politics, and Culture in France, 1981–2001*. New York: Palgrave Macmillan, 2003.

Chesnais, Jean-Claude. *The Demographic Transition: Stages, Patterns, and Economic Implications: A Longitudian Study of Sixty-Seven Countries Covering the Period 1720–1984*. Translated by Elizabeth Kreager and Philip Kreager. Oxford: Oxford University Press, 1992.

Christiansen, Rupert. *Paris Babylon: The Story of the Paris Commune*. New York: Penguin Books, 1994.

Clark, Linda. *Schooling the Daughters of Marianne: Textbooks and the Socialization of Girls in Modern French Primary Schools*. Albany: State University of New York Press, 1984.

Cole, Joshua. *The Power of Large Numbers: Population, Politics, and Gender in Nineteenth-Century France*. Ithaca, N.Y.: Cornell University Press, 2000.

Cook, Hera. *The Long Sexual Revolution: English Women, Sex, and Contraception 1800–1975*. Oxford: Oxford University Press, 2004.

Cova, Anne. "Féminisme et natalité: Nelly Roussel (1878–1922)." *History of European Ideas* 15, 4–6 (1992): 663–72.

———. *Maternité et droits des femmes en France: XIXe–XXe siècles*. Paris: Anthropos, 1997.

———. *"Au service de l'église, de la patrie et de la famille": Femmes catholiques et maternité sous la IIIe République*. Paris: L'Harmattan, 2000.

Coffey, Joan L. *Léon Harmel: Entrepreneur as Catholic Social Reformer*. Notre Dame, Ind.: University of Notre Dame Press, 2003.

Darrow, Margaret. *French Women and the First World War: War Stories of the Home Front*. Oxford: Berg, 2000.

Davidoff, Leonore, and Catherine Hall. *Family Fortunes: Men and Women of the English Middle Class, 1780–1850*. Chicago: University of Chicago Press, 1987.

Davy, Charlotte. *Une Femme*. Preface by Henri Barbusse. Paris: Eugène Figière, 1927.

De Giorgio, Michela. "The Catholic Model." In *A History of Women: Emerging Feminism from Revolution to World War*, ed. Geneviève Fraisse and Michelle Perrot, 4: 166–97. Cambridge, Mass.: Belknap Press of Harvard University Press, 1993.

Delumeau, Jean, and Yves Lequin, eds. *Les Malheurs des temps: Histoire des fléaux et des calamités en France*. Paris: Larousse, 1987.

Demeulenaere-Douyère, Christiane. *Paul Robin (1837–1912): Un Militant de la liberté et du bonheur*. Paris: Publisud, 1994.

———. "Être néo-malthusien à Paris à la Belle Époque: La Ligue de la Régénération Humaine." *Bulletin de la Société de l'histoire de Paris et de l'Île de France*, nos. 122–124 (1999).

Desan, Suzanne. "Constitutional Amazons: Jacobin Women's Clubs in the French Revolution." In *Recreating Authority in Revolutionary France*, ed. Bryant T. Ragan Jr. and Elizabeth Williams. New Brunswick, N.J.: Rutgers University Press, 1992.

———. *The Family on Trial in Revolutionary France*. Berkeley: University of California Press, 2004.

Dictionnaire des intellectuels français: Les Personnes, les lieux, les moments. Edited by Jacques Julliard, Michel Winock et al. Paris: Seuil, 1996, 2002.

Dizier-Metz. Annie. *La Bibliothèque Marguerite Durand: Histoire d'une femme, mémoire des femmes*. Paris: Mairie de Paris, 1992.

Drumont, Édouard. *La "France juive" devant l'opinion*. Paris: C. Marpon & E. Flammarion, 1886.

Dubois, Paul. *The Psychic Treatment of Nervous Disorders (The Psychoneuroses and Their Moral Treatment)*. Translated by Smith Ely Jelliffe and William A. White. 1905. 6th ed., rev. New York: Funk & Wagnalls, 1909.

Duchen, Claire. *Women's Rights and Women's Lives in France, 1944–1968*. New York: Routledge, 1994.

Eichner, Carolyn J. *Surmounting the Barricades: Women in the Paris Commune*. Bloomington: Indiana University Press, 2004.

Elosu, Dr. Fernand, *Amour infécond: Limitation raisonnée des naissances*. Bayonne: Action syndicale, 1908.

Elwitt, Sanford. *The Third Republic Defended: Bourgeois Reform in France, 1880–1914*. Baton Rouge: Louisiana State University Press, 1986.

Fassin, Eric. "The Purloined Gender: American Feminism in a French Mirror." *French Historical Studies* 22 (Winter 1999): 139–67.

Fierro, Alfred. *Histoire et dictionnaire de Paris*. Paris: R. Laffont, 1996. Translated by Jon Woronoff as *Historical Dictionary of Paris* (Lanham, Md.: Scarecrow Press, 1998).

Finney, Roy P. *The Story of Motherhood*. New York: Liveright, 1937.

Fisher, Kate, and Simon Szreter. "'They Prefer Withdrawal': The Choice of Birth Control in Britain, 1918–1950." *Journal of Interdisciplinary History* 23, 2 (Autumn 2003).

Fraisse, Geneviève, and Michelle Perrot, eds. *A History of Women: Emerging Feminism from Revolution to World War*. Vol. 3. Cambridge, Mass.: Belknap Press of Harvard University Press, 1993.

Frykman, Jonas, and Orvar Lofgren. *Culture Builders: A Historical Anthropology of Middle-Class Life*. Translated by Alan Crozier. New Brunswick, N.J.: Rutgers University Press, 1987.

Fuchs, Rachel G. *Abandoned Children: Foundlings and Child Welfare in Nineteenth-Century France*. Albany: State University of New York, 1984.

———. *Poor and Pregnant in Paris: Strategies for Survival in the Nineteenth Century*. New Brunswick, N.J.: Rutgers University Press, 1992.

Garelick, Rhonda K. *Rising Star: Dandyism, Gender, and Performance in the Fin de Siècle*. Princeton: Princeton University Press, 1998.

Gélis, Jacques. *History of Childbirth: Fertility, Pregnancy, and Birth in Early Modern Europe.* Boston: Northeastern University Press, 1991. Originally published as *L'Arbre et le fruit: La Naissance dans l'Occident moderne, XVIe–XIXe siècle* (Paris: Fayard, 1984).

Gemie, Sharif. *Women and Schooling in France, 1815–1914: Gender, Authority and Identity in the Female Schooling Sector.* Keele, UK: Keele University Press, 1995.

Giroud, Gabriel. *Paul Robin: Sa vie, ses idées, son action.* Paris: G. Mignolet & Storz, 1937.

Godineau, Dominique. *The Women of Paris and Their French Revolution.* Berkeley: University of California Press, 1998.

Goodman, Deena, ed. *Marie-Antoinette: Writings on the Body of a Queen.* New York: Routledge, 2003.

Gordon, Felicia A. *The Integral Feminist: Madeleine Pelletier, 1874–1939.* Minneapolis: University of Minnesota Press, 1990.

Gordon, Linda. *Woman's Body, Woman's Right: Birth Control in America.* New York: Penguin Books, 1990.

———. *The Moral Property of Women: A History of Birth Control Politics in America.* Urbana: University of Illinois Press, 2002.

Grayzel, Susan R. *Women's Identities at War: Gender, Motherhood, and Politics in Britain and France During the First World War.* Chapel Hill: University of North Carolina Press, 1999.

Great Britain. Ministry of Information. *Chronology of the War.* Edited by Major-General Lord Edward Gleichen et al. 3 vols. London: Constable, 1918–20. Reprinted as *Chronology of the Great War* (London: Greenhill Books, 1988).

Guerrand, Roger-Henri. *La Libre maternité, 1896–1969.* Paris: Casterman, 1971.

Guerrand, Roger-Henri, and Francis Ronsin. *Le Sexe apprivoisé: Jeanne Humbert et la lutte pour le control des naissances.* Paris: La Découverte, 1990.

Gulickson, Gay. *Unruly Women of Paris: Images of the Commune.* Ithaca, N.Y.: Cornell University Press, 1996.

Hanna, Martha. "A Republic of Letters: The Epistolary Tradition in France During World War I." *American Historical Review* 108 (December 2003): 1338–61.

Hargrove, June. *Les Statues de Paris: La Représentation des grands hommes dans les rues et sur les places de Paris.* Antwerp: Fonds Mercator; Paris: Albin Michel, 1989.

Harris, Ruth. "The 'Child of the Barbarian': Rape, Race and Nationalism in France During the First World War," *Past and Present* 141 (1993): 170–206.

Harvey, Joy Dorothy. *Almost a Man of Genius: Clémence Royer, Feminism, and Nineteenth Century Science.* New Brunswick, N.J.: Rutgers University Press, 1997.

Hause, Steven C., with Anne R. Kenney. *Women's Suffrage and Social Politics in the French Third Republic.* Princeton: Princeton University Press, 1984.

Hausser, Elizabeth. *Paris au jour le jour: Les Événements vus par la presse, 1900–1919.* Paris: Minuit, 1969.

Herzlich, Claudine, and Janine Pierret. *Illness and Self in Society.* Translated by Elborg Foster. Baltimore: Johns Hopkins University Press, 1987.

Hesse, Carla. *The Other Enlightenment: How French Women Became Modern.* Princeton: Princeton University Press, 2001.

Horne, John. "Soldiers, Civilians and the Warfare of Attrition: Representations of Combat in France, 1914–1918." In *Authority, Identity and the Social History of the Great War*, ed. Frans Coetzee and Marilyn Shevin-Coetzee, 223–49. Providence, R.I.: Berghahn Books, 1995.

Humbert, Jeanne. *Eugène Humbert: La Vie et l'oeuvre d'un néo-malthusien*. Paris: La Grande Réforme, 1974.

Humphries, M. J., and W. K. Lam. "Non-Respiratory Tuberculosis." In *Clinical Tuberculosis*, ed. P. D. O. Davies. London: Chapman & Hall Medical, 1998.

Hunt, Lynn. *The Family Romance and the French Revolution*. Berkeley: University of California Press, 1992.

———. "The Unstable Boundaries of the French Revolution." In *From the Fires of Revolution to the Great War*, ed. Michelle Perrot, vol. 4 of *A History of Private Life*, ed. Philippe Ariès and Georges Duby, 13–45. Cambridge, Mass.: Belknap Press of Harvard University Press, 1990.

Huss, Marie-Monique. "Pronatalism and the Popular Ideology of the Child in Wartime France: The Evidence of the Picture Postcard." In *The Upheaval of War: Family, Work, and Welfare in Europe, 1914–1918*, ed. Richard Wall and Jay Winter, 329–67. Cambridge: Cambridge University Press.

Iezzoni, Lynette. *Influenza 1918: The Worst Epidemic in American History*. New York: TV Books, 1999.

Iseman, Michael D. *A Clinician's Guide to Tuberculosis*. Philadelphia: Lippincott, Williams & Wilkins, 2000.

Ivimy, Alice M. *A Woman's Guide to Paris*. New York: Brentano's, 1910.

Jordanova, Ludmilla. *Sexual Visions*. Madison: University of Wisconsin Press, 1989.

Katznelson, Ira, and Aristide R. Zolbert, eds. *Working-Class Formation: Nineteenth-Century Patterns in Western Europe and the United States*. Princeton: Princeton University Press, 1986.

Kerber, Linda. *Women of the Republic: Intellect and Ideology in Revolutionary America*. Chapel Hill: University of North Carolina Press, 1980.

Klejman, Laurence, and Rochefort, Florence. *L'Égalité en marche: Le Féminisme sous la Troisième République*. Paris: Presses de la Fondation nationale des sciences politiques, 1989.

Knibiehler, Yvonne, and Catherine Fouquet. *Histoire des mères du moyen-âge à nos jours*. Paris: Montalba, 1980.

Kolata, Gina. *Flu: The Story of the Great Influenza Pandemic of 1918 and the Search for the Virus That Caused It*. New York: Simon & Schuster, 2001.

Koos, Cheryl. "'On les aura!' 'On les aura!' The Gendered Politics of Abortion and the Alliance nationale contre la depopulation, 1938–1944." *Modern and Contemporary France*, 7, 1 (February 1996).

———. "Gender, Anti-Individualism, and Nationalism: The Alliance nationale and the Pronatalist Backlash Against the Femme moderne, 1933–1940." *French Historical Studies* 19, 3 (Spring 1996).

———. "Fascism, Fatherhood, and the Family in Interwar France: The Case of Antoine Redier and the Legion." *Journal of Family History* 24, 3 (July 1999).

Lalouette, Jacqueline. *La Libre pensée en France, 1848–1940*. Paris: Albin Michel, 1997.

Landes, Joan B. *Women and the Public Sphere in the Age of the French Revolution*. Ithaca, N.Y.: Cornell University Press, 1988.

———*Visualizing the Nation: Gender, Representation, and Revolution in Eighteenth-Century France*. Ithaca, N.Y.: Cornell University Press, 2001.

Laqueur, Thomas. *Making Sex: Body and Gender from the Greeks to Freud*. Cambridge, Mass.: Harvard University Press, 1990.

Le Play, Fréderic. *On Family, Work, and Social Change*. Edited and translated by Catherine Bodard Silver. Chicago: University of Chicago Press, 1982.

Le Robert Dictionnaire historique de la langue française. Edited by Alain Rey et al. 3 vols. Paris: Dictionnaires Le Robert, 2000.

Lequin, Yves. *Les Ouvriers de la region lyonnaise (1848–1914)*. 2 vols. Lyon: Presses universitaires de Lyon, 1976.

Letourneau, Charles. *L'Évolution de la morale: Leçons professées pendant l'hiver de 1885–1886* Bibliothèque anthropologique, 3. Paris: A. Delahaye & E. Lecrosnier, 1887.

Loudon, Irvine S. L. *Death in Childbirth: An International Study of Maternal Care and Maternal Mortality, 1800–1950*. Oxford: Clarendon Press, 1992.

———. "Childbirth." In *Companion Encyclopedia of the History of Medicine*, ed. W. F. Bynum and Roy Porter, 1050–71. New York: Routledge, 1993.

MacKinnon, Catherine A. "Does Sexuality Have a History?" In *Discourses of Sexuality: From Aristotle to AIDS*, ed. Domna C. Stanton, 117–36. Ann Arbor: University of Michigan Press, 1992.

Magraw, Robert. *A History of the French Working Class*. 2 vols. Oxford: Blackwell, 1992.

Maitron, Jean, ed. *Dictionnaire biographique du mouvement ouvrier français*. 43 vols. Paris: Éd. ouvrières, 1964–97.

Mansker, Andrea. "'The Pistol Virgin': Feminism, Sexuality, and Honor in Belle Époque France." Ph.D. diss.. University of California, Los Angeles, 2003.

Margadant, Jo Burr. *Madame le Professeur: Women Educators in the Third Republic*. Princeton: Princeton University Press, 1990.

———. "Constructing Selves in Historical Perspective." In *The New Biography: Performing Femininity in Nineteenth-Century France*, ed. id., 1–32. Berkeley: University of California Press, 2000.

Martin-Fugier, Anne. *La Place des bonnes: La Domesticité féminine à Paris en 1900*. Paris: Bernard Grasset, 1979.

———. *La Bourgeoise: Femme au temps de Paul Bourget*. Paris: Bernard Grasset, 1983.

Mayeur, Françoise. *L'Enseignement sécondaire des jeunes filles sous la Troisième République*. Paris: Presses de la Fondation nationale des sciences politiques, 1977.

———. *L'Éducation des filles en France au XIXᵉ Siècle*. Paris: Hachette, 1979.

Mayeur, Jean-Marie. *La Vie politique sous la Troisième République, 1870–1940*. Paris: Seuil, 1984.

McCann, Carole R. *Birth Control Politics in the United States, 1916–1945*. Ithaca, N.Y.: Cornell University Press, 1994.

McLaren, Angus. *Birth Control in Nineteenth-Century England*. New York: Holmes & Meier, 1978).

———. "Revolution and Education in Late Nineteenth-Century France: The Early Career of Paul Robin." *History of Education Quarterly* 21, 3 (Fall 1981): 317–35.

————. *Sexuality and Social Order: The Debate over the Fertility of Women and Workers in France, 1770–1920.* New York: Holmes & Meier, 1983.

————. *A History of Contraception from Antiquity to the Present Day.* Oxford: Blackwell, 1992.

McMillan, James F. *Housewife or Harlot: The Place of Women in French Society, 1870–1940.* New York: St. Martin's Press, 1981.

————. *France and Women, 1789–1914: Gender, Society and Politics.* New York: Routledge, 2000.

Mercier, Lucien. *Les Universités populaires: 1899–1914: Éducation populaire et movement ouvrier au début du siècle.* Paris: Éducation Ouvrières, 1986.

Merriman, John M. *A History of Modern Europe: From the Renaissance to the Present.* New York: Norton, 1996.

Michaud, Stéphane. *Muse et madone: Visages de la femme de la Révolution française aux apparitions de Lourdes.* Paris: Seuil, 1985.

————. "Artistic and Literary Idolatries." In *A History of Women: Emerging Feminism from Revolution to World War,* ed. Geneviève Fraisse and Michelle Perrot, 3: 121–44. Cambridge, Mass.: Belknap Press of Harvard University Press, 1993.

Michelet, Jules. *L'Amour.* Paris: L. Hachette, 1858.

————. *La Femme.* Paris: L. Hachette, 1859.

Miller, Michael B. *The Bon Marché: Bourgeois Culture and the Department Store, 1869–1920.* Princeton: Princeton University Press, 1981.

Moses, Claire Goldberg. *French Feminism in the Nineteenth Century.* Albany: State University of New York Press, 1984.

Muel-Dreyfus, Francine. *Vichy et l'éternel féminin: Contribution à une sociologie politique de l'ordre des corps.* Paris: Seuil, 1996. Translated by Kathleen A. Johnson as *Vichy and the Eternal Feminine: A Contribution to a Political Sociology of Gender* (Durham, N.C.: Duke University Press, 2001).

Nye, Robert A. *The Origins of Crowd Psychology: Gustave Le Bon and the Crisis of Mass Democracy in the Third Republic.* Beverly Hills, Calif.: Sage, 1975.

————. "Degeneration and the Medical Model of Cultural Crisis in the French *Belle Époque.*" In *Political Symbolism in Modern Europe: Essays in Honor of George L. Mosse,* ed. Seymour Drescher, David Sabean, and Allan Sharlin. New Brunswick, N.J.: Transaction Books, 1982.

————. *Crime, Madness, and Politics in Modern France: The Medical Concept of National Decline.* Princeton: Princeton University Press, 1984.

————. "Medicine and Science as Masculine 'Fields of Honor.'" *Osiris* 12 (1997): 60–79.

————. *Masculinity and Male Codes of Honor in Modern France.* Berkeley: University of California Press, 1998.

————, ed. *Sexuality.* Oxford: Oxford University Press, 1999.

Offen, Karen. "Depopulation, Nationalism, and Feminism in Fin-de-Siècle France." *American Historical Review* 89 (June 1984): 648–76.

————. *European Feminisms, 1700–1950: A Political History.* Stanford: Stanford University Press, 2000.

Ozouf, Mona. *Les Mots des femmes: Essai sur la singularité française.* Paris: Fayard, 1995.

Translated by Jane Marie Todd as *Women's Words: Essay on French Singularity* (Chicago: University of Chicago Press, 1997).

Pateman, Carole. "Equality, Difference, Subordination: The Politics of Motherhood and Women's Citizenship." In *Beyond Equality and Difference: Citizenship, Feminist Politics and Female Subjectivity.* New York: Routledge, 1992.

Payer, Lynn. *Medicine and Culture.* New York: Holt, 1988.

Pedersen, Jean Elizabeth. *Legislating the French Family: Feminism, Theater, and Republican Politics, 1870–1920.* New Brunswick, N.J.: Rutgers University Press, 2003.

Perrot, Michelle. "On the Formation of the French Working Class." In *Working-Class Formation: Nineteenth-Century Patterns in Western Europe and the United States,* ed. Ira Katznelson and Aristide R. Zolbert. Princeton: Princeton University Press, 1986.

———. "The New Eve and the Old Adam: Changes in French Women's Condition at the Turn of the Century." In *Behind the Lines: Gender and the Two World Wars,* ed. Margaret Randolph Higonnet, Jane Jenson, Sonya Michel, and Margaret Collins Weitz, 51–60. New Haven: Yale University Press, 1987.

———. "The Family Triumphant." In *From the Fires of Revolution to the Great War,* ed. id., 99–129. Vol. 4 of *A History of Private Life,* ed. Philippe Ariès and Georges Duby. Cambridge, Mass: Belknap Press of Harvard University Press, 1990.

Pick, Daniel. *Faces of Degeneration: A European Disorder, c. 1848–c. 1918.* New York: Cambridge University Press, 1989.

Piot, Edmé-Georges. *La Question de la depopulation en France: Le Mal—ses causes—ses remèdes.* Paris: P. Mouillot, 1900.

Pollard, Miranda. *Reign of Virtue: Mobilizing Gender in Vichy France.* Chicago: University of Chicago Press, 1998.

Pope, Barbara Corrado. "Immaculate and Powerful: The Marian Revival in the Nineteenth Century." In *Immaculate & Powerful: The Female in Sacred Image and Social Reality,* ed. Clarissa W. Atkinson, Constance H. Buchanan, and Margaret R. Miles, 173–200. Boston: Beacon Press, 1985.

Popkin, Jeremy D. *A History of Modern France.* 2d ed. Upper Saddle River, N.J.: Prentice Hall, 2001.

Porter, Roy. "The Case of Consumption." In *Understanding Catastrophe,* ed. Janine Bourriau, 179–203. Cambridge: Cambridge University Press, 1992.

———. "Pain and Suffering." In *Companion Encyclopedia of the History of Medicine,* ed. W. F. Bynum and Roy Porter, 2: 1574–91. New York: Routledge, 1993.

Przyblyski, Jeannene M. "Between Seeing and Believing: Representing Women in Appert's *Crimes de la Commune.*" In *Making the News: Modernity and the Mass Press in Nineteenth-Century France,* ed. Dean de la Motte and Jeannene M. Przyblyski, 233–78. Amherst: University of Massachusetts Press, 1999.

Rearick, Charles. *Pleasures of the Belle Époque: Entertainment & Festivity in Turn-of-the-Century France.* New Haven: Yale University Press, 1985.

Rebérioux, Madeleine. *La République radicale? 1898–1914.* Paris: Seuil, 1975.

Reddy, William. *The Invisible Code: Honor and Sentiment in Postrevolutionary France, 1814–1848.* Berkeley: University of California Press, 1997.

Reed, James. *The Birth Control Movement and American Society: From Private Vice to Public Virtue.* Princeton: Princeton University Press, 1978.

Réquillard, Françoise Jupeau. *L'Initiation des femmes, ou, Le Souci permanent des francs-maçons français.* Monaco: Rocher, 2000.

Rich, Adrienne. *Of Woman Born: Motherhood as Experience and Institution.* New York: Norton, 1986.

Riddle, John M. *Contraception and Abortion from the Ancient World to the Renaissance.* Cambridge, Mass.: Harvard University Press, 1992.

———. *Eve's Herbs: A History of Contraception and Abortion in the West.* Cambridge, Mass.: Harvard University Press, 1997.

Roberts, Mary Louise. *Civilization Without Sexes: Reconstructing Gender in Postwar France, 1917–1927.* Chicago: University of Chicago Press, 1994.

———. "Acting Up: The Feminist Theatrics of Marguerite Durand." *French Historical Studies* 19 (Fall 1996): 1103–38.

———. "Feminist Journalism in Fin-de-Siècle France." In *Making the News: Modernity and the Mass Press in Nineteenth-Century France,* ed. Dean de la Motte and Jeannene M. Przyblyski, 302–50. Amherst: University of Massachusetts Press, 1999.

———. *Disruptive Acts: The New Woman in Fin-de-Siècle France.* Chicago: University of Chicago Press, 2002.

Rochefort, Florence. "L'Antiféminisme: Une Rhétorique réactionnaire." In *Un siècle d'antiféminisme,* ed. Christine Bard, 133–47. Paris: Fayard, 1999.

Ronsin, Francis. *La Grève des ventres: Propagande neo-malthusienne et baisse de natalité en France (XIXe–XXe siècles).* Paris: Aubier Montaigne, 1980.

Sanger, Margaret. *Margaret Sanger: An Autobiography.* New York: Norton, 1938.

Scarry, Elaine. *The Body in Pain. The Making and Unmaking of the World.* Oxford: Oxford University Press, 1985.

Schiebinger, Londa. *The Mind Has No Sex? Women in the Origins of Modern Science* Cambridge, Mass.: Harvard University Press, 1989.

———. *Nature's Body: Gender and the Making of Modern Science.* Boston: Beacon Press, 1993.

Schwartz, Vanessa R. *Spectacular Realities: Early Mass Culture in Fin-de-Siècle Paris.* Berkeley: University of California Press, 1998.

Scott, Joan Wallach. *Only Paradoxes to Offer: French Feminists and the Rights of Man.* Cambridge, Mass.: Harvard University Press, 1996.

———. "Language, Gender, and Working-Class History." In *Class,* ed. Patrick Joyce, 154–67. Oxford: Oxford University Press.

———. "'L'Ouvrière! Mot impie, sordide . . . ': Women Workers in the Discourse of French Political Economy, 1840–1860." In id., *Gender and the Politics of History.* New York: Columbia University Press, 1988.

Sewell, William, Jr. *Work and Revolution in France: The Language of Labor from the Old Regime to 1848.* Cambridge: Cambridge University Press, 1985.

Sherman, Daniel J. *The Construction of Memory in Interwar France.* Chicago: University of Chicago Press, 1999.

Shorter, Edward. *From Paralysis to Fatigue: A History of Psychosomatic Illness in the Modern Era.* New York: Free Press, 1992.

Simon, Jules. *L'Ouvrière*. Paris: Hachette, 1861.

Smith, Bonnie. *Ladies of the Leisure Class: The Bourgeoises of Northern France in the Nineteenth Century*. Princeton: Princeton University Press, 1981.

Smith, Leonard V. "Masculinity, Memory, and the French First World War Novel." In *Authority, Identity and the Social History of the Great War*, ed. Frans Coetzee and Marilyn Shevin-Coetzee, 251–74. Providence, R.I.: Berghahn Books, 1995.

Smith, Leonard V., Stéphane Audoin-Rouzeau, and Annette Becker. *France and the Great War, 1914–1918*. Cambridge: Cambridge University Press, 2003.

Sohn, Anne-Marie. *Chrysalides: Femmes dans la vie privée (XIXe–XXe siècles)*. 2 vols. Paris: Publications de la Sorbonne, 1996.

———. *Du premier baiser à l'alcôve: La Sexualité des Français au quotidien, 1850–1950*. Paris: Aubier, 1996.

Soloway, Richard Allen. *Birth Control and the Population Question in England, 1877–1830*. Chapel Hill: University of North Carolina Press.

Sonn, Richard D. *Anarchism and Cultural Politics in Fin de Siècle France*. Lincoln: University of Nebraska Press, 1989.

Sontag, Susan. *Illness as Metaphor and Aids and Its Metaphors*. New York: Anchor Books, 1990.

Sowerwine, Charles. *Sisters or Citizens? Women and Socialism in France since 1876*. Cambridge: Cambridge University Press, 1982.

———. *France since 1870: Culture, Politics and Society*. New York: Palgrave, 2001.

Sowerwine, Charles, and Claude Maignien. *Madeleine Pelletier: Une Féministe dans l'arène politique*. Paris: Éd. ouvrières, 1992.

Steinbrugge, Lieselotte. *The Moral Sex: Woman's Nature in the French Enlightenment*. New York: Oxford University Press, 1995.

Stewart, Mary Lynn. *For Health and Beauty: Physical Culture for French Women, 1880s–1930s*. Baltimore: Johns Hopkins University Press, 2001.

Stone, Judith. "The Republican Brotherhood: Gender and Ideology." In *Gender and the Politics of Social Reform in France, 1870–1914*, ed. Elinor A. Accampo, Rachel G. Fuchs, and Mary Lynn Stewart, 28–58. Baltimore: Johns Hopkins University Press, 1995.

———. *Sons of the Revolution: Radical Democrats in France, 1862–1914*. Baton Rouge: Louisiana State University Press, 1996.

Stora-Lamarre, Annie. *L'Enfer de la IIIe République: Censeurs et pornographes, 1881–1914*. Paris: Imago, 1990.

Sussman, George. "The Wet-Nursing Business in Nineteenth-Century France." *French Historical Studies* 9 (1975): 304–28.

———. "The End of the Wet-Nursing Business in France, 1874–1914." *Journal of Family History* 2 (Fall 1977): 237–58.

Thébaud, Françoise. *Quand nos grand-mères donnaient la vie: La Maternité en France dans l'entre-deux-guerres*. Lyon: Presses universitaires de Lyon, 1986.

———. *La Femme au temps de la guerre de 14*. Paris: Stock, 1988.

Thompson, Victoria. "Creating Boundaries: Homosexuality and the Changing Social Order in France, 1830–1870." In *Feminism and History*, ed. Joan Wallach Scott, 398–428. Oxford: Oxford University Press, 1996.

Tiersten, Lisa. *Marianne in the Market: Envisioning Consumer Society in Fin-de-Siècle France.* Berkeley: University of California Press, 2001.

Tilburg, Patricia Ann. "Reimagining the Republican Ideal: Work, Art, and the Body in Colette's Belle Époque." Ph.D. diss., University of California, Los Angeles, 2002.

Valici-Bosio, Sabine. *La Mère et l'enfant dans l'ancienne France.* Etrepilly: C. de Bartillat, 1988.

Villani, Sue Lanci, with Jane E. Ryan. *Motherhood at the Crossroads: Meeting the Challenge of a Changing Role.* New York: Plenum Press, 1997.

Waelti-Walters, Jennifer, and Steven C. Hause, eds. *Feminisms of the Belle Epoque: A Historical and Literary Anthology.* Lincoln: University of Nebraska Press, 1994.

Waldberg, Patrick. *Eros in La Belle Époque.* New York: Grove Press, 1969.

Warner, Marina. *Joan of Arc: The Image of Female Heroism.* New York: Knopf, 1981.

Weisz, George. *The Emergence of Modern Universities in France, 1863–1914.* Princeton: Princeton University Press, 1983.

Williams, Rosalind H. *Dream Worlds: Mass Consumption in Late Nineteenth-Century France.* Berkeley: University of California Press, 1982.

Winock, Michael. "Jeanne d'Arc." In *Les Lieux de mémoire,* ed. Pierre Nora, 3: 4427–73. Paris: Gallimard, 1997.

Winter, Jay. *The Great War and the British People.* London: Macmillan, 1985.

———. *Sites of Memory, Sites of Mourning: The Great War in European Cultural History.* Cambridge: Cambridge University Press, 1995.

Wright, Gordon. *Notable or Notorious? A Gallery of Parisians.* Cambridge, Mass.: Harvard University Press, 1991.

———. *France in Modern Times: From the Enlightenment to the Present.* 1981. 5th ed. New York: Norton, 1995.

Zeldin, Theodore. *France, 1848–1945: Ambition and Love.* Oxford: Oxford University Press, 1979.

———. *France, 1848–1945: Anxiety and Hypocrisy.* Oxford: Oxford University Press, 1981.

Zylberman, Patrick. "A Holocaust in a Holocaust: The Great War and the 1918 'Spanish' Influenza Epidemic in France." In *The Spanish Influenza Pandemic of 1918–19: New Perspectives,* ed. Howard Phillips and David Killingray, 191–201. New York: Routledge, 2003.